Amsterdam's Anatomy Lessons Dissected

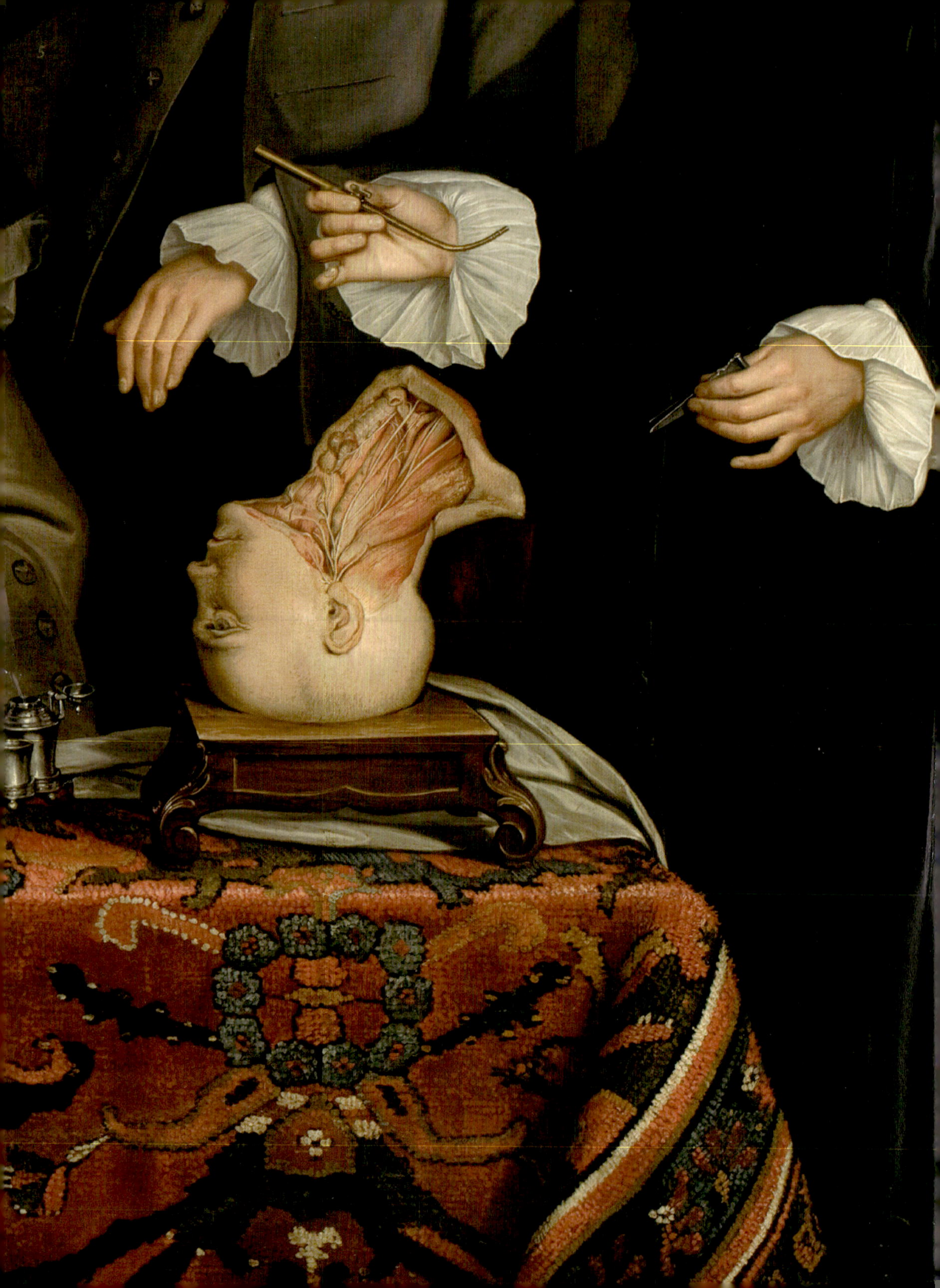

Frank IJpma & Thomas van Gulik

Amsterdam's Anatomy Lessons Dissected

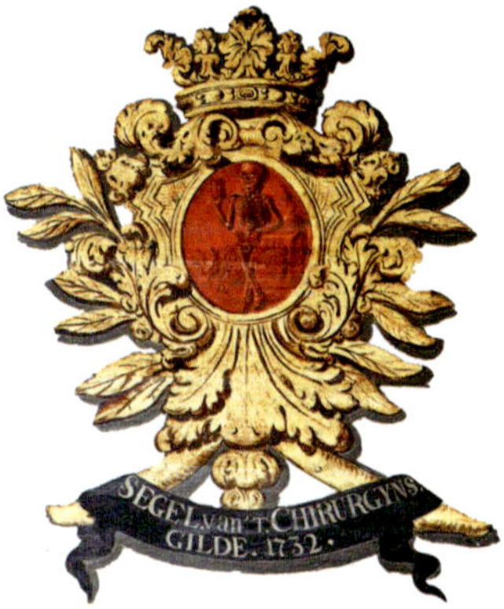

Routledge
Taylor & Francis Group
LONDON AND NEW YORK

Frank IJpma & Thomas van Gulik
Amsterdam's Anatomy Lessons Dissected

First published in Dutch by Boom,
Amsterdam, 2013.
Japanese edition published by University
of Tokyo Press, 2020.

Published 2025 by Routledge
4 Park Square, Milton Park, Abingdon, Oxon OX14 4RN
605 Third Avenue, New York, NY 10158

Routledge is an imprint of the Taylor & Francis Group, an informa business

ISBN: 9789048568284 (hbk)
ISBN: 9781041175506 (pbk)
ISBN: 9781003690726 (ebk)

NUR 694

Translation Rosemary Robson, Joyce Bergvelt
Book design René van der Vooren

DOI 10.5117/ 978 90 4856 828 4

Front cover
Detail of Rembrandt, *The Anatomy Lesson of Jan Deijman*, 1656 (see Chapter 5)

Back Cover
Detail of Rembrandt, *The Anatomy Lesson of Nicolaes Tulp*, 1632 (see Chapter 4)

Fly-leaf left
Detail of Jan van Neck, *The Anatomy Lesson of Frederik Ruysch*, 1683 (See Chapter 4)

Fly-leaf right
Detail of Thomas de Keyser, *The Osteological Lesson of Sebastiaen Egbertszn*, 1619 (see Chapter 2)

Frontispiece
Detail of Tibout Regters, *The Anatomy Lesson of Petrus Camper*, 1758 (Chapter 9)

Image on Title Page
Coat-of-arms of the Amsterdam Surgeons' Guild, in the vault of the dome of the Anatomy Theatre in The Weighing House, on the Nieuwmarkt in Amsterdam (see p. 18)

Contents

Introduction

Healthcare in Amsterdam in the seventeenth and eighteenth centuries

During the seventeenth and eighteenth centuries, the responsibility for Amsterdam's healthcare was shared among various authorities. The *Doctores medicinae* and apothecaries were registered with the *Collegium Medicum* (Medical Supervisory Board), while the *Doctores Medicinae* were academically trained physicians whose principal concern was the internal ailments of patients. They wrote prescriptions and, if a surgical intervention was deemed necessary, they consulted a surgeon.

The meaning of the word 'surgery' is derived from the Greek word χειρἑργον (*cheirergon*), which means 'working with the hand'. Indeed, surgeons were primarily involved in dealing with external physical ailments which could be treated 'by hand': or in other words, by operations. Besides barbering, their work consisted of bloodletting, bandaging, treating wounds and ulcers, draining abscesses, the setting of broken bones and performing small operations such as repairing inguinal hernias and the removal of bladder stones. In contrast to physicians, surgeons were traditionally trained by a master surgeon as apprentices, and were not academically trained. In 1600, there were approximately thirty practising surgeons in Amsterdam, serving a population of 100,000 inhabitants. By 1670, the population had grown to around 200,000, while the number of surgeons expanded to around 240 in 1688.

▸ **The Amsterdam Surgeons' Guild** Initially, the surgeons in Amsterdam belonged to one single guild that also included barbers, patten-, frame- and skate-makers. In 1551, the latter three set up their own guild. The surgeons detached themselves from the barbers a year later, upon which the territories of these various professions were indelibly defined.

The Amsterdam Surgeons' Guild was an extremely well-organized professional body; it monitored surgical care, and organised the surgeons' training and examination. The board consisted of six governors. Every year in September, the Municipal Council of Amsterdam would choose two new governors from a list of four candidates. Usually, a governor remained in office for three years, after which he was not permitted to serve in any other capacity on the board for at least one year. The dean and the Chief Tutor (*proef-meester*) were president and vice-president of the guild, while the chief tutor was responsible for preparing candidates to take the guild examinations, the rules of which were meticulously recorded in the Guild Regulations. The Board of Governors regularly met to discuss routine — and financial matters and also awarded (membership) tokens — also known as presentation tokens — by which fellow guild members could identify themselves at official guild gatherings. Sometimes, tokens were issued to mark special occasions. The Surgeon's Guild activities were diligently recorded by the Board in the minute books, the majority of which are still preserved in the Amsterdam City Archives.

The municipal council appointed a *praelector anatomia* (literally: a reader in anatomy), an academically trained physician (*doctor*

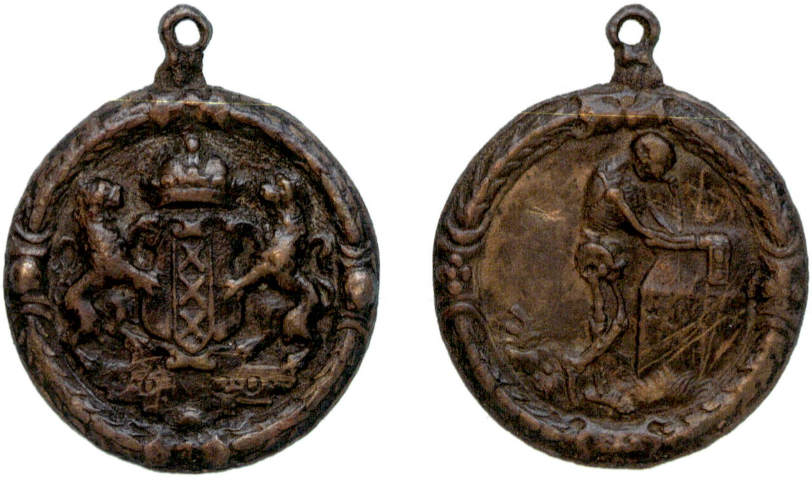

Oldest extant membership token of the Amsterdam Surgeons' Guild, dating from 1620. Private Collection.

medicinae) whose task was to provide the Surgeons' Guild with theoretical knowledge instruction twice a week. To supplement this instruction, the Surgeons' Guild also organised anatomy lessons — initially once a year. In order to teach empirical anatomy, the *praelector* dissected the body of a criminal who had been condemned to death. During his anatomical dissections, the *praelector* was assisted by the Assistant Tutor, whose tasks included rotating the dissection table and handing the *praelector* his surgical instruments.

▸ **The Surgeon's Shop** The surgeons practised their craft in surgeon's shops, which were located throughout Amsterdam. A 1669 painting by Egbert van Heemskerck gives us a glimpse of the surgeon's shop of Jacob Franszn, a practising surgeon in Amsterdam at that time. Jacob is depicted performing a blood-letting as his son Thomas, catches the blood in a bowl, while his wife sits on the right with his other son and daughter. In the background, an

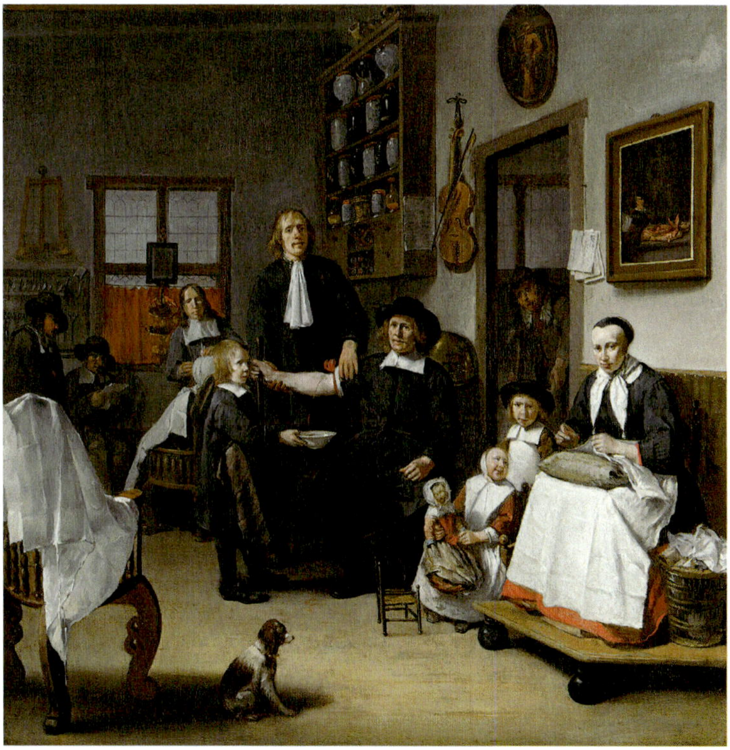

Egbert van Heemskerck, *Jacob Franszn (c. 1635–1708) and His Family in the Surgeon's Shop*, 1669. Detail. Collection Amsterdam Museum.

apprentice is seen shaving a customer. In the background on the left, two other customers are awaiting their turn and a fourth customer is leaning on crutches as he stands in the doorway on the right. The shop is furnished with several distinctive items that are indicative of Jacob Franszn's profession. A wall cabinet containing surgical instruments and jars containing medications. A skull adorns the top of one cabinet, and a stuffed swordfish is suspended from the ceiling. There is a painting on the right wall showing a miniature reproduction of an anatomical dissection of the abdominal and thoracic cavities. Van Heemskerck's painting of the interior allows us a unique opportunity to go back to the conditions in which a surgeon practised his profession at that time.

▸ **The Surgeon's Education** For centuries, surgeons were traditionally trained according to the master-apprentice principle. Pupils learned their craft by serving as an apprentice in a surgeon's shop for a number of years -usually five- during which they were taught by a master surgeon. The quality of the training depended heavily on the knowledge, skills and dedication of the master surgeon concerned. At the beginning of their training period, apprentices were registered in the guild book, paying a registration fee of 12 to 20 *stuyvers* (a Dutch copper coin worth 5 cents, or one-twentieth of a guilder) to the Surgeons' Guild. At the successful conclusion of an apprenticeship, the master provided his pupil with a certificate (*leerbrief*). In this certificate, the master declared that the apprentice had worked in his surgeon's shop for a certain number of years in a satisfactory manner, having shown both diligence and dedication.

Apart from having to work in the surgeon's shop, the apprentices had to attend compulsory lectures given by the *praelector anatomiae,* which were held at the Anatomy Theatre (*Theatrum Anatomicum*). When they embarked on their training, the apprentices were given a so-called letter of permission, confirming that they had been granted permission by their masters to attend the lectures. Failure to attend could result in an apprentice being barred from partaking in the final practical examination, the masterpiece.

The final practical examination — the masterpiece —, took place at the very end of the surgeon's training and was the ultimate test of a surgeon's competence. It was prepared and conducted by the Chief Tutor in the presence of the *praelector anatomiae* and the Guild's Board of Governors. The exam commenced with the candidate having

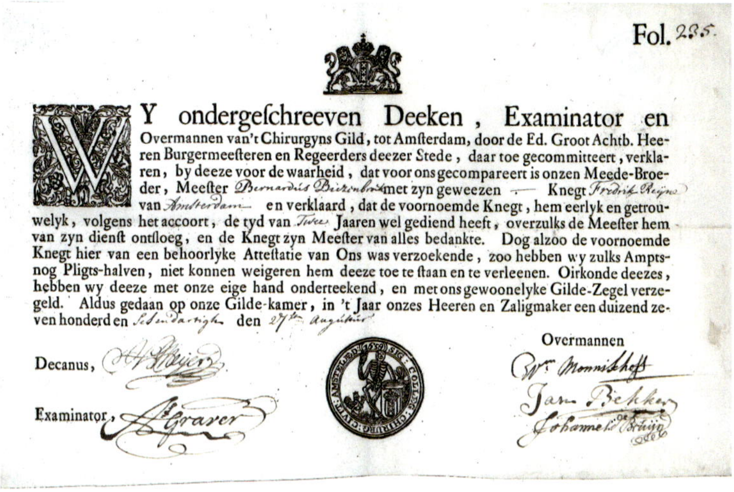
Fol. 285.

WY ondergeſchreeven Deeken, Examinator en Overmannen van't Chirurgyns Gild, tot Amſterdam, door de Ed. Groot Achtb. Heeren Burgermeeſteren en Regeerders deezer Stede, daar toe gecommitteert, verklaren, by deeze voor de waarheid, dat voor ons gecompareert is onzen Meede-Broeder, Meeſter Bernardus Biezenbrink met zyn geweezen — Knegt Frederik Reijne van Amsterdam en verklaard, dat de voornoemde Knegt, hem eerlyk en getrouwelyk, volgens het accoort, de tyd van Twee Jaaren wel gediend heeft, overzulks de Meeſter hem van zyn dienſt ontſloeg, en de Knegt zyn Meeſter van alles bedankte. Dog alzoo de voornoemde Knegt hier van een behoorlyke Atteſtatie van Ons was verzoekende, zoo hebben wy zulks Ampts- nog Pligts-halven, niet konnen weigeren hem deeze toe te ſtaan en te verleenen. Oirkonde deezes, hebben wy deeze met onze eige hand onderteekend, en met ons gewoonelyke Gilde-Zegel verzegeld. Aldus gedaan op onze Gilde-kamer, in 't Jaar onzes Heeren en Zaligmaker een duizend zeven honderd en Sesendartigh den 27th Augustus

Decanus,

Examinator,

Overmannen

Certificate of apprenticeship issued by the Amsterdam Surgeons' Guild granted by Master Surgeon Bernardus Biezenbrink for his apprentice Frederik Reijne (1736). Municipal Archive Amsterdam.

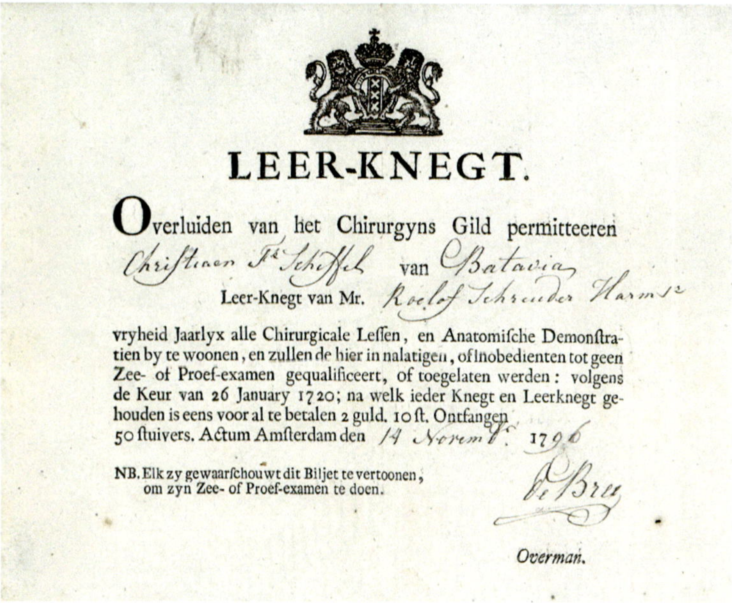
LEER-KNEGT.

Overluiden van het Chirurgyns Gild permitteeren Christiaan Fr. Scheffel van Batavia Leer-Knegt van Mr. Roelof Schreuder Harms vryheid Jaarlyx alle Chirurgicale Leſſen, en Anatomiſche Demonſtratien by te woonen, en zullen de hier in nalatigen, of Inobedienten tot geen Zee- of Proef-examen gequalificeert, of toegelaten werden: volgens de Keur van 26 January 1720; na welk ieder Knegt en Leerknegt gehouden is eens voor al te betalen 2 guld. 10 ſt. Ontfangen 50 ſtuivers. Actum Amſterdam den 14 Novemb. 1796

NB. Elk zy gewaarſchouwt dit Biljet te vertoonen, om zyn Zee- of Proef-examen te doen.

De Bree

Overman.

Certificate of apprenticeship for apprentice C.F. Scheffel (1796). Municipal Archive Amsterdam.

to produce three lancets which would be able to cut through a piece of leather 'soundlessly and without so much as a creak'. If the lancets were approved, the candidate would be examined on 'the question of phlebotomy' (bloodletting). Bloodletting was often used at the time to treat illnesses in the belief that it would restore an imbalance of the bodily fluids. If the candidate answered these questions correctly, his bloodletting skills were put to the test. Using the three prepared lancets, he had to 'let the median vein in the arm, the main vein in the hand and the liver vein'. The practical examination also entailed the bandaging of wounds on patients who were brought in from the poorhouses, as well as the execution of a 'trepan on a skull', the drilling of a hole through the skull. During the theoretical section of his final exam, the apprentice was tested on his knowledge of surgical instruments, 'unnatural growths' (tumours), humoralism (knowledge of Hippocratic theory of bodily fluids), wounds, fractures, dislocations, and medications. Over time, the number of examination questions gradually increased. Once an apprentice passed his final examination, he was granted his certificate of learning and admitted to the

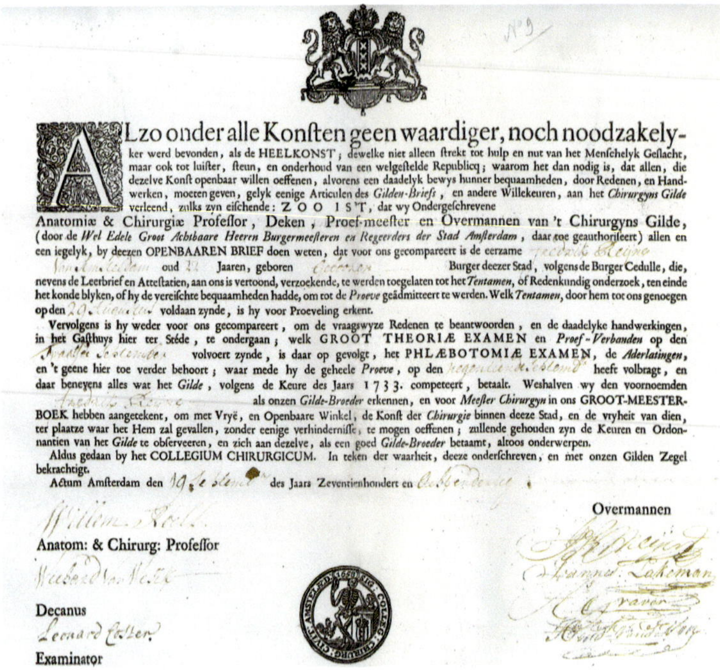

ALzo onder alle Konsten geen waardiger, noch noodzakelyker werd bevonden, als de HEELKONST; dewelke niet alleen strekt tot hulp en nut van het Menschelyk Geslacht, maar ook tot luister, steun, en onderhoud van een welgestelde Republicq; waarom het dan nodig is, dat allen, die dezelve Konst openbaar willen oeffenen, alvorens een daadelyk bewys hunner bequaamheden, door Redenen, en Handwerken, moeten geven, gelyk eenige Articulen des *Gilden-Briefs*, en andere Willekeuren, aan het *Chirurgyns Gilde* verleend, zulks zyn eischende: ZOO IST, dat wy Ondergeschrevene Anatomiæ & Chirurgiæ Professor, Deken, Proef-meester en Overmannen van 't Chirurgyns Gilde, (door de *Wel Edele Groot Achtbaare Heeren Burgermeesteren en Regeerders der Stad Amsterdam*, daar toe geauthoriseert) allen en een iegelyk, by deezen OPENBAAREN BRIEF doen weten, dat voor ons gecompareert is de eerzame [illegible] oud [illegible] Jaaren, geboren [illegible] Burger deezer Stad, volgens de Burger Cedulle, die, nevens de Leerbrief en Attestatien, aan ons is vertoond, verzoekende, te werden toegelaten tot het *Tentamen*, of Redenkundig onderzoek, ten einde het konde blyken, of hy de vereischte bequaamheden hadde, om tot de *Proeve* geädmitteert te werden. Welk *Tentamen*, door hem tot ons genoegen op den [illegible] voldaan zynde, is hy voor Proeveling erkent.

Vervolgens is hy weder voor ons gecompareert, om de vraagswyze Redenen te beantwoorden, en de daadelyke handwerkingen, in het Gasthuys hier ter Stéde, te ondergaan; welk GROOT THEORIÆ EXAMEN en *Proef-Verbanden* op den [illegible] volvoert zynde, is daar op gevolgt, het PHLÆBOTOMIÆ EXAMEN, de *Aderlatingen*, en 't geene hier toe verder behoort; waar mede hy de geheele *Proeve*, op den [illegible] heeft volbragt, en daar beneyens alles wat het *Gilde*, volgens de Keure des Jaars 1733. competeert, betaalt. Weshalven wy den voornoemden [illegible] als onzen *Gilde-Broeder* erkennen, en voor *Meester Chirurgyn* in ons GROOT-MEESTER-BOEK hebben aangetekent, om met Vryë, en Openbaare Winkel, de Konst der *Chirurgie* binnen deeze Stad, en de vryheit van dien, ter plaatze waar het Hem zal gevallen, zonder eenige verhindernisse, te mogen oeffenen; zullende gehouden zyn de Keuren en Ordonnantien van het *Gilde* te observeeren, en zich aan dezelve, als een goed *Gilde-Broeder* betaamt, altoos onderwerpen.

Aldus gedaan by het COLLEGIUM CHIRURGICUM. In teken der waarheit, deeze onderschreven, en met onzen Gilden Zegel bekrachtigt.

Actum Amsterdam den [illegible] des Jaars Zeventienhondert en [illegible]

Willem Röell

Anatom: & Chirurg: Professor

Decanus

Examinator

Overmannen

Frederik Reijne's graduation certificate, presented by Amsterdam Surgeons' Guild, also signed by Willem Röell, *Praelector Anatomiae* (1738). Municipal Archive Amsterdam.

Guild as a qualified surgeon. He would then be granted permission to open up his own surgeon's shop in the city, where he could train a new generation of aspiring surgeons.

Taking the final surgeon's exam was a relatively costly affair for the aspiring-surgeons. In 1676, the examination fee was 155 guilders (equivalent to 1,500 Euros today), and by 1733 the costs had increased to 250 guilders (equivalent to 2,800 Euros). Of this amount, 10 guilders were meant for the *praelector anatomiae*, 60 guiders went to the Board of Governors, 6 guilders were given to the Guild servants, 1 guilder was donated to the poor, and 173 guilders were reserved for the banquet the Guild would hold upon the completion of the exam.

▸ **The Anatomy Theatre at the Weighing House (*Waag*), the dissection room of Amsterdam's surgeons** The Guild of Surgeons looked after the interests of Amsterdam's surgeons, defined the scope of their profession, organised their education as well as their further training. The Board of Governors held their gatherings at the guildhall: this was where they held their meetings and where the surgeon's examinations took place. They also had a dissection room at their disposal here. Since the end of the seventeenth century, this *Theatrum Anatomicum* (Anatomy Theatre), was located at the city's Weighing House. In this way, the guildhall and the dissection room became the very centre of the Amsterdam surgeons' existence.

The very first anatomical dissections took place at what had previously been the St.-Ursula Convent on the Oudezijds Achterburgwal, which would later become a house of correction for women. In 1578, they relocated the dissection room to the former Convent of Saint Margaret above the Lesser Meat Market on the Nes. The surgeons eventually moved to the newly constructed Weighing House on the Nieuwmarkt (New Market) in 1619. At first, this was solely used as their guildhall, but a few years later in 1624, they also set up a small dissection-room there. When in 1639 these premises became too small, they returned to their previous location on the first floor of the St.-Margaret's convent on the Nes, while the surgeons' guildhall remained at the Weighing House. As time passed, the upper floor of the former St.-Margaret's convent also became overcrowded. Due to the lack of space, compounded by the dilapidated state of the building, the surgeons were forced to search for another location. To this end, they submitted a request for suitable premises to the municipal council. This led to the decision to construct a proper

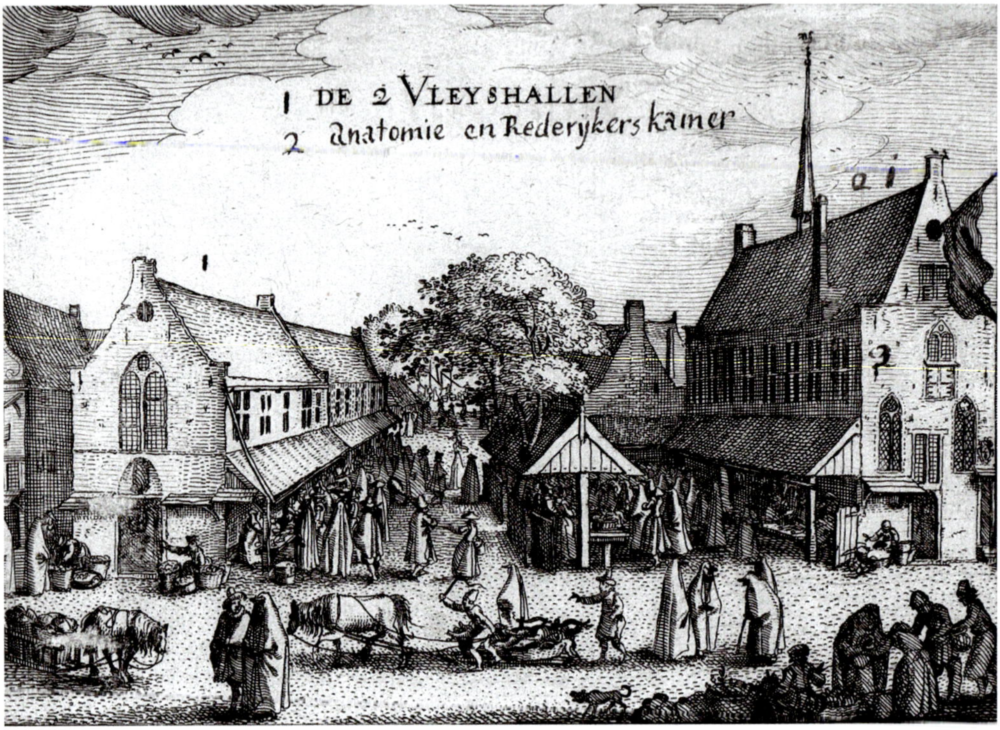

An engraving from 1611 shows the Greater and Lesser Meat Markets on either side of the Nes in Amsterdam (The latter was the former St.-Margaret's Convent). The upper storey of the building on the right, where a flag is seen hanging, housed the guildhall and the dissection room of the Amsterdam Surgeons' Guild. The surgeons shared the upper storey with the *rederijkers* (rhetoricians; poets and professional orators). Municipal Archive Amsterdam.

anatomy lecture theatre for the surgeons. This new *Theatrum Anatomicum,* as the dissection room of the surgeons' guild was called, was specifically built for the purpose inside an octagonal dome at the centre of the Weighing House. Once the building was finally completed and equipped in 1691, the Surgeons' Guild settled there for good.

For more than five centuries, the Weighing House was the most iconic building on the Nieuwmarkt, at the old centre of Amsterdam. It originally served as a city gate (St Anthony's Gate), and was part of the medieval city wall. After the wall was dismantled at the beginning of the seventeenth century, the building was designated as Weighing House. On the ground floor, all manner of merchandise ranging from iron, lead, timber, rope, wool and beer was weighed before it was readied for sale. The municipal council made the upper floor available to a number of guilds, including those of the ironsmiths, painters, masons and surgeons. Each guild had its own entrance at one of the

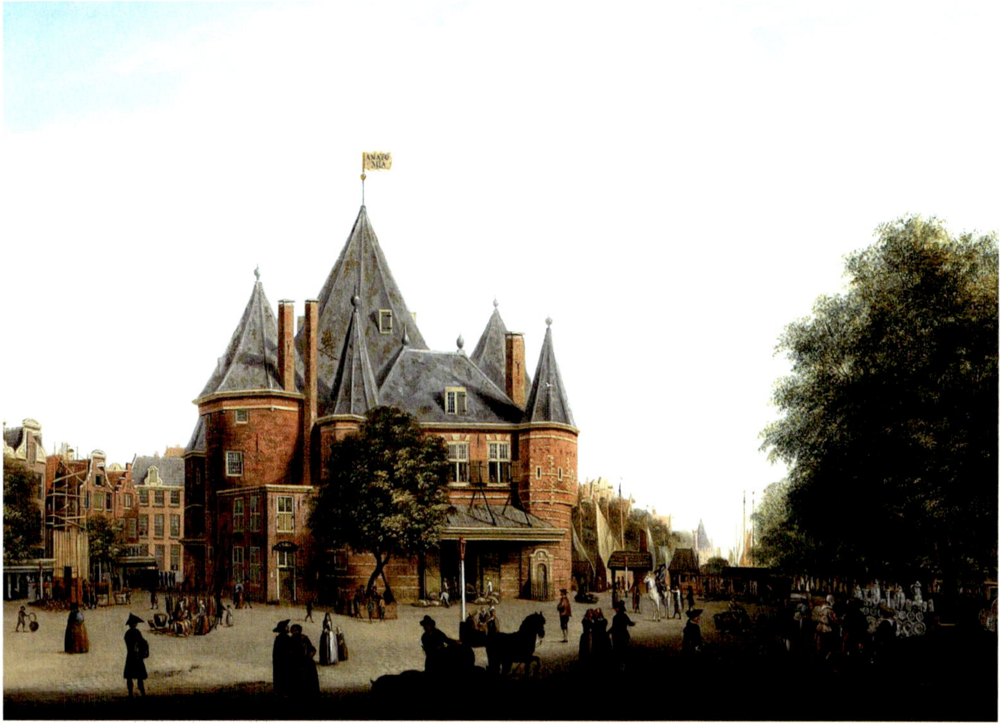

Isaac Ouwater, *View of the Weighing House on the Nieuwmarkt (New Market) in Amsterdam*, c. 1775. The gate at the right turret was the entrance to the Guild Hall and the *Theatrum Anatomicum* (Anatomy Theatre) of the Surgeons' Guild. The high central tower, under which the anatomy lecture theatre was located, is shown by a small weather-vane bearing the word ANATOMIA.

building's corner-towers. The entrance to the surgeon's guildhall and the dissection room was to the right of the old front gate located at the southeastern tower of the Weighing House, now the entrance to the cafe-restaurant *In de Waag*. In the façade above the entrance, a stone inscription still proclaims *Theatrum Anatomicum* (Anatomy Theatre).

In the guildhall's antechamber stood a cabinet containing surgical instruments, while the guild's archives and collection of medical books were kept in a specially constructed chest or book cabinet. The sandstone mantlepiece was decorated with the carved-out coats-of-arms that belonged to the members of the board of the Surgeons' Guild. For the rest, the remarkable interior boasted all kinds of curiosities which had been collected by the surgeons. The walls were hung with paintings the guild had commissioned to be made for them during the seventeenth and eighteenth centuries. Next to the guildhall was the anatomy lecture theatre (*Theatrum Anatomicum*) – at

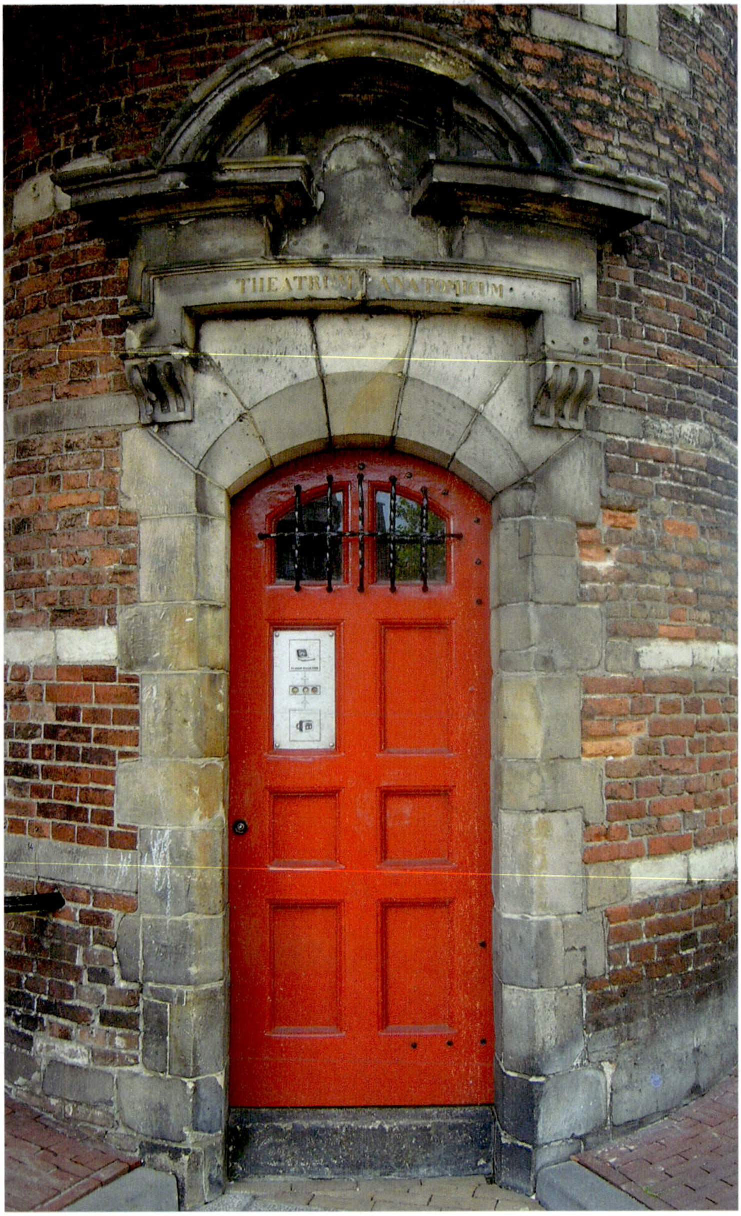

Entrance at the southeastern turret of the Weighing House (*Waag)* on Nieuwmarkt, what was once the front entrance to the guildhall and the Anatomy Theatre of the Amsterdam Surgeons' Guild. The words THEATRUM ANATOMICUM can still be seen inscribed above the door.

Introduction

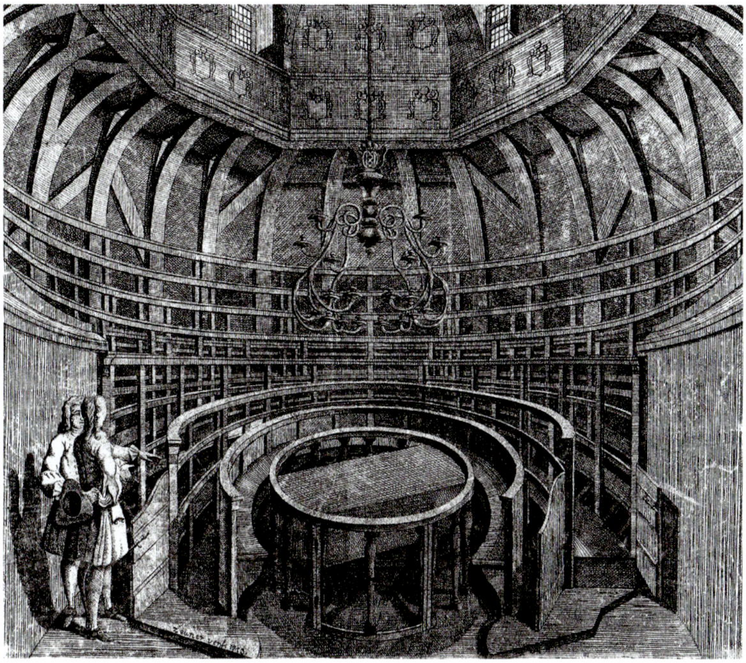

Jonas Zeuner, *Theatrum Anatomicum in the Weighing House*, c. 1775–1799. The dissection table stands at the centre, surrounded by circular tiers of seats. The room is lit by a chandelier suspended from the vault of the dome. Collection Amsterdam Museum.

that time the largest Anatomy Theatre in the country –, which could accommodate an audience of several hundreds. On top of the tower's spire, sat a gilded weather-vane which was inscribed with the word ANATOMIA, announcing the location of the Anatomy Theatre, the pride of the Amsterdam Guild of Surgeons.

The dissections, which were so fundamental for the anatomical instruction of the surgeons and apprentice surgeons, were carried out in this anatomy lecture theatre. The design of the dissection room was based on that of Europe's oldest anatomy lecture theatre in Padua in Northern Italy. It is shaped like an amphitheatre with a dissection table at its centre. The octagonal dome's four windows were placed in such a way that light fell directly onto the dissection table. The members of the board would commission painters to have their family coats-of-arms painted on the dome vault. Centrally placed is that of Frederik Ruysch, who was associated with the surgeons' guild as *praelector anatomiae* from 1666 until his death in 1731. Painted in three concentric rows, Ruysch's coat of arms is surrounded by thirty-six others, all belonging to surgeons who had

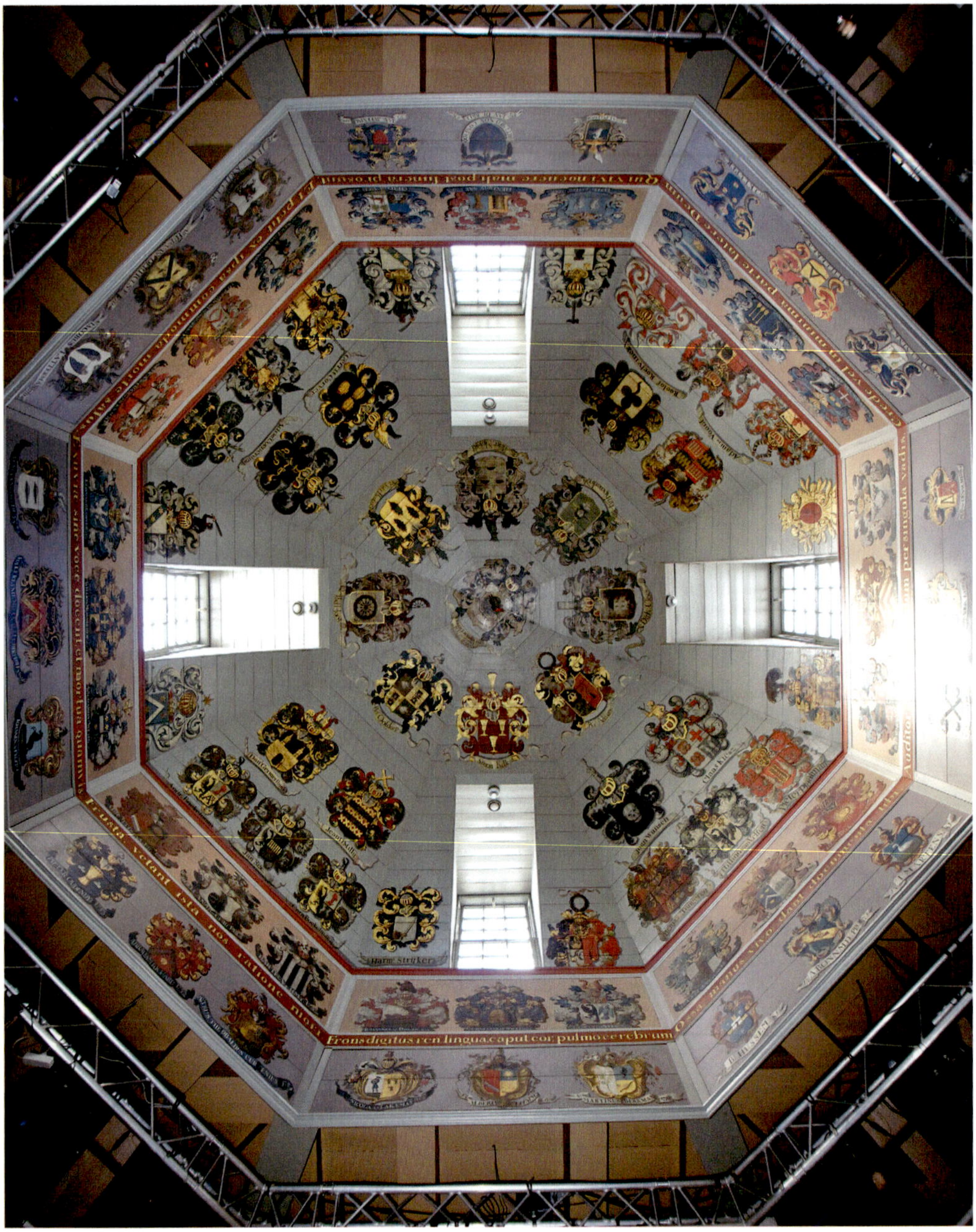

The coats of arms of the Amsterdam Surgeons' Guild Members of the Board, displayed on the circular wooden vault of the *Theatrum Anatomicum* in the Weighing House in Amsterdam.

Introduction

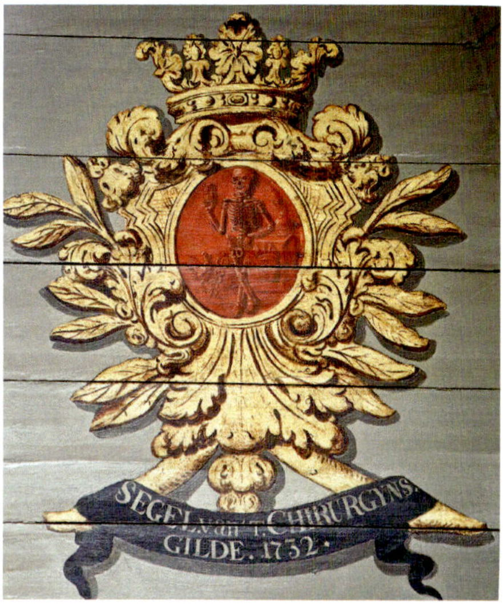

The coat-of-arms of the Amsterdam Surgeons' Guild painted on the vault of the *Theatrum Anatomicum* in the Weighing House. The human skeleton is a reference to the centuries-old *memento mori* "remember you must die" a theme with which surgeons were regularly confronted in their professional lives. A human skeleton as a symbol of the 'transience of existence' was also featured on the tokens of the surgeons' guild (see p. 8). The skeleton still serves as a symbol on the present-day Netherlands Association of Surgeons' medal of honour.

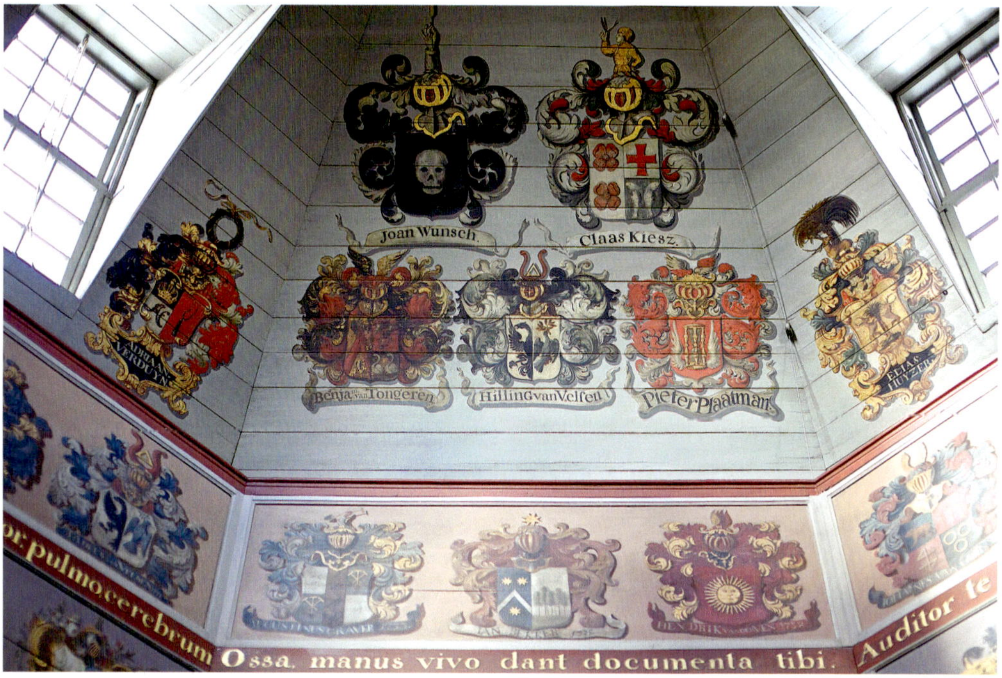

Family coats of arms of the Amsterdam surgeons in the vault of the *Theatrum Anatomicum* inside the Weighing House.

served as chairman of the Guild's board. One notable exception is that of the 'Seal of the Surgeon's Guild' in the third row. It was clear that these chairmen greatly valued having their coats of arms displayed in the dome vault. When they ran out of space for new coats of arms, wooden partitions were mounted on the banisters under the dome, to which another forty-eight coats of arms were added. Of all the surgeons whose coat of arms are displayed on the dome, the functions they fulfilled on the guild's board (chairman, dean or Chief Tutor) are known. A number of them became famous either for their surgical skills, or for their contributions to the guild. The room remained in use for anatomical instruction at the University of Amsterdam until 1869, its painted dome vault beautifully restored in 1992. The dissection table and the circular tribunes gradually disappeared, but the coats of arms displayed on the vault dome remain as a constant reminder of the hall's original function.

▸ **The Anatomy Lessons** The Amsterdam Surgeons' Guild took pride in its right to organise the anatomy lessons. Amsterdam was one of the first cities in the Netherlands where anatomy lectures were given as part of the training and where the stipulations for surgical training were properly laid down. Halfway through the sixteenth century, the members of the Amsterdam Surgeons' Guild recognised that anatomical instruction was an essential part of a surgeon's proper education. Moreover, a solid knowledge of anatomy was imperative for acquiring the practical skills required of a surgeon. Even before the guild had been granted official permission to carry out anatomical dissections, at least one anatomy lesson had taken place in Amsterdam. According to the guild's Anatomy Book, in which dissection reports were registered, the first lecture was given in 1550, using the corpse of the notorious thief 'Suster Luyt', the first woman to be condemned to death. Apparently, the surgeons kept the body's carefully preserved skin as a trophy of their very first lecture in anatomy for many years.

In 1555, King Philip II of Spain (technically still the sovereign of the Netherlands) granted the Amsterdam Surgeons' Guild official permission to instruct its members and the apprentices in anatomy by using corpses of criminals of those condemned to death for dissection purposes. Initially, the guild was given approval to organise one 'anatomy lesson' a year. This lecture was to be given at a location designated by the guild for the dissection by the *praelector anatomiae* (lecturer in anatomy). As time passed, it became clear that lessons were given more regularly throughout the year. However, in some years no lectures were held at all, due to the fact that the guild did not have any corpses at its disposal.

The corpse which was to be the subject of the dissection was referred to as the *subjectum anatomicum*. During the anatomy lessons, the surgeons usually used corpses of criminals who had been condemned to death. In the Anatomy Book of the Surgeons' Guild as well as the Amsterdam judicial archives, we often come across the names of the condemned criminals in the dissection reports, as well as the crime he or she had committed, and the manner in which he or she had been executed. Other bodies that were available for dissection were the bodily remains of 'strangers': those who had died in Amsterdam's hospitals and poorhouses and who had no family to mourn for them.

Anatomy lessons were held at the dissection room of the guild: originally at the former St.-Ursula Convent, then at St.-Margaret's Convent and after 1691, at the *Theatrum Anatomicum* in the Weighing House. The dissection table stood at the centre of the room, encircled by tribunes for anyone interested. The central figure during these lessons on whom all eyes were focused, was the *praelector anatomiae*. Usually, the lecturer began his lecture with a moral argument which justified the dissection of a human body. On the one hand, the spectators would be reminded of the transience of existence and on the other, that the acquisition of anatomical knowledge was a divine path towards knowledge. Once he had finished his speech, he would commence dissecting the corpse on the table.

Most anatomical dissections took place in the winter, as perishable organs did not decompose as quickly at lower temperatures. In fact, the speed at which the organs decomposed dictated the order in which the dissection took place. This requirement ensured that it followed strict guidelines. The first organs to be dissected were those in the abdominal cavity, followed by those in the thoracic cavity, the brain and finally the limbs. Including the customary intermissions, these anatomical lessons generally required a number of days.

At the beginning of the seventeenth century, various rules were introduced to ensure that instruction in dissection for surgeons proceeded in an orderly manner. In 1606, these rules were laid down in an official document called The Anatomy Ordinance (*Ordonnantie voor de Anatomie*) and incorporated in the Surgeons' Guild's regulations. The Ordinance listed nine requirements of conduct for the surgeons during the course of their education, as well as the protocol which they were expected to follow:

Article I Regular lessons are given on Tuesdays and Fridays. All surgeons must attend and pay a 3-*stuyver* lecture fee each time. Lessons in osteology (the study of bones), anatomy, physiology, the theory or practice of surgery — or any another subject related to the science of dissection which the lecturer might happen to select — are held on Tuesday for the apprentices and aspirant surgeons and on Friday for the master surgeons. The time is not always fixed, but is determined by the lecturer. On the occasion of public dissections, weekly lessons will be cancelled.

Article II On lecture days, the guild servant must be present half an hour in advance to ensure that all is prepared for the anatomy lesson. The guild servant has a key to both the guildhall and the anatomy lecture theatre.
* After 1723, the guild servant was no longer in possession of a key, because a fire that had broken out in the ante-room of the guildhall as a result of a servant's carelessness.

Article III Talking, laughing and walking around the lecture theatre during lessons are forbidden.

Article IV Surgeons have to pay the guild 6 *stuyvers* in order to attend a lecture in anatomical dissection.

Article V Members of the audience will take their seats on the benches surrounding the dissection table in order of arrival. However, the innermost benches are reserved for the city's administrators and doctors aged fifty and older. The second and third rows are designated for doctors, the guild's members of the board, and master surgeons aged fifty and older. The next three rows are assigned to master surgeons, while the remaining, outer rows are meant for *knechten* (trainee-surgeons) and any other spectators.

Article VI The Assistant Tutor (*collegemeester*) will assist the lecturer in both the weekly lessons as well as the lessons in dissection. His duties might include rotating the dissecting-table or handing over specific instruments. Generally, his tasks are to provide the assistance necessary to ensure that the lecture will run smoothly. The presence of the chief tutor is required at all the lessons given by the *praelector*. Another task is to take a note

→
Andries Stock, after a design by Jacob de Gheyn II, *Anatomy Lesson*, 1615. Collection Rijksmuseum Amsterdam.

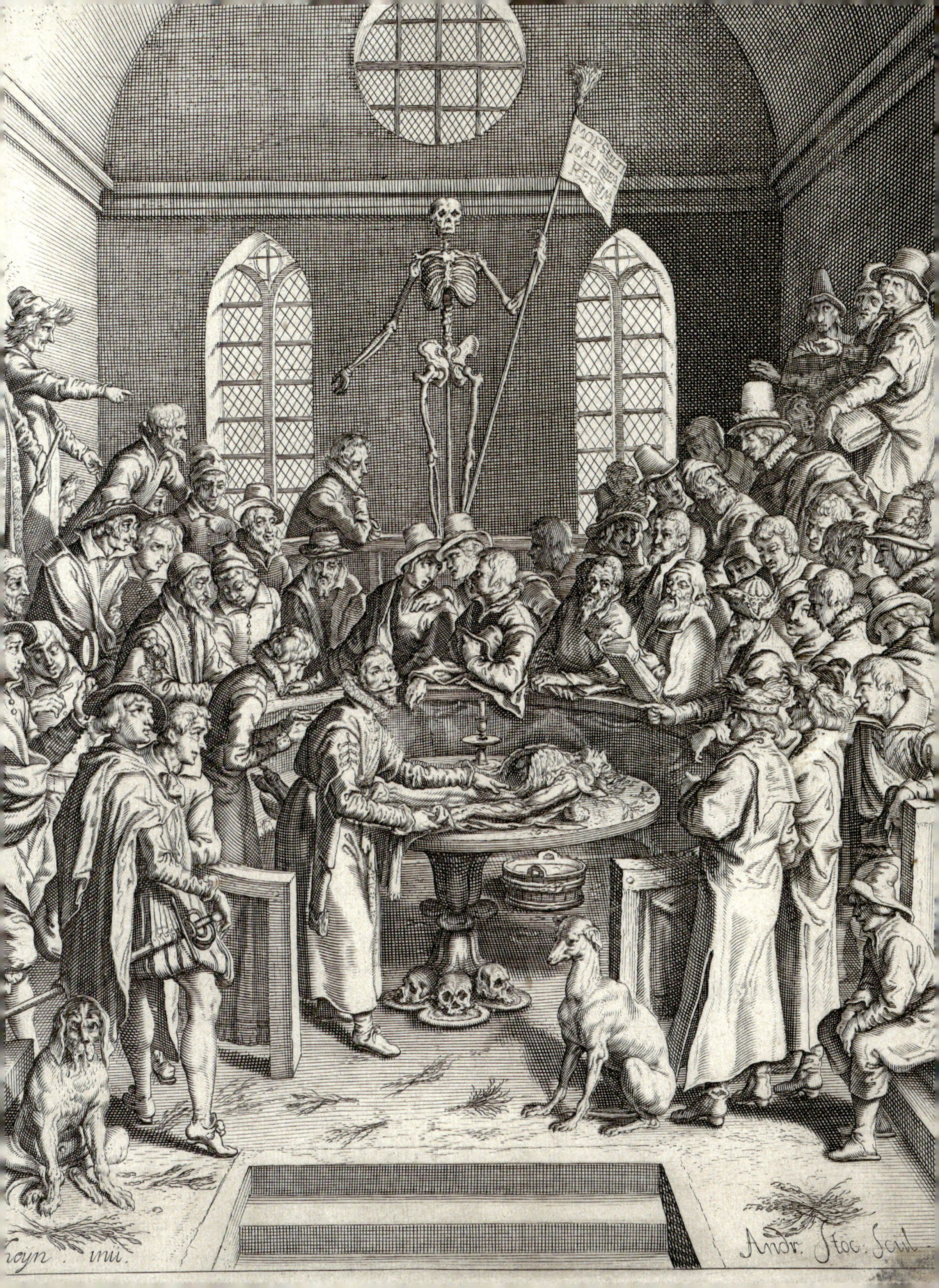
MORS ULTI
MA LINEA
RERUM
Andr. Stoc. Scul.

of the surgeons' attendance. The attendance roll is to be handed over to the Board of Governors once a year so that those who have been absent can be fined.

Article VII None of the spectators are permitted to remove any part of the dissected corpse. Anyone stealing a part of the corpse will be imposed with a fine of at least 6 guilders (present value 100 Euros).

Article VIII Should anyone among those present have a question about the anatomy, he can ask the *praelector* after the lesson. Before this rule was implemented in 1606, the number of surgeons amounted to no more than thirty, so it was still possible to ask questions during the demonstration. As time passed and the number of surgeons grew, this was no longer possible.

Article IX During question-and-answer sessions, as well as during all other discussions, it is forbidden to humiliate or ridicule one another.

This set of regulations provides some insight as to how the anatomy lessons were organised. The weekly 'theoretical' lectures provided the basis of the surgeons' education. The anatomy lessons were observational of character, during which the *praelector anatomiae* instructed students who followed the demonstration from their benches. Opportunities during which the surgeons were able to do any actual practical dissection themselves were very limited. Attending a public anatomical dissection remained an exceptional event for the surgeons for years, however. The ability to observe an actual human body during these lessons provided them with a unique opportunity to supplement the knowledge they had obtained from their anatomy textbooks.

An engraving dating from 1615 (see preceding page) gives an impression of what took place during an anatomy lesson at the time. It shows a *praelector* standing at the dissection-table as he lectures to a modest group of about fifty spectators The image probably shows an anatomy lesson given in Leiden, but the situation will not have been very different from the lectures given at the time in the dissection room above the Lesser Meat Hall in Amsterdam.

In the course of the seventeenth century, the anatomy demonstrations grew to become well-attended events that increasingly drew the attention of the bourgeoisie. In the Guild Statutes of 1625, it is expressly stated that, 'from now on, anyone interested in anatomy [...] will have to pay an entrance fee of 4 *stuyvers*, and guild members had to pay 6 *stuyvers*, for each body that is dissected.' Anatomy lessons were not just confined to guild members but — for the payment of 4 *stuyvers* — open to anyone interested in attending a lecture on the subject. A glance at the Surgeons' Guild Anatomy Book reveals that an anatomy lesson in the seventeenth century could last, over several days, attracting hundreds of spectators. It prompts the question to what extent such a throng of visitors negatively affected the educative value of the exercise for the surgeons. According to Article V of the 1606 regulation as cited above, the surgical apprentices, who were there to actually learn, had to sit in the back rows of the Amsterdam Anatomy Theatre, together with the general public. A picture showing an anatomical lecture at the Anatomy Theatre in Leiden gives a good impression of the high attendance and the wide public interest for such an event (see next page). The situation in the Amsterdam Weighing House would not have been very different. The income generated by the lessons was used to pay the expenses incurred by the lesson and for the burial of what remained of the corpse. Any money that still remained was usually spent on an extensive guild banquet — held after the anatomy lesson.

▸ **The *praelector anatomiae* (reader in anatomy)** From 1550 to 1578, the anatomical dissections were performed by the Guild's governors. In 1578, a *praelector anatomiae* was appointed to ensure that the lectures ran smoothly and to raise the standard of quality. These lecturers were academically trained physicians (*doctores medicinae*) who enjoyed a high social standing. Martin Janszn Coster, alias Martin Aedituus (c. 1520–1592) was the first *praelector anatomiae* to be appointed by the Amsterdam Surgeons' Guild. He had studied medicine at the University of Bologna in Italy and had previously worked as court physician to Frederick II of Denmark. Unfortunately, little is known of his career as lecturer. He was succeeded by Sebastiaen Egbertszn (1563–1621), who held the function from 1595 until his death in 1621. Just as his predecessor Coster, Egbertszn also occupied a number of other important functions, including the position of burgomaster of Amsterdam. Johan Fonteijn (1574–1628), also known as Johannes Fontanus, followed in Egbertszn's footsteps as *praelector* in 1621. Apart from his medical

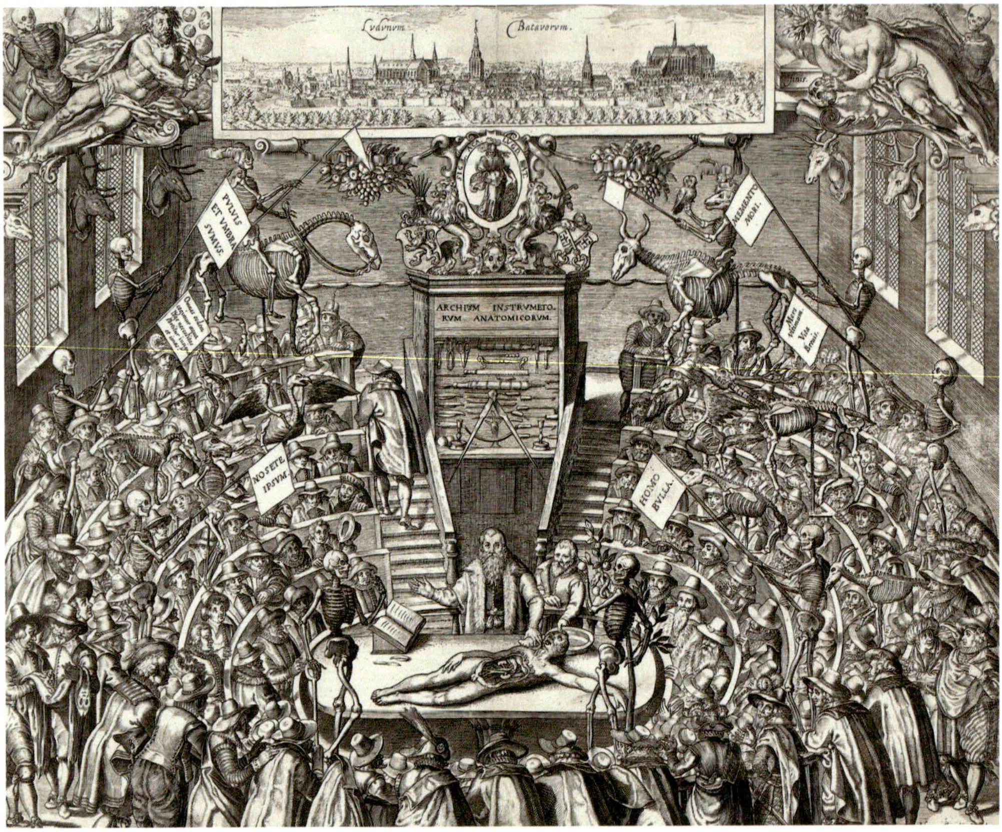

Bartholomeus Dolendo, after a drawing by Jan Corneliszn van 't Woud, *The Theatrum Anatomicum in Leiden*, 1619. Collection Rijksmuseum Amsterdam.

achievements, he was also known as a connoisseur of culture and the arts.

Nicolaes Tulp (1593–1674) succeeded Fonteijn in 1628. Of course, Tulp is best known for his being portrayed in *The Anatomy Lesson of Nicolaes Tulp*, the world-famous group portrait painted by Rembrandt for the Amsterdam Surgeons' Guild in 1632. During his career as a medical doctor, he built up an impressive track record. Among other achievements, he took the initiative in the founding of the *Collegium Medicum* (College of Medicine), a body which supervised the quality of health care in Amsterdam, and he compiled a manual on the preparation and use of medications. Tulp was one of the first *praelectors* to record the findings during anatomical dissections. His *Observationes Medicae* contains descriptions of the medical histories of more than two hundred patients. Tulp's meticulous anatomical observations irrefutably led to medical discoveries. In 1653, he resigned from the position to become a burgomaster of Amsterdam, and he was succeeded by Jan Deijman (1619–1666). Like Tulp before him, Deijman was also portrayed by Rembrandt in another prestigious portrait of the members of the guild: *The Anatomy Lesson of Jan Deijman* (1656). Unfortunately, the painting was badly damaged by the fire which broke out in the guildhall in 1723. In 1667, Deijman was succeeded as *praelector* by Frederik Ruysch (1638-1731), under whom great progress was made in anatomical education. He successfully preserved cadavers by injecting the blood vessels with a warm, waxlike substance which solidified as it cooled. He built up an imposing collection of at least 2,000 (preserved) anatomical preparations, the bulk of which is still kept at the Peter the Great Museum for Anthropology and Ethnography (*Kunstkamera*) in St Petersburg. Ruysch, who was *praelector* for sixty years, made a significant contribution to the education of surgeons in that period. From 1731 to 1755, Willem Röell held the position of *praelector*. This was a period in which the guild was plunged into difficulties due to the fraudulent practices perpetrated by members of the board. In 1755, Petrus Camper was appointed Röell's successor. Anatomical education under Camper was valued highly. He also played a prominent role academically, he was particularly renowned for his publication of a series of finely illustrated anatomical atlases of the pelvis, groin and arm, based on the finding from his dissections. In his farewell speech to the guild, Camper declared that he had dissected the bodies of more than fifty adults and children. Folkert Snip (1733–1771), Camper's successor, held the position from 1762–1771. Finally, Andreas Bonn (1738–1818) was the last *praelector anatomiae* of the Amsterdam Surgeons' Guild. He wrote a detailed description of the collection of bones bearing pathological features, which was kept at the guildhall in the Weighing House. This task culminated in the publication of *Tabulae Ossium Morbosorum* (Atlas of Morbid Bones) (1785). The collection is now on display at the Vrolik Museum at the Amsterdam University Medical Center (location Academic Medical Centre) in Amsterdam.

In the final decades of the eighteenth century, the Amsterdam Surgeons' Guild went through a particularly difficult time. Naturally, the number of surgeons in the city had increased manyfold, but there was increased dissent among the guild members while the educational standards deteriorated. After two and a half centuries of striving for progress for surgical care in Amsterdam, all these factors contributed to the surgeons' guild's demise. In 1798, the Surgeons' Guild was disbanded and incorporated into the Board of Medical Supervision. In the last decade of the eighteenth century, a number of surgeons already felt the need to be able to exchange knowledge and experiences on a regular basis. This led to the establishment of the *Genootschap ter Bevordering der Heelkunde* (Society for the Advancement of Surgery) in Amsterdam in 1790, under the direction of Andreas Bonn, the *praelector* of the Surgeons' Guild. This society organized public lectures and focused on training surgeons.

▸ **The Portrayal of Amsterdam's Surgeons** In the course of the seventeenth and eighteenth centuries, the Amsterdam Surgeons' Guild commissioned a large number of group portraits by famous Dutch artists, such as Rembrandt, Pickenoy, Backer, Van Neck, Troost and Quinkhard. The paintings concerned were carefully composed group portraits, painted to commemorate those portrayed in the solidarity of their profession. Each person who wished to be included in a painting had to pay a fee to the artist. No doubt, the commissions for such paintings also stem from the desire to raise the status of the surgeon's profession, as well as to line the guildhall's walls with masterpieces.

In the period between 1601–1758, no fewer than eighteen group portraits were painted for the guild. In nine of these portraits, a lesson in anatomy is the main subject, in which the leading roles are played by the *praelector anatomicum* and the *subjectum anatomicum* (the anatomical subject). For this reason, these group portraits — dating from 1601–1603, 1619, 1621, 1632, 1656, 1670, 1683, 1728 and 1758 — are also referred to as 'the anatomy lessons' or 'the anatomy works of art' (see also Chapters 1 to 9). At the end of the seventeenth century, the anatomy lesson began to lose its importance as the surgeons' group portraits' main theme. Paintings of the *praelectors* and the cadavers on the dissecting-table were gradually replaced by portraits of the members of the board seated around a conference table. Paraphernalia such as medical manuals, anatomical illustrations and surgical instruments were strategically placed on the table to indicate the profession of the portrayed men. For this reason, these later portraits (totaling nine) are referred to as 'the portraits of the guild governors' (see Chapter 10). These portraits were hung in the guildhall where they formed the guild's unique art collection. Nowadays most of the paintings are kept at the Amsterdam Museum.

This book will focus on these nine anatomical lessons. Important events in the surgeons' guild's history — such as the first anatomy lesson delivered by a new *praelector* or the opening of a new guildhall — were reason enough to commission a new painting of an anatomy lesson. Obviously, the artist and surgeons chose to have the theme of an anatomy lesson incorporated into their group portrait, as the anatomical demonstrations organized by the guild played a vital role in the lives of the surgeons. Besides, the dissections inspired the artist to create unique compositions. However, the paintings were primarily carefully composed group portraits, and were not realistic depictions of the anatomical demonstrations that were held in the surgeons' dissection room.

Almost all of the nine anatomy lessons exhibit a number of recurring characteristics: a dissector (the *praelector anatomiae*) surrounded by a group of surgeons, a human cadaver and one dissected body part. Every anatomy lesson contains a story just waiting to be told. Who is the *praelector anatomiae?* What was his background and what lessons did he give? Who are the surgeons portrayed and what did they do? Who is the silent witness in the painting, the executed criminal on the dissection table, and what crime had he committed? Furthermore: what anatomical structures are shown in the dissected body part and to what extent is the anatomy accurately depicted? Is there some underlying symbolic significance? The anatomical lessons will come to life when one immerses oneself in the lives and work of those portrayed. With this purpose in mind, Amsterdam's anatomy lessons will be dissected in the following chapters.

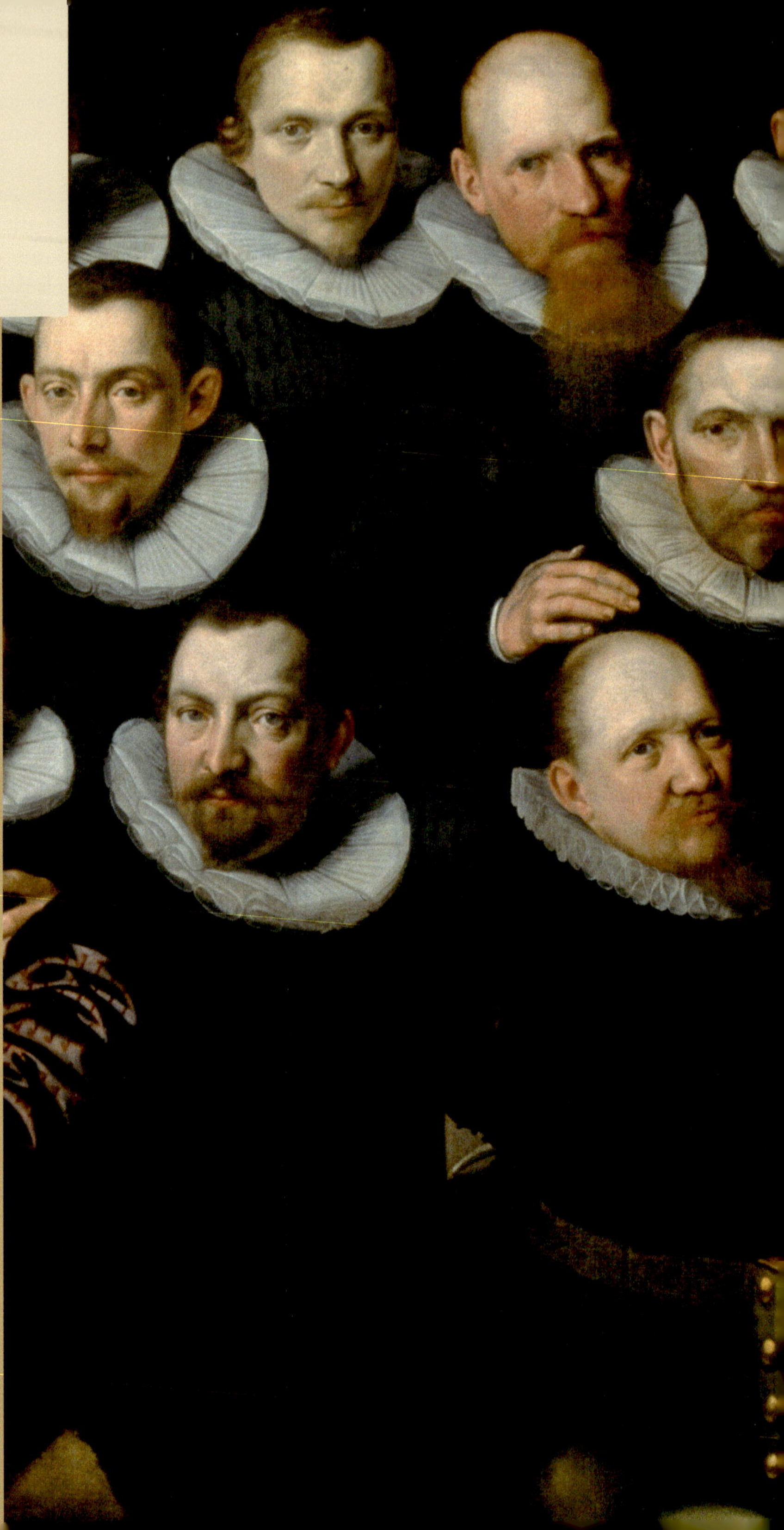

Aert Pieterszn, *The Anatomy Lesson of Sebastiaen Egbertszn,* 1601–1603. Detail. Collection Amsterdam Museum.

1

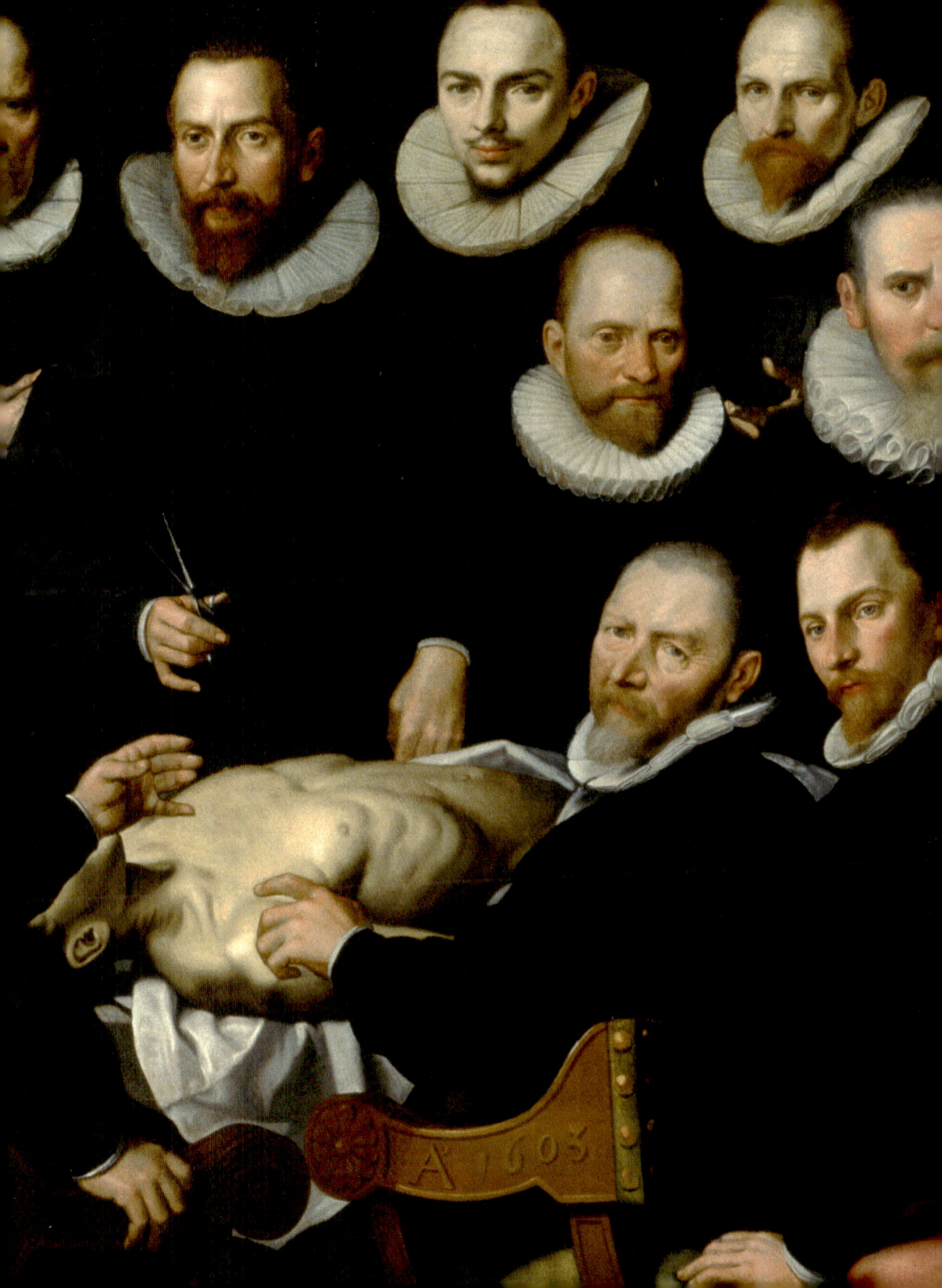
A° 1603

Sebastiaen Egbertszn [1]

The Anatomy Lesson of Sebastiaen Egbertszn,
painted by Aert Pieterszn in 1601–1603

▸ **The Painting** *The Anatomy Lesson of Sebastiaen Egbertszn*, which dates from 1601–1603, is the oldest in the series of the nine so-called 'Anatomy Lessons' or 'Anatomy Works of Art', painted for the Amsterdam Surgeons' Guild during the seventeenth and eighteenth centuries. It laid the foundation for a tradition in portrait painting which would last for a hundred and fifty years. The theme of the 'anatomy lesson' was masterfully combined to create a series of carefully composed group portraits of the guild's surgeons. The guild members obviously chose for the anatomy lesson theme to be included in the composition. After all, the anatomy demonstrations given by the *praelector* were of great importance to the surgeons.

In the *Anatomy Lesson of Sebastiaen Egbertszn*, painted between 1601 and 1603, the *praelector anatomiae* and the surgeons are shown gathered around a corpse that has been placed on a table in front of them. Egbertszn, who had been *praelector anatomiae* of the Surgeons' Guild since 1595, is instructing the surgeons. From the way he clasps the surgical forceps in his right hand, it seems as if he is about to commence his demonstration. What is remarkable in this painting, is the way the men's focus is not on the dissected body as one might expect, but directed at something beyond the scope of the painting, this allows their features and their facial expressions to be accurately depicted. In this composition, the anatomical dissection in question has been reduced in significance. The real focus of attention is the portrayals of the individual surgeons. The *Anatomy Lesson of Sebastiaen Egbertszn* was never intended to be an exact reproduction of a documented dissection. Just as the other paintings in the anatomy lesson series, it is a group portrait whose purpose was to glorify the *praelector* and the surgeon-members of the Amsterdam Surgeons' Guild, and to emphasize their importance. Due to the rapid growth in numbers of the surgeons' guild members in the course of the seventeenth century, the privilege of being portrayed in later years was usually limited to the *praelector* and Board of Governors.

▸ **The Artist** Aert Pieterszn (1550–1612) came from an artistic family. He was the son of the famous painter Pieter Aertsen, known as "Tall Pier" (1509-1575), who was noted for his magnificent still-life and genre paintings in which he depicted scenes from everyday life. Aert had an older brother, Pieter Pieterszn, and a younger brother, Dirck Pieterszn, who were both painters. Sometime around 1562, when Aert was about twelve, the Pieterszn family lived on Oudekerksplein 62 in Amsterdam. At this time, many gold-smiths, painters and sculptors lived in the vicinity of the Oude Kerk.

The Oudekerksplein is situated in the oldest part of town in the heart of what is now known as "the Wallen", between the Warmoesstraat and the Oudezijds Voorburgwal. When Aert Pieterszn married, he moved to a house on the Oude Doelenstraat 2. Around 1598, he moved back to his old family neighbourhood, where he bought a house on the Prinsenhofsteeg (nr. 191 or 193), a side-street of the Oudezijds Voorburgwal, where he lived for the rest of his life. If he

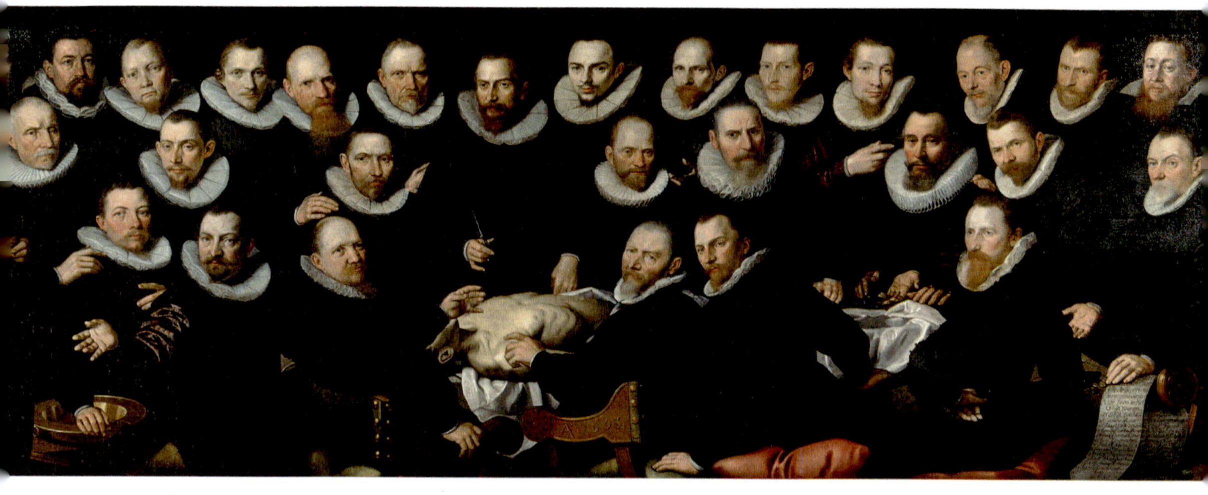

Aert Pieterszn, *The Anatomy Lesson of Sebastiaen Egbertsz*, 1601–1603. Collection Amsterdam Museum.

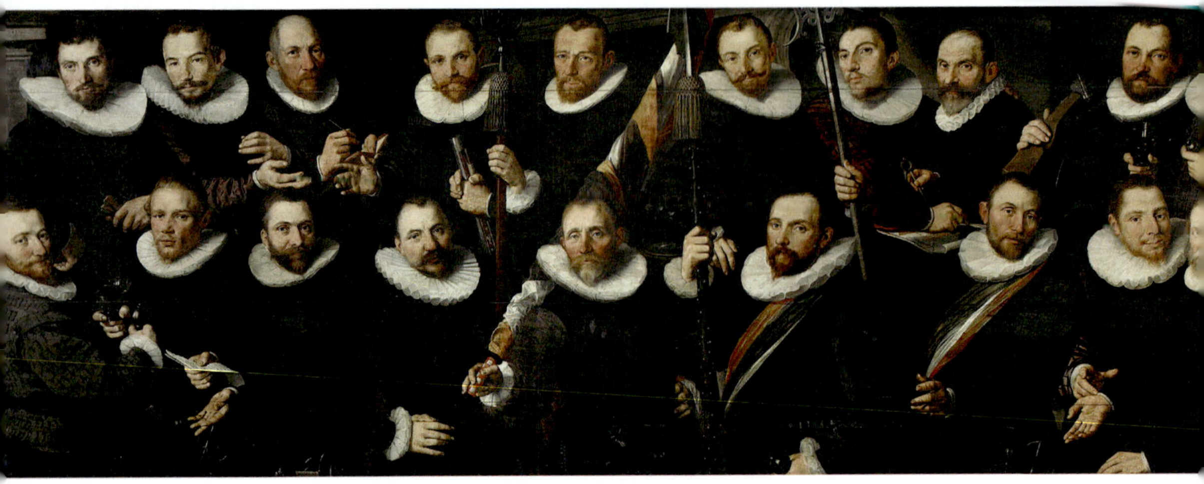

Aert Pieterszn, *Musketeers from Captain Jan de Bisschop and Ensign Pieter Egbertszn Vinck's Civic Guard*, 1599. Collection Amsterdam Museum.

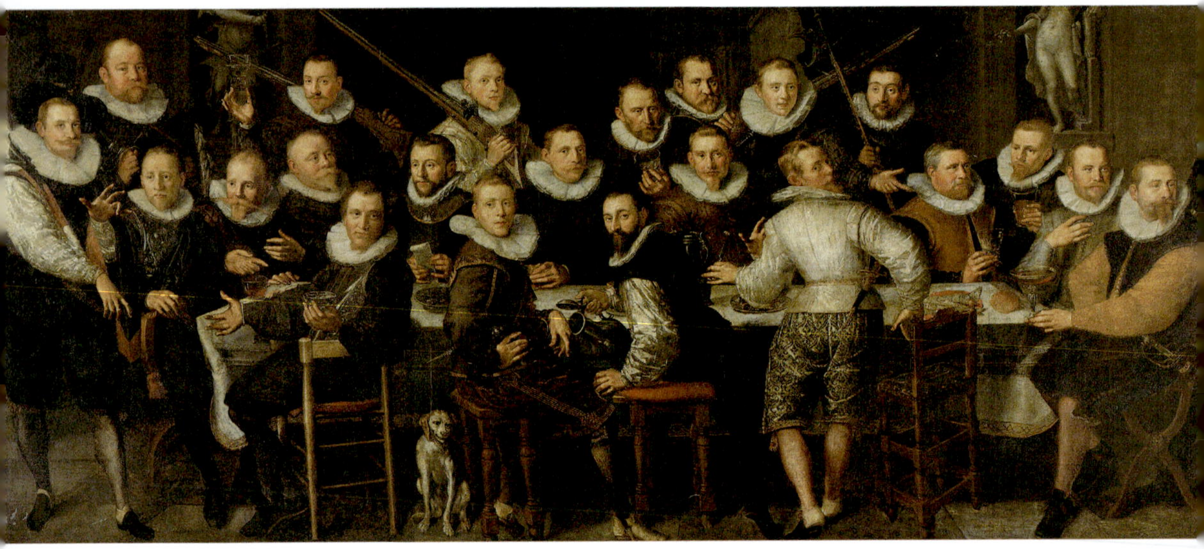

Pieter Isaacszn, *Musketeers from Captain Gillis Janszn Valckenier and Lieutenant Pieter Jacobszn Bas's Civic Guard*, 1599. Collection Amsterdam museum.

1

Sebastiaen Egbertszn[1] *1601–1603*

did have an artist's studio at home, this might have been the place where he painted *The Anatomy Lesson of Sebastiaen Egbertszn* between 1601–1603.

It is not unlikely that Aert Pieterszn obtained the commission to paint a group portrait of Egbertszn and the surgeons due to the success of his portrait of a group of the Amsterdam civil militia, *The Musketeers of Captain Jan de Bisschop and Ensign Pieter Egbertszn Vinck's Squadron,* painted in 1599. Pieterszn had completed this magnificent group painting of this Amsterdam civil militia a few years before. The militia, later referred to as 'the civic guard' (*burgerwacht*), consisted of groups of citizens who had taken it upon themselves to keep law and order and, when necessary, to defend the city. One of the most famous *schuttersstukken* (militia group portraits) in history is *Captain Frans Banning Cocq and Lieutenant Willem van Ruytenburgh's squadron* also known as *The Night Watch,* painted by Rembrandt van Rijn in 1642. If the musketeers were shown whilst enjoying a guild banquet, these paintings were called a 'Banquet of the Civic Guard'. Those who were portrayed in the painting each had to pay the artist an individual fee.

Pieterszn's *Anatomy Lesson of Sebastiaen Egbertszn* of 1603 displays several similarities to his earlier militia painting of 1599. He probably used it for inspiration when he received the commission from the surgeons. In both paintings, the subjects have been portrayed next to each other in an orderly fashion, ensuring that they are equally displayed. The faces are shown at a slight angle on a flat surface. The surgeons' group portrait also shares a striking similarity with *The Civic Guard of Captain Gillis Janszn Valckenier and Lieutenant Pieter Jacobszn Bas,* a scene from a banquet of the Civic Guard, painted by Pieter Isaacszn, also from 1599. Although the subjects are arranged in the same manner, the musketeers' dining table has been replaced by the surgeons' dissection table. The composition of the first group portrait of the surgeons was most probably inspired by these two slightly earlier group portraits of the civil militia, and marks the beginning of a unique portrait tradition in the Amsterdam Surgeons' Guild.

▸ **The Dissector** Sebastiaen Egbertszn (1563–1621) was the son of the rich Amsterdam merchant Egbert Meynertszn. His mother was Dieuwer Jacobsdr. Meynertszn was a fervent supporter of the Reformation and he was arrested for his religious beliefs and

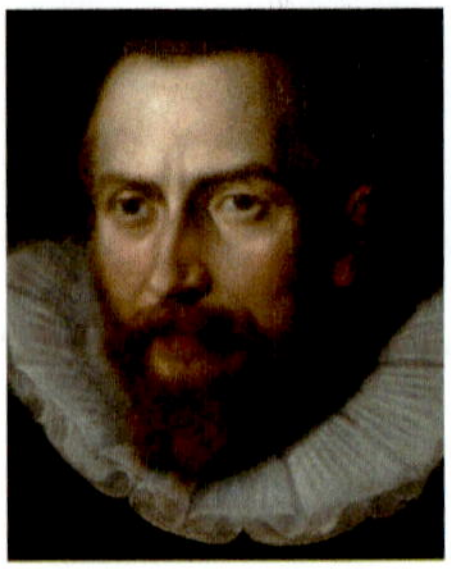

Sebastiaen Egbertszn (1563–1621)

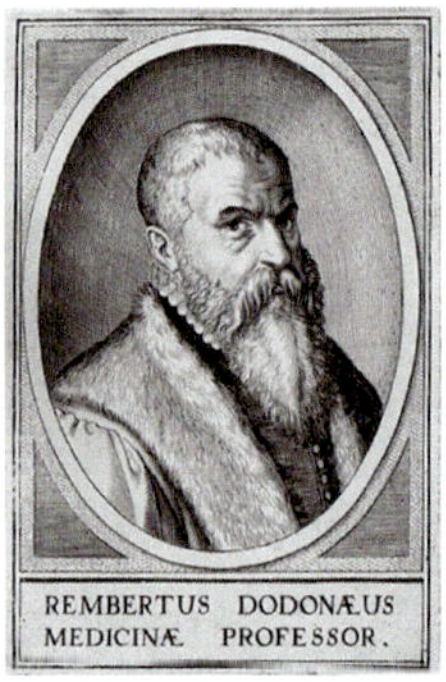

Rembertus Dodonaeus (1517–1585). Museum Boerhaave, Leiden.

condemned to death. However, he died in prison under atrocious conditions the night before he was due to be executed. Sebastiaen was only five years old at the time, and had to grow up without a father. He studied medicine at the prestigious universities of Leiden and Padua in Northern Italy and, at the age of twenty-five, he obtained his doctorate in medicine as a physician. He then returned to Amsterdam and in 1596 he married Agnieta Jacobsdr. She must have died a few years later because, in 1606, Egbertszn married again, this time to Margriete van Dronckelaer. They lived in the vicinity of the Oudezijds Cemetery.

In 1595 Egbertszn was appointed *praelector anatomiae* of the Amsterdam Surgeons' Guild, as the successor to Martin Coster. No doubt, he was well-acquainted with medical literature. While he was still a student in Leiden, Egbertszn attended the lectures of Rembertus Dodonaeus (1517–1585), who was the professor of medicine in Leiden at that time. Dodonaeus' medical career had been impressive. He started his career in 1541 as the town physician of Mechelen in Belgium, which he left in 1574 for Vienna to take up the post of personal physician to Emperor Maximilian II. In 1582 he was offered a chair in Leiden. Dodonaeus published several influential books, including the *Cruydt-boeck* (Book of Herbs) in 1554 and *Stirpium historiae pemptades sex* (Description of Plants in Six Volumes) in 1583. His *Praxis Medica* (Medical Practice), a collection of his lectures in Latin, was published posthumously in Amsterdam in 1616. Egbertszn annotated his former professor's book with notes and explanatory captions which were based on his own empirical observations. This was followed six years later by an edited Dutch version, entitled *Ars Medica, ofte Ghenees-kunst. (The Art of Medicine, or the Art of Healing).* This book consists of seventy-three chapters, and 423 pages. The title page shows that a great diversity of internal and external ailments are covered in the book, and that these have been further explained by the Highly Learned 'Doctor Sebastiaen Egbertszn'.

Egbertszn also intended to make medical literature accessible to surgeons. At that time, the majority of medical books was written in Latin. In contrast to the academically schooled *doctores medicinae* (physicians), most surgeons had not been taught Latin, and were therefore not proficient in the language. A year after his appointment as *praelector*, Egbertszn translated an important work by Doctor Johannes Fernelius (Fernel) from Latin into Dutch, titled *De*

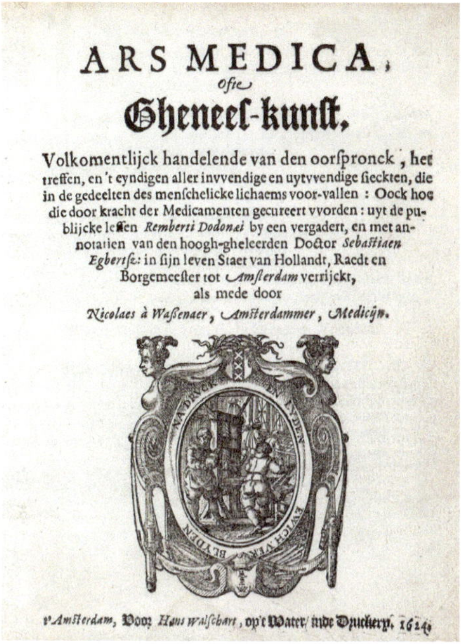

ARS MEDICA,
ofte
Gheneeſ-kunſt,

Volkomentlijck handelende van den oorſpronck, het treffen, en 't eyndigen aller invvendige en uytvvendige ſieckten, die in de gedeelten des menſchelicke lichaems voor-vallen : Oock hoe die door kracht der Medicamenten gecureert vvorden : uyt de publijcke leſſen *Remberti Dodonæi* by een vergadert, en met annotatien van den hoogh-gheleerden Doctor *Sebaſtiaen Egbertſz:* in ſijn leven Staet van Hollandt, Raedt en Borgemeeſter tot *Amſterdam* verrijckt, als mede door

Nicolaes à Waſsenaer, Amſterdammer, Medicijn.

t'*Amſterdam*, Door *Hans walſchart*, op't Water/ inde Druckery. 1624.

Title page of *Ars Medica, ofte Ghenees-kunst* with the legend: 'Complete Treatment of the origin, diagnosis and termination of all internal and external illnesses, which occur in the parts of the human body. Also, how these can be cured by the efficacy of medications: from the public lessons of Rembert Dodonaeus, collected and annotated by the highly learned Doctor Sebastiaen Egbergtszn: during his lifetime a member of the States of Holland, Councilor and Alderman of Amsterdam, and also by Nicholaes à Wassenaar, citizen of Amsterdam, Physician.' Special Collections, Universiteit Amsterdam [OTM: O 62-7274].

beschrijvinge der deelen des lichaems van den mensche; in 't Latijn door D. Johannem Fernelium ghemaeckt: ende nu in Neder-duytsche spraecke overghezettet (The Description of the Parts of the Human Body; compiled in Latin by D. Johannem Fernelium: now translated into the Low German language). This reference work consisted of 132 pages. Around fifty years later, Fernelius and Egbertszn's book still attracted considerable interest and was republished.

Fernelius (1497–1558) was one of the most prominent medical doctors of the sixteenth century. He grew up in France and, from an early age, he schooled himself in philosophy, astronomy and mathematics. He had a successful medical practice in Paris and was appointed Professor of Medicine at the University of Paris in 1534. One of his best students was Andreas Vesalius who would later achieve great fame. In his foreword to the book, Egbertszn writes that, 'a sound knowledge of anatomy lays the foundation for medicine'. He believed that the work would serve 'for the benefit and convenience, primarily for the Guild of Surgeons here at this place'. He then addresses the reader stating: 'How imperative it is, gracious reader, that surgeons should master the knowledge of human bodies,

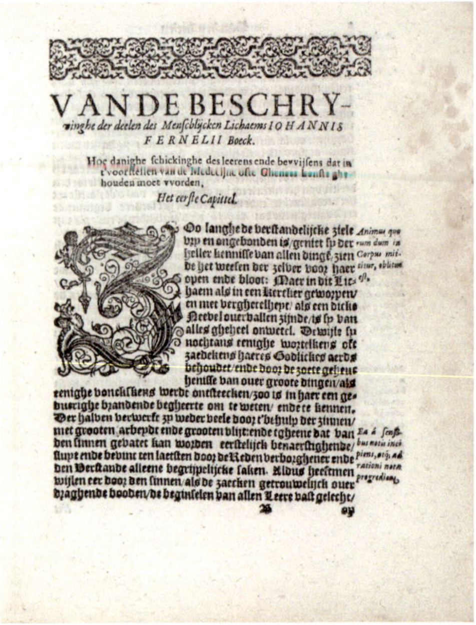

VANDE BESCHRY-
vinghe der deelen des Menschlijcken Lichaems IOHANNIS FERNELII Boeck.

Hoe danighe schickinghe des leerens ende bewijsens dat in t'voorstellen van de Medicijne ofte Ghenees konste ghehouden moet worden,

Het eerste Capittel.

Zo langhe de verstandelijcke ziele vry en ongebonden is/geniet sy der heller kennisse van allen dinge/ziende het weesen der zelver door haer open ende bloot: Maer in dit Lichaem als in een kercker geworpen/en met verghetelheyt/als een dicke Neevel overvallen zijnde/is sy van alles gheheel onwetel. Dewijle sy nochtans eenighe wortelkens ofte zaedekens haeres Godlickes aerds behoudet/ende door de zoete gheheugenisse van over groote dingen/als eenighe vonckskens werdt ontsteecken/zoo is in haer een gedurighe brandende begheerte om te weten/ ende te kennen. Der halven verwerckt zy weder veele door t'behulp der zinnen/met grooten arbeydt ende grooten vlijt: ende tgheene dat van den sinnen gevatet kan worden eerstelijck benaerstighende/ sluyt ende bevint ten laetsten door de Reden verborghener ende den Verstande alleene begrijpelijcke saken. Aldus heeftmen wijlen eer door den sinnen/als de zaecken getrouwelijck over draghende boden/de beginselen van allen Leere vast gelecht/

Animus quorum dum in Corpus mittitur, oblitus est.

Ea à sensibus notis incipiens, atq; ad rationi notam progrediens.

B

op

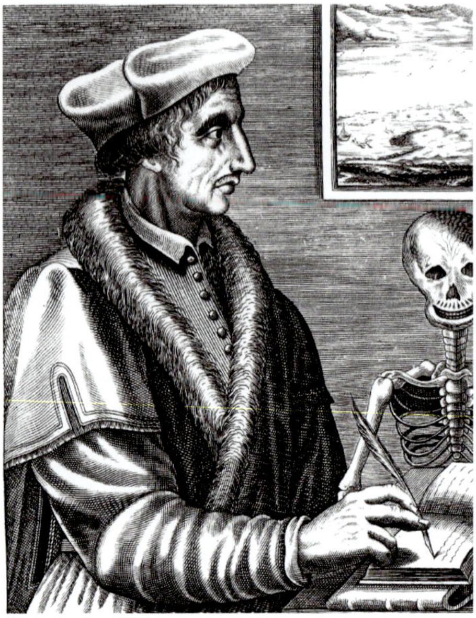

Johannes Fernelius (1497–1558)

Title page of the first chapter of the book *Description of the Parts of the Human Body* (1596). The work was translated from Latin into Dutch for surgeons by Sebastiaen Egbertszn. Special Collections, Universiteit Amsterdam [OTM: O 73-16].

through which they will be able to exercise their skill and hand.' He tries his utmost to translate the difficult Latin terminology into Dutch. Egbertszn signed his petition for providing surgeons with medical literature, and sealed it with his coat of arms.

The book by Fernelius and Egbertszn covers a wide-range of subjects including 'bones, cartilage, joints and ligaments, muscles, the internal parts enabling the enjoyment of food (digestive system), abdominal parts supporting life [*heart and lungs*], the head, the nervous system, arteries and the skin.'

In the sixteenth and final chapter, Fernelius and Egbertszn give a detailed description of the 'method for dissecting bodies' in anatomy lessons. According to him, these lectures should be delivered at a high dissection table set at the centre of the dissection room. Spectators could take their seats around this table. The person doing the dissection should have ready at hand: 'scissors, scalpels, cloths, awls, saws, hammers, needles, bandages, buckets and sponges.' The *praelector* – in the Amsterdam Surgeons' Guild this would be Sebastiaen Egbertszn – would begin his lesson with a short homily on the 'dignity' of the body. After that, he would set to work on the dissection and name all the anatomical structures in the human body in a fixed sequence.

During the period in which Egbertszn was *praelector*, a number of different rules were introduced to regulate and improve the surgeons' education in dissection. In 1606, the Ordinance for Anatomy was issued and incorporated into the statutes of the surgeons' guild. This ordinance announced nine requirements for monitoring the education of surgeons bearing on the conduct of the lessons and the protocol to be observed (see p. 22). These regulations give an insight as to how the lectures under Egbertszn's guidance were organized. He held his lectures in a small dissection room above the former chapel of the St.-Margaret's Convent on the Nes (see p. 14). At that time the ground floor was being used as a meat market.

It is now impossible to trace the exact number of lessons Egbertszn gave. No detailed reports of the first anatomy lessons have survived. This hiatus can in part be explained by the fact that the oldest guild documents were lost in a fire in 1597. This fire broke out in the home of Guild director Claes Claeszn Kist, 'having most of the Guild's old papers and documents at his house at that time, these were consumed by the flames.'

On top of his medical duties, Sebastiaen Egbertszn also held a number of public offices. Among other achievements, he was one of the founders of the Amsterdam House of Correction (*Tuchthuis*) in 1589. The opening of this institution marked a fundamental change in thought on criminality at that time. In earlier times, criminals had been subjected to severe corporal punishments, such as flogging, branding, amputation of limbs and hanging, or they were banished from the city (which would mean a loss of their citizen's rights). However, by this time attitudes to punishment were gradually changing and it was thought that those who had committed 'petty' crimes or misdemeanors should be spared these severe punishments. The idea behind these houses of correction was to provide a place in which they would be spared these harsh penalties. Instead, the goal was to rehabilitate them in an institutional setting so that they could return to society as better citizens. In these prisons, in regimes designed to instill order and regularity into their lives, convicted petty criminals would be put to work. Male offenders were sent to the *Rasphuis* on the Heiligeweg, in which they were set to work

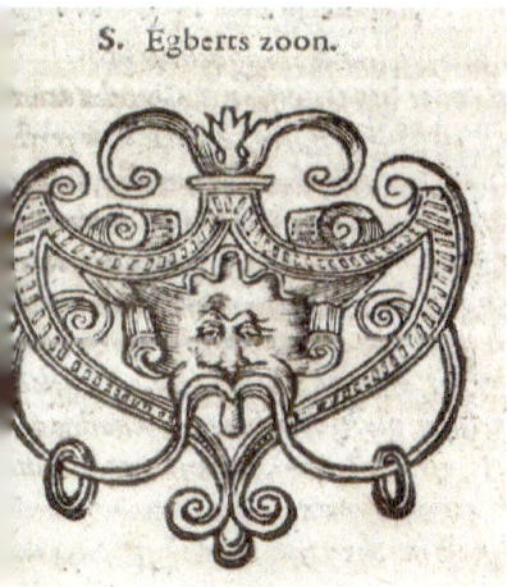

Coat of arms of Sebastiaen Egbertszn. Special Collections, Universiteit Amsterdam [OTM: O 73-16]

pulverizing Brazilian hardwood into powder that was subsequently used in the production of paint. Female delinquents were put to work in the *Spinhuis* in the former St.-Ursula Convent on the Oudezijds Achterburgwal. The women sat in a large hall where they were made to spin wool and sew.

At the early age of thirty, Egbertszn already held an important position on the Amsterdam municipal council. In 1593, he was appointed as *schepen* (alderman), and from 1606 to 1611 he was a member of the standing committee of the States of Holland (the parliament). In 1618 he was dismissed from the city administration of Amsterdam by Prince Maurits of Nassau (the stadtholder) because of his sympathies for the Remonstrant Movement, a more modern variant of the Dutch Reformed Church. Egbertszn died during the plague outbreak of 1621. He was clearly a respected, influential man. When he died in the Kalverstraat, he left a fortune of 206,000 guilders. He was buried in the Oosterkerk (East Church) in Amsterdam.

▸ **The Surgeons** The surgeon standing on the far-right of the painting holds a list of names declaring that 'All the Master Surgeons of the Guild in the Year 1603' are depicted in the painting. In 1600, there were about thirty practising surgeons in Amsterdam, serving a population of 100,000 inhabitants. This means that *The Anatomy Lesson of Sebastiaen Egbertszn*, which dates from 1603, is the only painting on which all the members of the guild can be seen. At the time, they were the ones who attended Egbertszn's anatomy lesson. A few of them are supplied with the instruments which they used to exercise their profession, such as, scissors and a barbers' shaving bowl.

The majority of these surgeons painted in 1603 can be identified by the number on the name list shown. The numbers correspond to those written above the heads of the surgeons on the original canvas. During the last restoration of the painting, eighteen of the twenty-eight numbers could be identified, allowing some of the names on the list to be linked to the men in the painting. This led to the discovery that for various men portrayed, surgery was a passion that was shared by more members of the same family. For instance, there are two pairs of fathers and sons, Roos (Nrs 2 and 23) and Kist (Nrs 3 and 22). There are also three sets of brothers: Sybrantszn de Bont(e) (Nrs 4 and 20), Adriaenszn Koorenkint (Nrs 7 and 13) and Wiggertszn (Nrs 9 and 15). Although the names of those depicted are known,

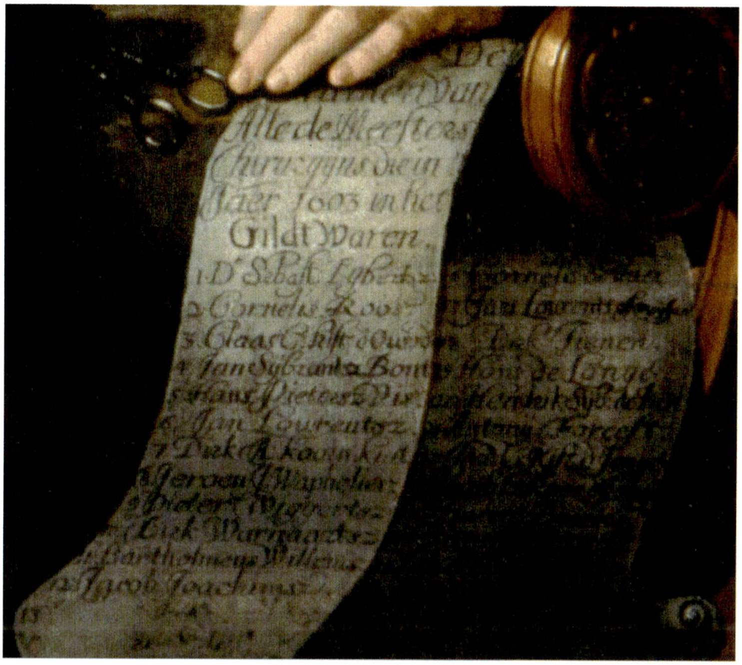

List of Names of the Surgeons depicted in *The Anatomy lesson of Sebastiaen Egbertszn.*

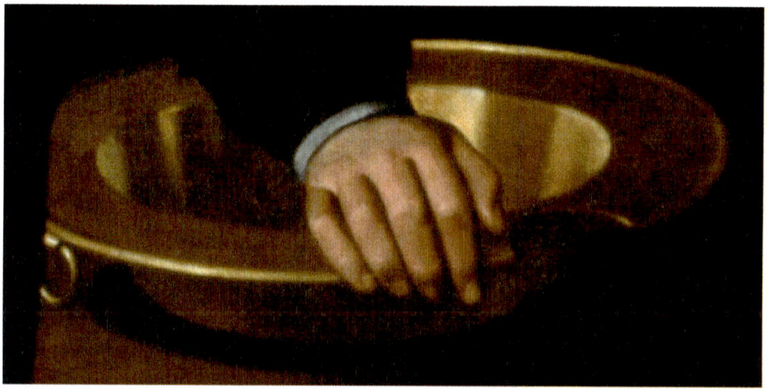

Shaving bowl held by the surgeon in the left foreground of the painting.

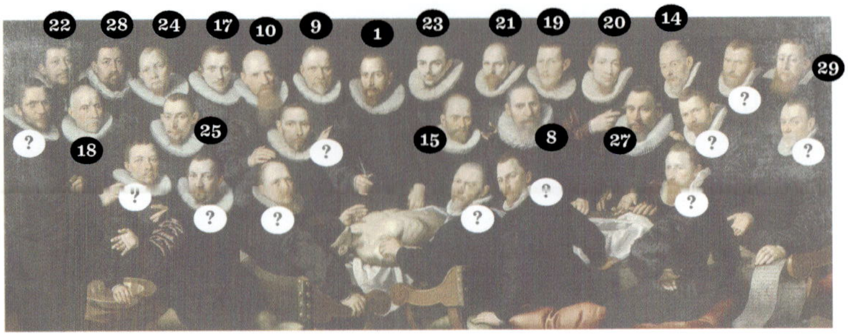

1 Sebastiaen Egbertszn
2 Cornelis Symonszn Roos
3 Claes Claeszn Kist de Oude
4 Jan Sybrantszn Bont(e)
5 Hans Pieterszn Vis
6 Jan Lourentszn
7 Dirck Adriaenszn Koorenkint
8 Jeroen Joriszn Wa(p)felier
9 Pieter Wiggertszn
10 Dirck Warnaers
11 Bartholomeus Willemszn
12 Jacob Joachimszn
13 Albert Adriaenszn Koorenkint
14 Pieter Gelliszn Splinter
15 Jan Wiggertszn
16 Cornelis Hendrickszn van Triest
17 Jan Laurentszn
18 Dirck Janszn Tienen
19 Hans (de) Langhe
20 Hendrick Sybrantszn de Bont(e)
21 Anthony Foreest
22 Claes Claeszn Kist de Jonge
23 Jacob Corneliszn Roos
24 Barent Beenes
25 Barent Janszn Potgieter
26 Albert Janszn Scherm
27 Coenraet Andrieszn Stangerus
28 Cornelis Bartholo (of Bartelszn)
29 Albert Gerritszn Hop

no detailed records survived of the operations these men performed more than four hundred years ago.

In 1601, the artist Aert Piertszn was commissioned to paint a portrait of Egbertszn, centrally positioned among the other master surgeons. Shortly after he had begun working on this masterpiece, Amsterdam was struck by plague. In 1602 this dreadful disease claimed more than 11,000 lives in the city and beyond. As a result of the subsequent upheavals in the city, Pieterszn was forced to put his artistic activities on hold. When the painting was finally handed over in 1603, five of the portrayed surgeons had died of the plague. The likeness of one of them, Bartholomeus Willemszn, was even captured on canvas by the painter as he lay on his death bed. The likenesses of two other surgeons who did not survive the epidemic, Pieter Gelliszn Splinter (No. 14) and Hans (de) Langhe (No. 19), have also been identified. They had already succumbed to the disease before the painting was finished.

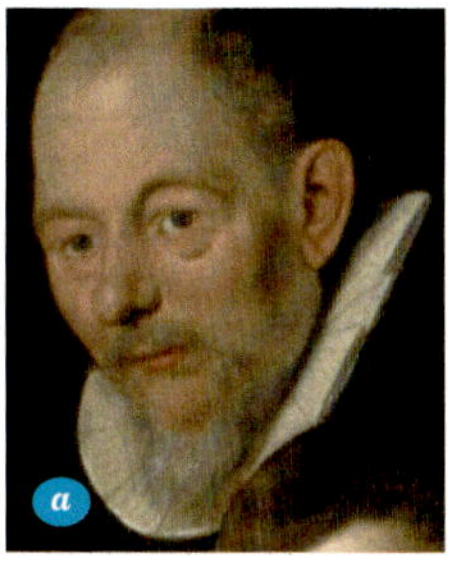

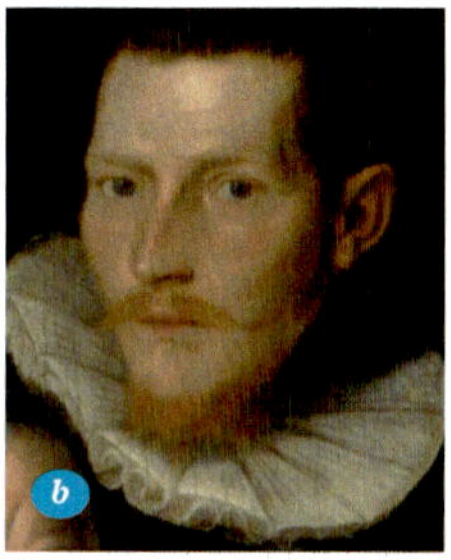

Two victims who died of the plague before the painting was completed: Pieter Gelliszn Splinter [a] and Hans (de) Langhe [b].

Just before the artist was ready to hand over the painting in 1603, three more surgeons were added. These surgeons had joined the guild that same year. At the last moment, he added the likenesses of Cornelis Bartholo (or Bartelszn) (No. 28), Albert Gerritszn Hop (No. 29) and Claes Claeszn Kist Jr (No. 22) to the composition. The name 'Kist' is one that was already mentioned in connection with the fire in 1597 in the house of Claes Claeszn Kist Senior, in which a large proportion of the guild archives was destroyed. After the painting was finished, Aert Pieterszn signed his masterpiece on the two chairs which are shown in the foreground.

One unusual detail in this painting is the unexplained, an additional left hand shown next to the hands of Coenraet Andrieszn Stangerus (No. 27), who is seated at the right of the table. The hand is not his, nor that of any of the surgeons next to or opposite him. An X-ray examination of the painting suggests that the portraits of Strangerus (No. 27) and Wa(p)felier (No. 8) were added to the canvas a few years after it had been completed. Perhaps this was an update of their portraits after they had been re-appointed governors in 1619. There is a strong possibility that the 'extra hand' crept into the picture unintentionally at that time.

▸ **The Corpse** The identity of the man's body on Egbertszn's dissection-table is unknown. Only the trunk is visible. The face is concealed by the arm of the surgeon seated at the dead man's head. None of the guild documents contains any specific details about the dead man. The bodies usually used for anatomy lessons were those of executed criminals who had been condemned to death. Any records

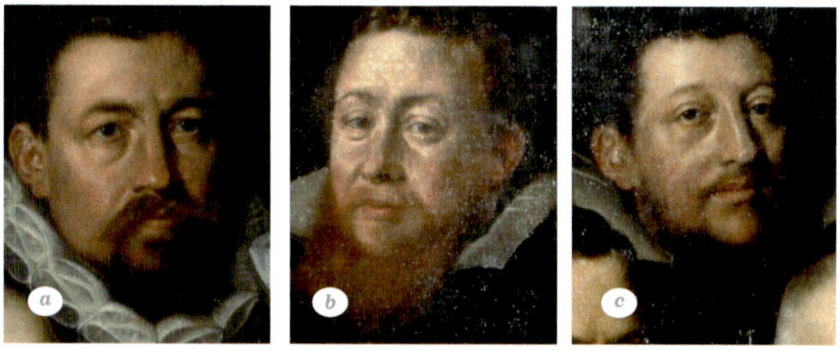

The surgeons who became members of the Guild in 1603 and were added to the composition at the last moment by the artist: Cornelis Bartholo (or Bartelszn) [a], Albert Gerritszn Hop [b] and Claes Claeszn Kist de Jonge [c].

about Egbertszn's anatomy lesson which might have offered some clues on this, have also disappeared. It is not beyond the bounds of possibility that the artist did not use a real body for a model. After all, the most important reason for the painting was to produce a group portrait, and not to give a realistic reproduction of one of Egbertszn's anatomy lessons. Therefore, the question of how the corpse on the dissection-table came to be painted remains a mystery.

▸ **Anatomy** In *The Anatomy Lesson of Sebastiaen Egbertszn*, the *praelector* has not yet begun the dissection. Hence, the anatomical secrets of the human body still remain hidden in the as yet unscathed corpse on the table.

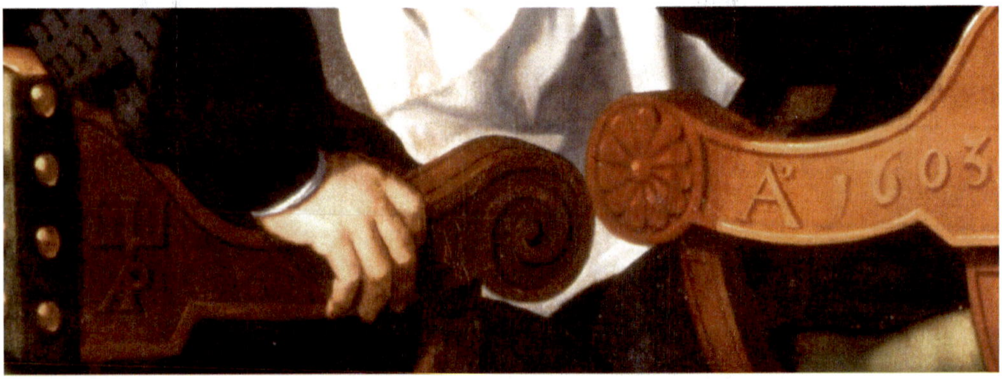

Signature of Aert Pieterszn dated 1603, shown on the chair back.

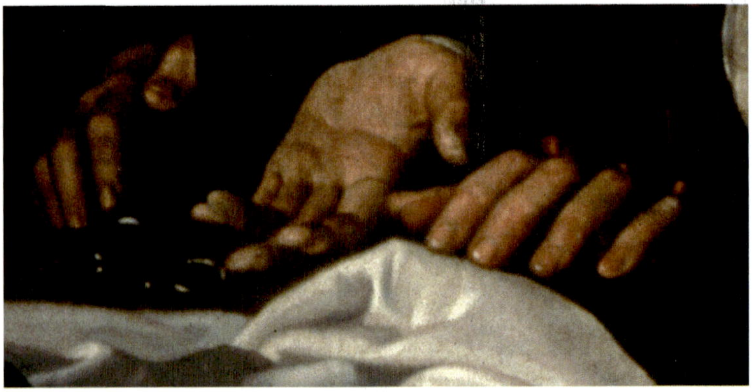

Unexplained hand on the far right of the painting's detail as shown. The pair of hands near the surgical clamp belong to Coenraet Andrieszn Stangerus.

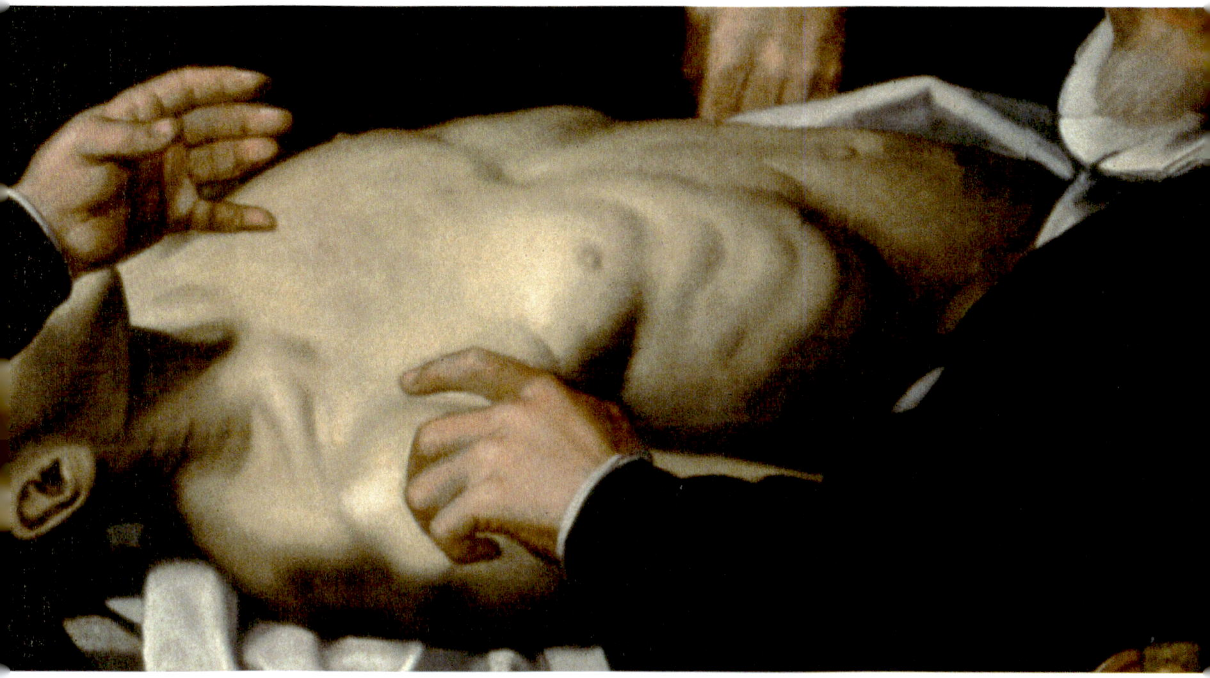

The corpse on Sebastiaen Egbertszn's dissection table.

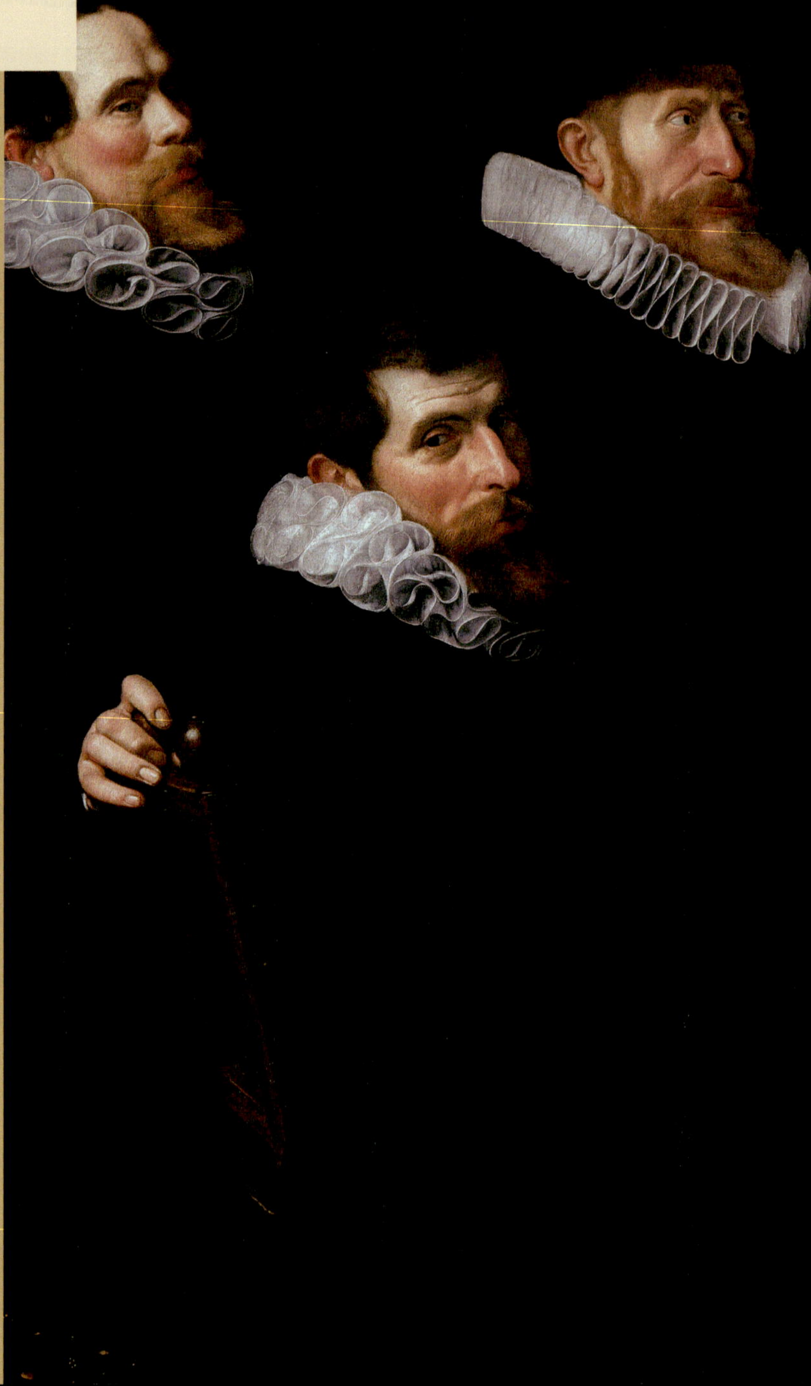

The Osteology Lesson of Sebastiaen Egbertszn by Thomas de Keyser, 1619. Collection Amsterdam Museum.

2

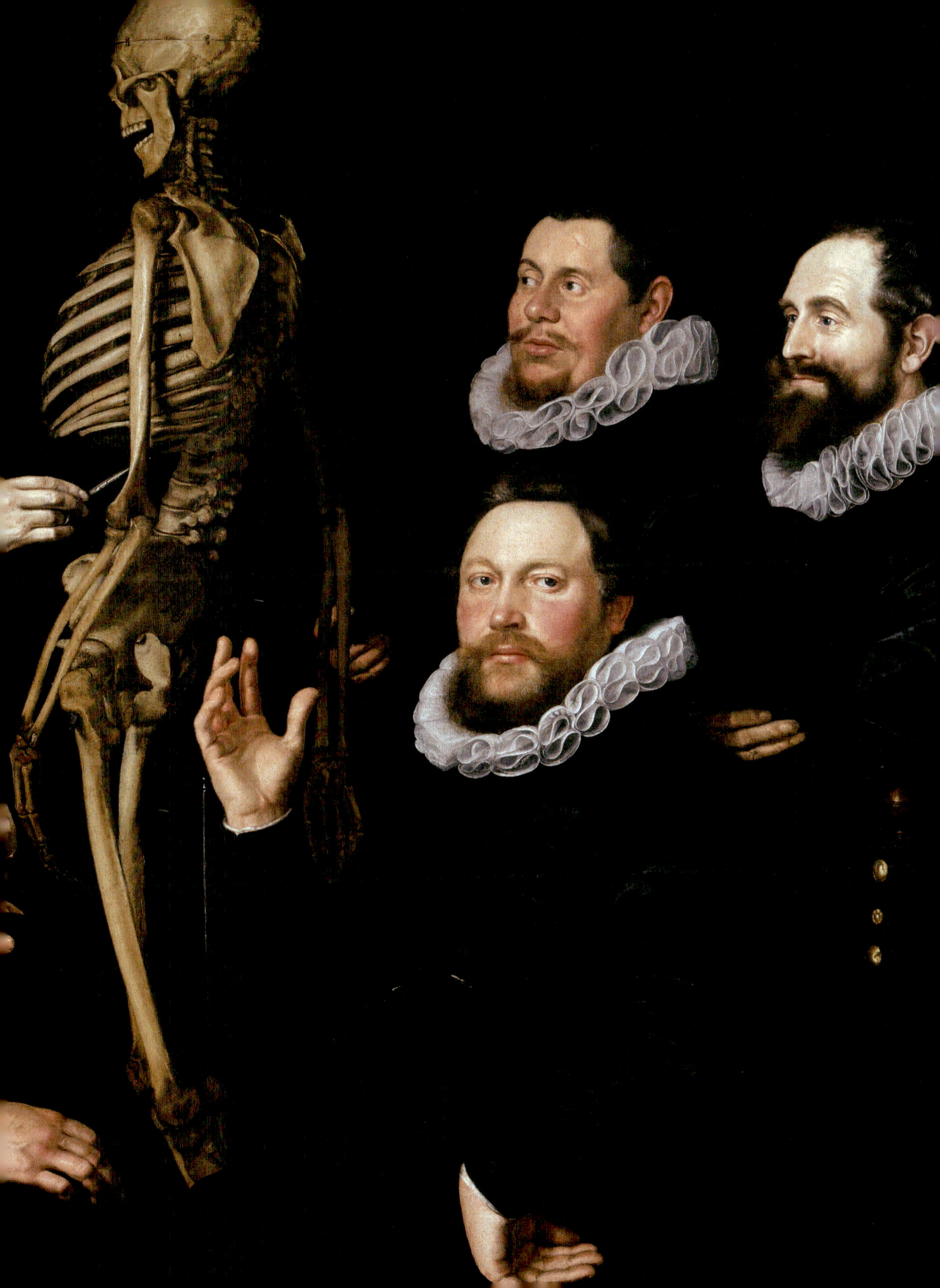

Sebastiaen Egbertszn [2]

The Osteology Lesson of Sebastiaen Egbertszn,
painted by Thomas de Keyser in 1619

▸ **The Painting** The second group painting of the Amsterdam Surgeons' Guild, *The Osteology Lesson of Sebastiaen Egbertszn,* was painted at the end of Dr Egbertszn's term as *praelector*. He is shown on the painting as he gives an explanation of the human skeleton. For no less than twenty-four years, Egbertszn had given his anatomy lessons in the 'Lesser Meat Hall' situated on the upper floor of the former chapel of the St.-Margaret Convent on the Nes. However, in 1619, the surgeons moved to the New Weighing House on Nieuwmarkt, and on April 19th of that same year, Sebastiaen Egberstzn opened the new guildhall at that location. In honour of the occasion, he held a lecture about one of the most outstanding works on medicine dating from Classical Antiquity, *De Medicina*, written by the Roman physician Aulus Cornelius Celsus (c. 25 BC to AD 50). In this classic work consisting of eight volumes, various aspects of medicine are discussed, including anatomy and surgery.

Taking up residence at their new guildhall in the Weighing House must have been an important occasion for the Amsterdam surgeons. This second group portrait was probably commissioned by the Amsterdam Surgeons' Guild to commemorate this change of premises. Another possible reason for the commission could have been the ample wall space that would become available to them at the new guildhall. This painting was given a prominent place above the mantlepiece, where it would remain for many years. It is now housed at the Amsterdam Museum.

▸ **The Painter** *The Osteology Lesson of Sebastiaen Egbertszn* was never signed. The question of who actually painted this masterpiece has been a topic of debate among art historians for quite some time. One older, trustworthy source from around 1750 suggests that 'Thomas de Kijzer' (Thomas de Keyser) was the creator of this group portrait.

This information was based on the notes of the surgeon Monnikhoff, who had copied older text segments from the now lost *Groot-Memoriael Gildeboek* (Great Commemorative Guild Book) of the surgeons at that time.

Thomas de Keyser (1596/97–1667) was the son of the famous Dutch sculptor and architect, Hendrick de Keyser, and one of the most sought-after portrait painters in the years between 1625 and 1635. His work was innovative because he usually painted his subjects carrying out a certain activity, while set at a location suited for that activity. By doing so, he created a portrait style that was less formal than had hitherto been the case. De Keyser produced a large number of superb portraits. One of his most ambitious group portraits is the militia piece *Het korporaalschap van kapitein Allaert Cloeck en luitenant Lucas Jacobszn Rotgans* (The Corporalship of Captain Allaert Cloeck and Lieutenant Lucas Jacobszn Rotgans) from 1632. Other well-known works by him are *Een musikant met zijn dochter* (A Musician and his daughter) (1629), *De schutters van de compagnie van kapitein Jakob Symonszn de Vries en luitenant Dirck de Graeff* (The Musketeers of the Company of Captain Jakob Symonszn de Vries and Lieutenant Dirck de Graeff) (1633) and *De Amsterdamse burgermeesters vernemen de aankomst of Maria de Medici* (The Amsterdam Burgomasters Learn of the Arrival of Maria de Medici) (1628). After 1640, the De Keyser received fewer com-

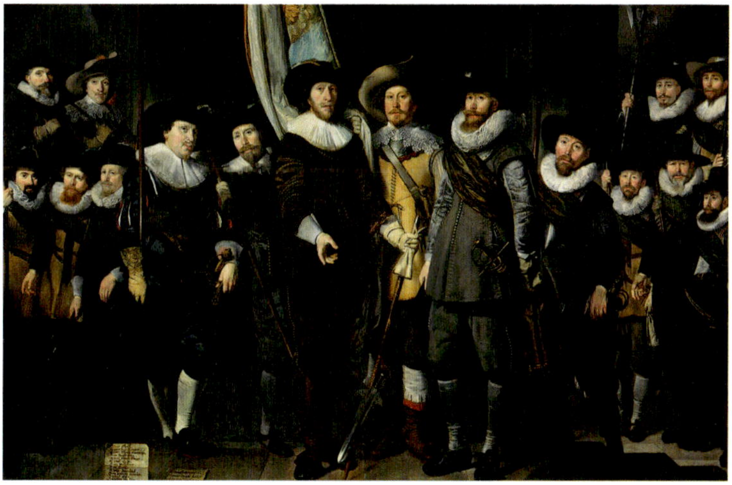

Thomas de Keyser, *The Corporalship of Captain Allaert Cloeck and Lieutenant Lucas Jacobszn Rotgans of the Harquebusiers' Butts Amsterdam* (Kloveniersdoelen), 1632. The painting shows the officers and other ranks of Amsterdam's District III led by Cloeck and Rotgans. Collection Rijksmuseum Amsterdam.

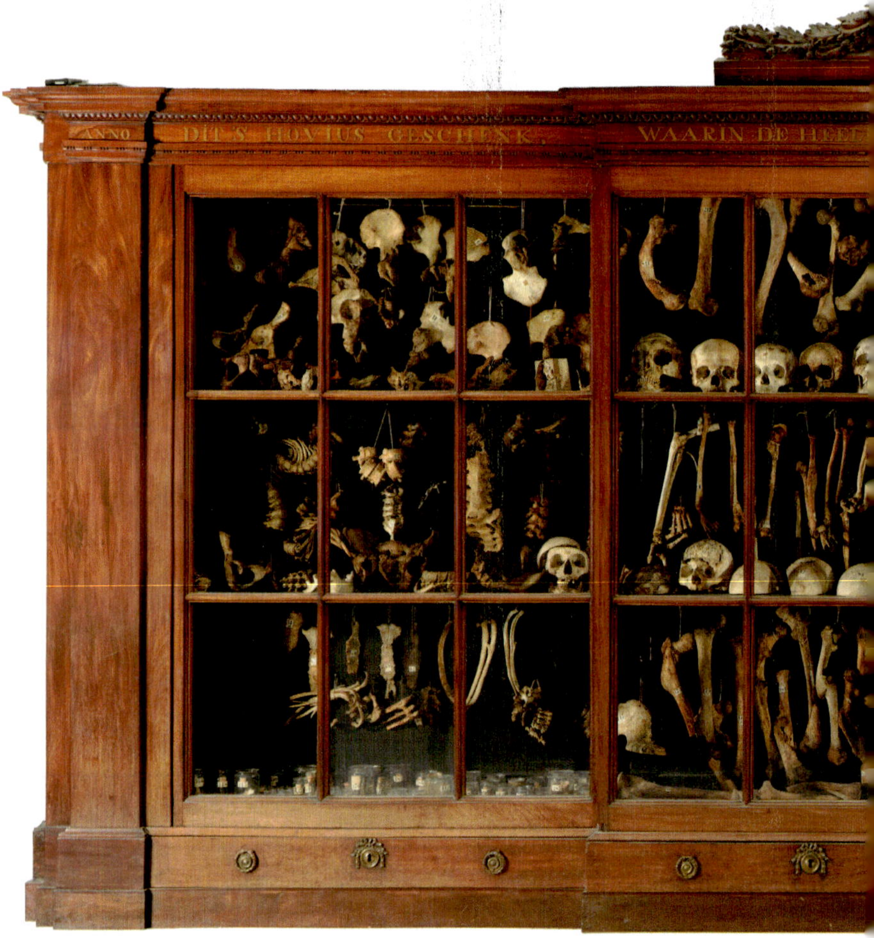

Hovius' Cabinet with its unique osteological collection. Jacob Hovius presented the collection of bones to the Amsterdam Surgeons' Guild in 1773 for the benefit of the education offered by the Guild. Museum Vrolik, Amsterdam University Medical Center (AMC), Amsterdam.

2

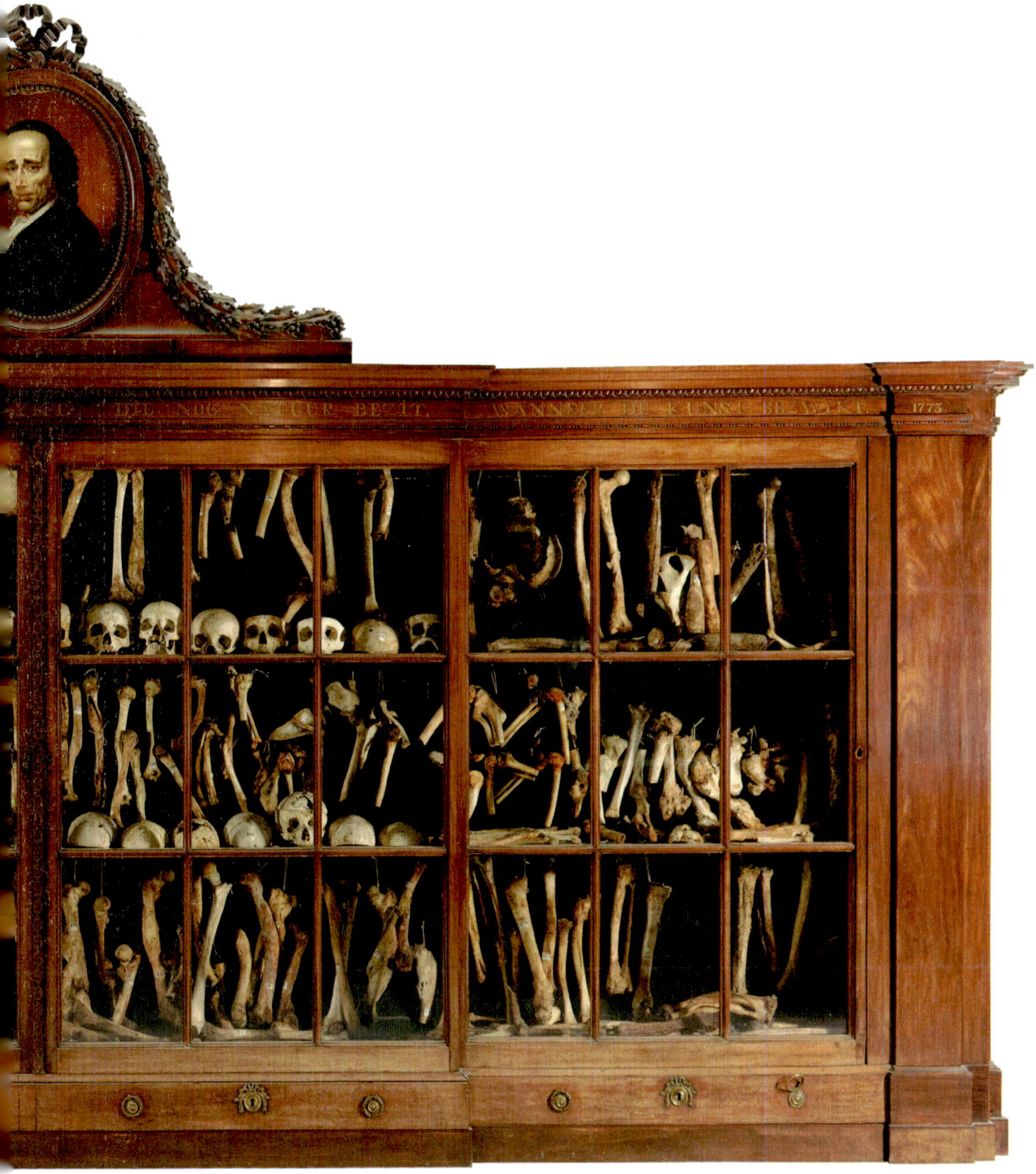
1773

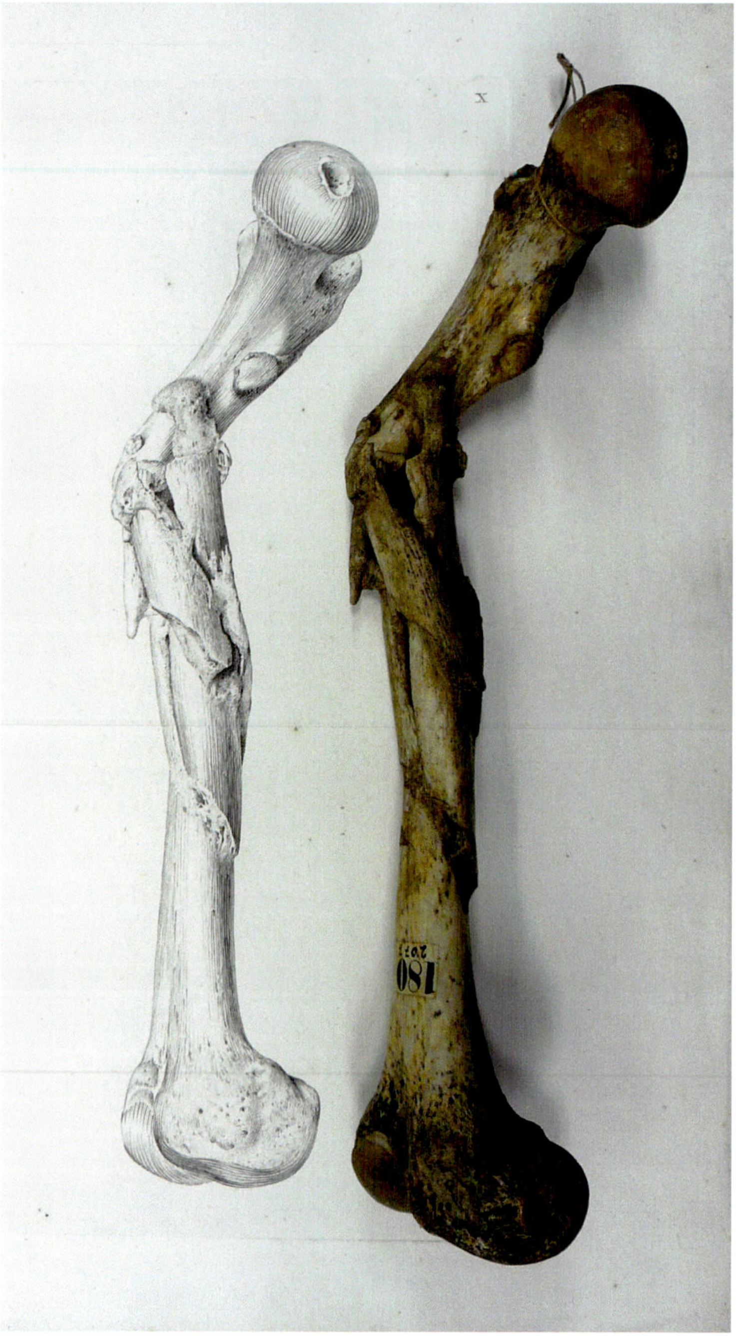

2

Sebastiaen Egbertszn[2] *1619*

The bone collection was expanded upon by the last *praelector anatomiae*, Andreas Bonn (1738–1817), at the end of the eighteenth century. In 1785, he also published an anatomical atlas entitled *Tabulae Ossium Morbosorum* (Atlas of Diseased Bones), containing descriptions and illustrations of the 'diseased bones' in the Hovius Cabinet. The Hovius Cabinet and its contents are still preserved at the Museum Vrolik in Amsterdam, now part of the Amsterdam University Medical Center, location Academic Medical Center (AMC). Many of the specimens in the cabinet exhibit the advanced stages of certain diseases which we rarely come across in the modern world because of improved medical treatments. The Hovius' Cabinet still evokes awe and wonder, just as must it have done for surgeons at that time.

▸ **The Surgeons** In contrast to the first anatomy lesson of Sebastiaen Egbertszn painted in 1603 in which all the master surgeons appear, only five apprentice surgeons — besides Egbertszn himself — are portrayed in *The Osteology Lesson of Sebastiaen Egbertszn* of 1619. Due to the great increase in the number of guild members, it was probably no longer possible to include them all in one painting. Those portrayed in 1619 were all members of the board. One of the governers, namely Albert Janszn Scherm (see p. 42), had already been immortalized in the first painting commissioned by the Amsterdam Surgeons' Guild. In this second group portrait, the surgeons are grouped less formally. The way in which the artist shows the surgeons looking in different directions was quite novel at that time, giving the scene a more dynamic character. The surgeons could be identified using the numbered name list in the upper left corner of the painting, the

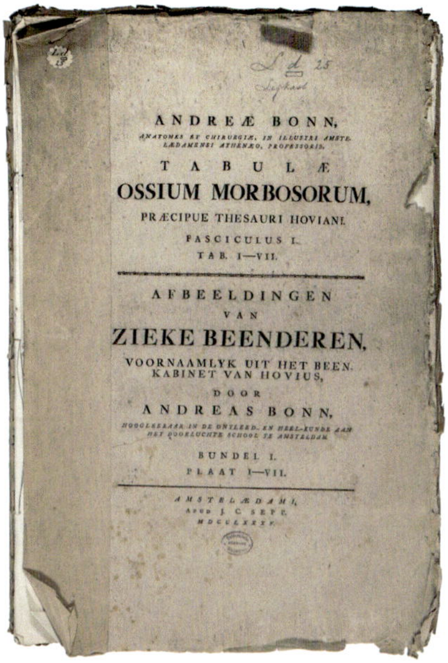

ANDREÆ BONN,
ANATOMES ET CHIRURGIÆ, IN ILLUSTRI AMSTELÆDAMENSI ATHENÆO, PROFESSORIS.
TABULÆ
OSSIUM MORBOSORUM,
PRÆCIPUE THESAURI HOVIANI.
FASCICULUS I.
TAB. I—VII.

AFBEELDINGEN
VAN
ZIEKE BEENDEREN,
VOORNAAMLYK UIT HET BEEN. KABINET VAN HOVIUS,
DOOR
ANDREAS BONN,
HOOGLEERAAR IN DE ONTLEED- EN HEEL-KUNDE AAN HET DOORLUCHTE SCHOOL TE AMSTELDAM.
BUNDEL I.
PLAAT I—VII.

AMSTELÆDAMI,
APUD J. C. SEPP.
MDCCLXXXV.

Title page of the *Tabulae Ossium Morbosorum* by Andreas Bonn (1785). The work contains illustrations and descriptions of 'diseased bones' from the Hovius Cabinet. Library University of Groningen.

←
Specimen of a broken thigh bone (*femur*) from Hovius' Cabinet. It corresponds to a description of the specimen from the *Tabulae Ossium Morbosorum* (Atlas of Diseased Bones, 1785) by Andreas Bonn: 'A right thigh bone, broken into ten or more pieces by the wheel of a heavily laden wagon. Even though the muscles must have been torn by the crushing violence, the skin remained intact. The loose fragments of bone, although severely displaced, formed new bone tissue so that once again they formed a sturdy limb, which was only slightly truncated. [...] An excellent example of the healing power of nature. Osteological Cabinet nr. 209.' Museum Vrolik, Amsterdam University Medical Center (AMC), Amsterdam.

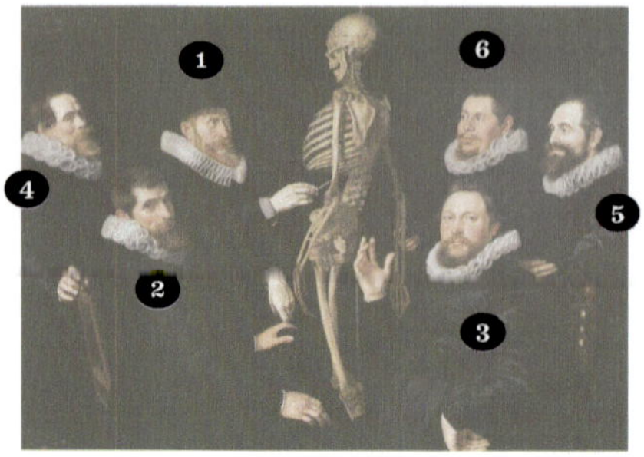

1 Sebastiaen Egbertszn
2 Anthoni Janszn Uytdenhooven
3 Hendrick Claeszn Koolvelt
4 Lambert Jacobszn
5 Gerrit Indies
6 Jan Arentszn de Wees

numbers corresponding to those numbers shown next to the surgeon concerned.

▸ **The Corpse** The skeleton which takes centre stage on the painting is probably that of an executed English pirate. In 1615, The Anatomy Book of the Surgeons' Guild reports that, Egbertszn dissected the body of an English pirate for the surgeons. From the bones that remained, the surgeons reconstructed the skeleton. The painting clearly shows that the skeleton is being held up center by an iron rod. The left hip is attached to the pelvis by a pin. The ribs are bound to each other by a wire. The cranial vault has been trepanned and later reattached using a number of small clasps. Egbertszn used the skeleton regularly in his osteological lesson for the surgeons. In this painting, the skeleton is not being used as a symbol of vanity, which was often the case in seventeenth-century art. Using such symbols as skulls, skeletons, hour-glasses, wilted flowers or candles that had been extinguished, artists would refer to the transience of our earthly existence. On the contrary: this accurately re-assembled skeleton was clearly intended to provide instructional material for the surgeons.

Around 1615, a man called Daniel Sylvester wrote a eulogy in Latin in praise of the renowned and illustrious doctor 'Sebastianum Egbertsonum', obviously with reference to the skeleton shown in *The Osteological Lesson of Sebastiaen Egbertszn*. The English translation runs as follows:

> *To the widely renowned and most illustrious Doctor Sebastiaen Egbertszn, burgomaster and treasurer of Amsterdam and praelector of the anatomy theatre in that same place.*

The skeleton of an executed English pirate used in *The Osteology lesson of Sebastiaen Egbertszn.*

Cranial vault has been sawn through and then re-attached using a number of small clamps.

The ribs are held together by a metal wire.

The hip has been attached to the pelvis by a pin.

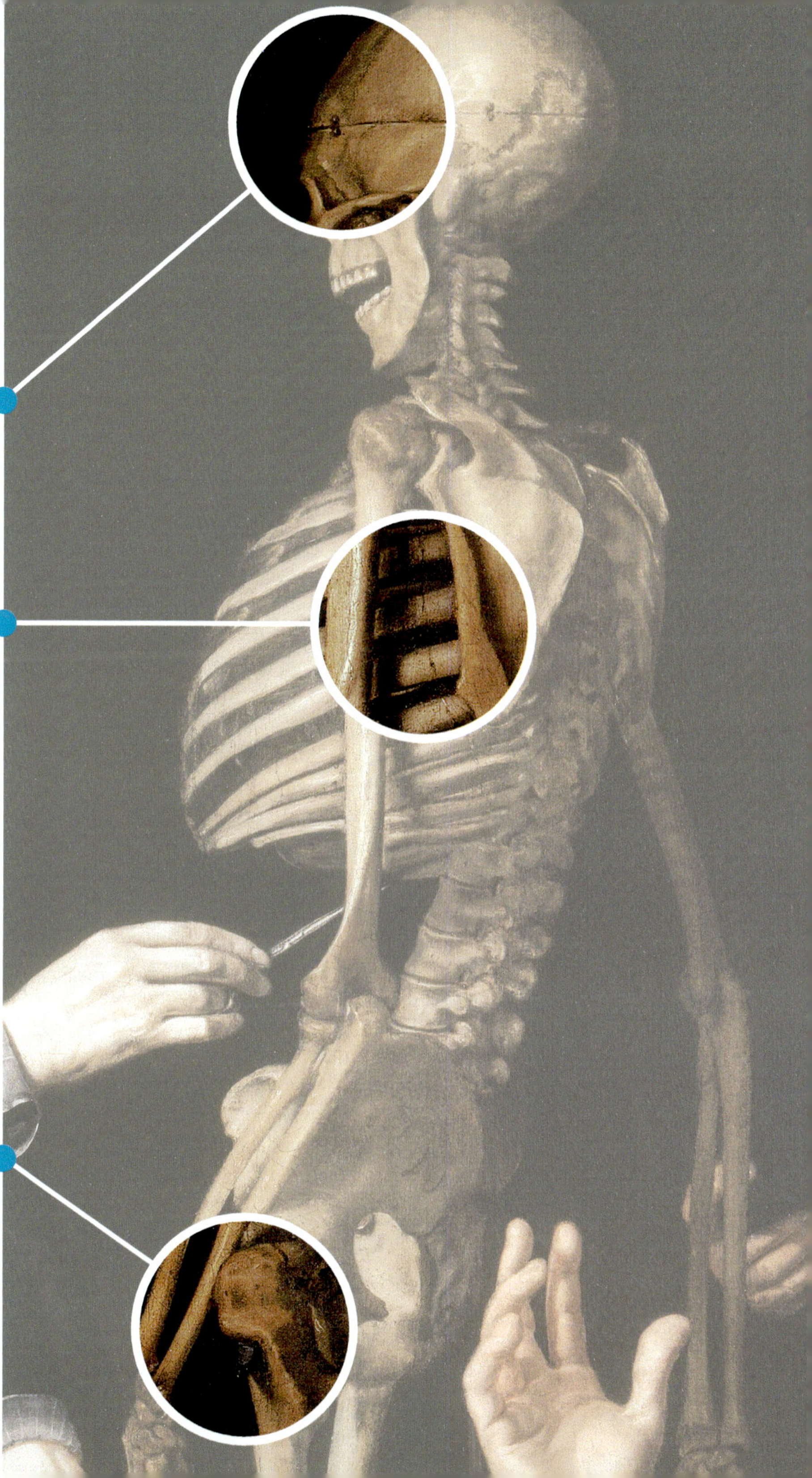

When during your professorship, I assembled the bones of the dissected body with a practiced hand and to much applause, the praise you bestowed upon me based on your assessment, and the tangible evidence of your laudatory words on the skeleton as assembled by me: How great a pleasure this was for me! A man of substance, a celebrated man, worthy of the Muses and Apollo, expressed his appreciation of the work of the craftsman with words of deserved commendation. Therefore, as an abiding testimony of my efforts and with the most honorouble of hearts, I dedicate the following sentiments to you: May your city be contented with you as burgomaster, the surgeons with you as praelector *and all the Netherlands with such a great man.*

Daniel Sylvester

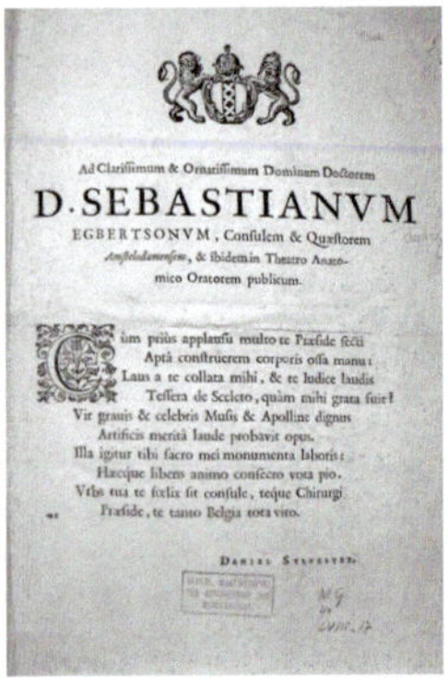
Ad Clarissimum & Ornatissimum Dominum Doctorem
D·SEBASTIANVM
EGBERTSONVM, Consulem & Quæstorem
Amstelodamensem, & ibidem in Theatro Anato-
mico Oratorem publicum.

Cùm priùs applausu multo te Præside feci
Aptà construerem corporis ossa manu:
Laus a te collata mihi, & te Iudice laudis
Tessera de Sceleto, quàm mihi grata fuit!
Vir grauis & celebris Musis & Apolline dignus
Artificis meritâ laude probavit opus.
Illa igitur tibi sacro mei monumenta laboris:
Hæcque libens animo consecro vota pio.
Vrbs tua te fœlix sit consule, teque Chirurgi
Præside, te tanto Belgia tota viro.

Daniel Sylvester.

Eulogy for Sebastiaen Egbertszn by Daniel Sylvester dated c. 1615. Special Collections Universiteit Amsterdam [UBM: Br. M.G. 4 to 58: 17].

From this eulogy, we can deduce that Sylvester was among those present at the dissection of the English pirate and probably involved in the skeleton's re-assembly. Egbertszn had complimented Sylvester profusely on his anatomical skills and his contribution to the restructuring of the bones. Naturally, Egbertszn's words of praise were music to Sylvester's ears. In turn, Sylvester honours Egbertszn by mentioning his name alongside that of Apollo and the Nine Muses (daughters of Zeus and sisters of Apollo). In Greek mythology they were the patrons of the arts and sciences. Sylvester regarded Egbertszn as a cultivated man who was highly learned in the sciences. Sylvester dedicated this eulogy to him as a token of his appreciation and as a tangible reminder of his efforts in the field of anatomy. He concludes by expressing his hope that the city of Amsterdam, the Surgeons' Guild and the entire Netherlands will prosper greatly under the guiding hand of Sebastiaen Egbertszn.

▸ **Anatomy** The skeleton in the painting is depicted quite accurately and fairly realistically. Four years later, it is more than likely that the English pirate's skeleton of 1615 served as the model for the skeleton in the painting. The anatomy of the skull, vertebrae, pectoral girdle and hip are reproduced in the finest detail. Using his dissecting forceps, Egbertszn draws attention to the lowest rib of the skeleton. In total the human body has twelve ribs on either side of the breastbone. The muscles and joints between the ribs allow the rib cage to expand and contract in rhythm while breathing. At the back, the ribs are connected to the spine. At the front, the upper ribs are connected to the breastbone (*sternum*). The eighth, ninth and tenth front ribs are connected to the upper ribs by cartilage. The eleventh and twelfth ribs do not continue through to the sternum and are therefore called "floating ribs". Why is Egbertszn drawing attention to these floating ribs? After all, the floating ribs are not the most interesting bones in the human body.

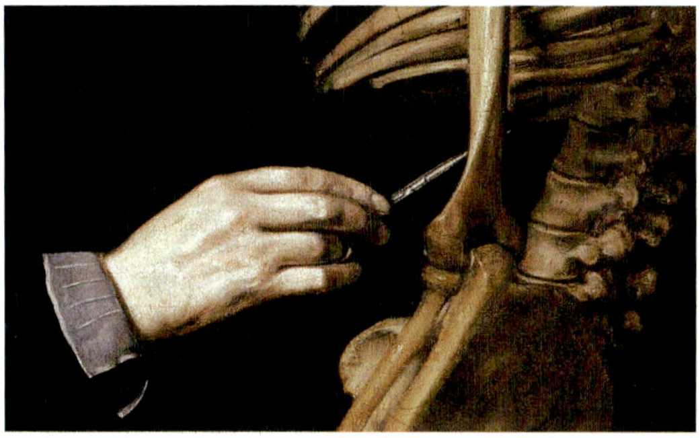

Sebastiaen Egbertszn demonstrates the anatomy of the lowest ribs.

Although they do not have an important function, they can cause severe pain in the flanks in the case of floating rib syndrome. One possible cause is that the connective tissue between the bottom-most ribs slacken in the course of time, resulting in the nerves between the floating ribs becoming irritated. With every intake of breath, the floating rib can press on the iliac crest, which irritates floating ribs' periosteum and causes pain as a result. However, it is unlikely that there was an awareness of floating rib syndrome in those days. Perhaps the floating rib had a symbolic significance and Egbertszn's indicating gesture towards it is a subtle reference to the story of the Creation, in which Eve was made from Adam's rib. The relevant biblical passage goes as follows:

> *And thus, God caused the man to fall into a deep sleep, and while he was sleeping, He took one of his ribs, filling the cavity it left with flesh. From the rib he had taken from the man the Lord God created a woman, and He brought her to the man.*

The myth that men have one less rib than women could possibly have been based on this biblical story, but it is highly unlikely that it would have escaped Egbertszn's attention during his osteology lessons that men and women have, in fact, got the same number of ribs. However, there are no solid arguments to back up such a symbolic interpretation for Egbertszn's indication of the floating rib.

▸ **Anatomical Perspective** Anatomical education formed the basis of surgical training. In the seventeenth century, osteology was an important section of surgical education and actually laid the foundation for modern orthopedics and trauma surgery. The book *Ulhoorns Osteologia,* written by the Amsterdam surgeon Hendrik Ulhoorn (1687–1746) indicates that master surgeons gradually began to spend more time on the instruction of osteology. The book contains a detailed account of osteology lessons and it was said that 'there is no book that is as concise, precise and readable available to aspiring surgeons in our mother tongue than this'. Osteology was not just taught: the apprentice surgeons were also examined on the subject at their final examination, the masterpiece. The examination records reveal that various aspects of osteology were covered in the oral exams that took place.

A sound knowledge of osteology was of great benefit to the surgeons in their daily work, because they could apply it when dealing with broken bones. Throughout the ages, this knowledge was passed down by means of atlases of anatomy and textbooks. Atlases of Anatomy usually came to fruition due to close co-operation between a medical doctor and an artist. In the case of an anatomical drawing, the draughtsman or engraver would draw what the anatomist pointed out during a dissection or a demonstration in osteology. These anatomical illustrations eventually led to an art specialism, the works of which sometimes included symbolic allusions of the transience of earthly life. What is remarkable is the often exceptional high quality of the illustrations. In the anatomical atlases of famous doctors like Andreas Vesalius (Andries van Wesel), Govard Bidloo, William Cheselden and Bernard Siegfried Albinus, the osteology is illustrated to an extremely high standard. These leading illustrated works are based on accurate anatomical observations, and offer an insight into the field of knowledge of osteology during the sixteenth, seventeenth and eighteenth centuries.

Andreas Vesalius (1514–1564) was professor of anatomy and practiced as a surgeon in the north Italian city of Padua in the middle of the sixteenth century. The first edition of his *De humani corporis fabrica* (On the Fabric of the Human Body) was published in 1543. In this academic work, he describes the compete anatomy of the human body. This pioneering work was considered to be 'the most important of all the books [...] which have so far been written about anatomy' and a few years later, he was rewarded for his outstanding achievement, by being elevated to the aristocracy. The book ushered in a new era in anatomy and was based on personal observations made during the dissection of the human body. *De humani corporis fabrica* consists of seven volumes. In roughly 80,000 words, forty chapters and 140 illustrations, the first volume covers all the bones in the human body. It was provided with accurate anatomical illustrations by Jan Stefan Kalkar (1499–1545). These drawings went far beyond the scope of just osteology. Set against the undulating landscape of Padua, we are treated to scenes

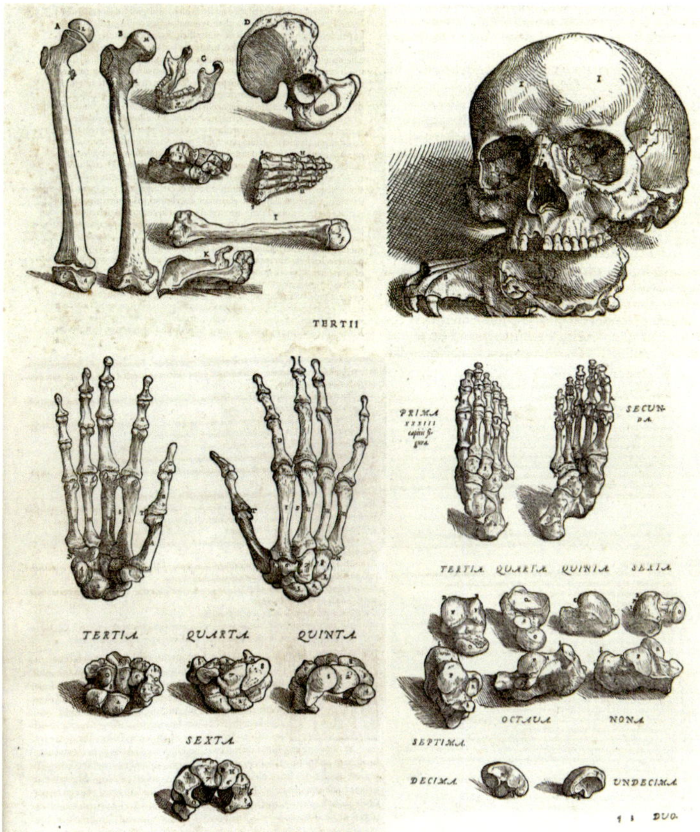

Anatomical illustrations relating to osteology from *De humani corporis fabrica libri primus* (On the Fabric of the Human Body Book One) (1555) by Andreas Vesalius. Library University of Groningen.

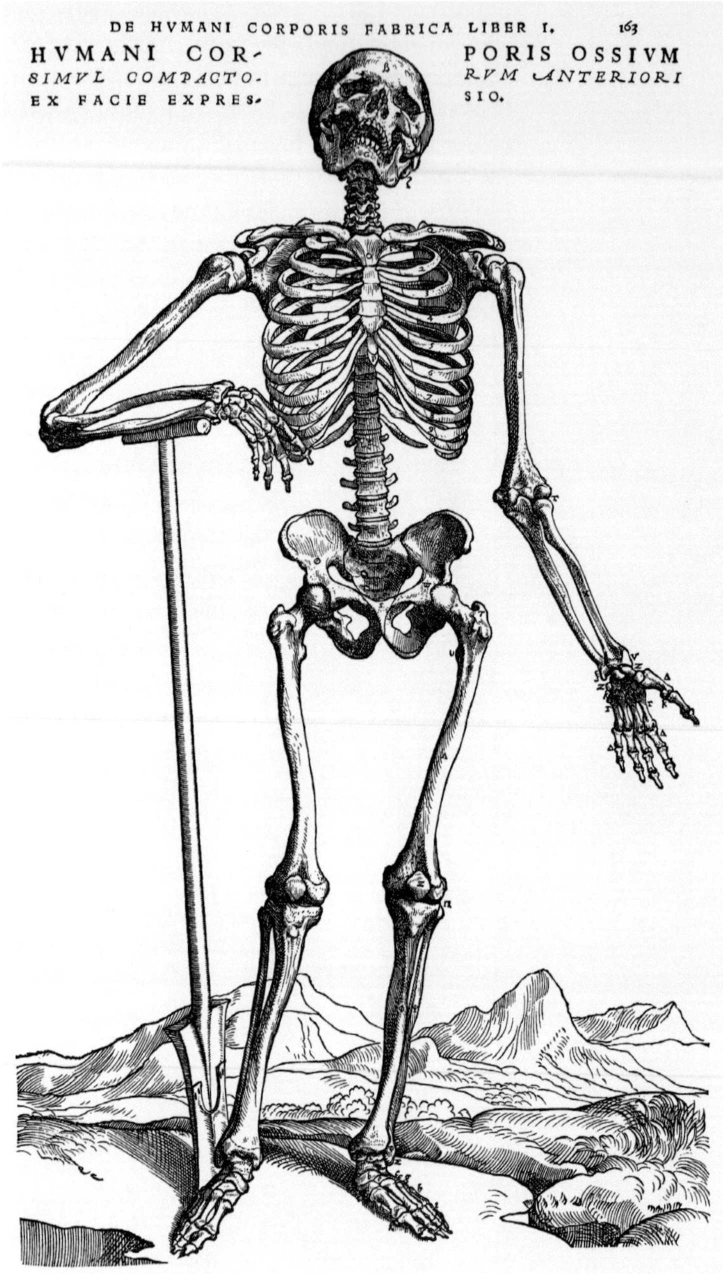

2

Sebastiaen Egbertszn[2] *1619*

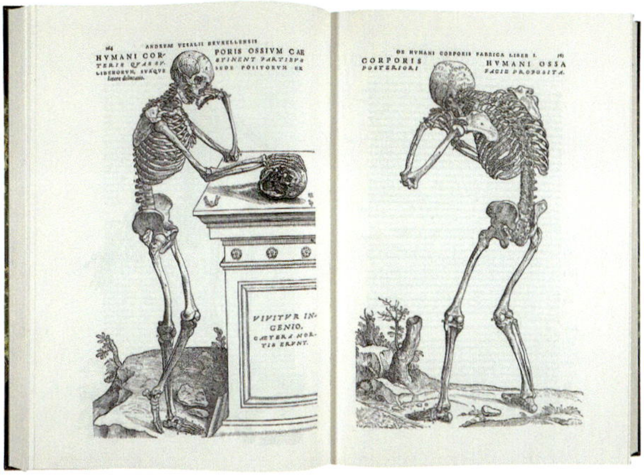

Left and right
Illustrations of skeletons from *De humani corporis fabrica libri primus* (1555) by Andreas Vesalius.

of skeletons, brought back to life to mourn their own deaths. These are *memento mori,* reminding us of our mortality. Vesalius describes how he dissected a body and boiled the bones to get rid of the remaining flesh. In order to study the mutual relationship between the bones, he would reconstruct the entire skeleton using copper wire. The ribs of the skeleton in *The Osteology Lesson of Sebastiaen Egbertszn* were also held together by a wire. Vesalius seriously questioned a number of false notions surrounding osteology that dated back to the traditional Greek and Roman writings on medicine. In many ways, Vesalius' sixteenth-century work laid the foundation for osteology in Europe.

Govard Bidloo (1649–1713) was trained as a surgeon at the Amsterdam Surgeons' Guild. In the course of his education there, he attended the osteology lessons. Later on in his career, he was appointed professor of anatomy in Leiden (1694). In 1690, Bidloo, an admirer of Vesalius' work, published his own anatomical atlas entitled *Ontleding des Menschelijken Lichaams* (Dissection of the Human Body), which included beautiful osteological illustrations. The work was intended as a textbook for surgeons. Bidloo collaborated with the artist Gerard de Lairesse (1640-1711), one of the most successful artists in Amsterdam at that time, who owed at least some of his success to the support he was given by the Amsterdam art dealer Gerrit van Uylenburgh, whose father was a friend of

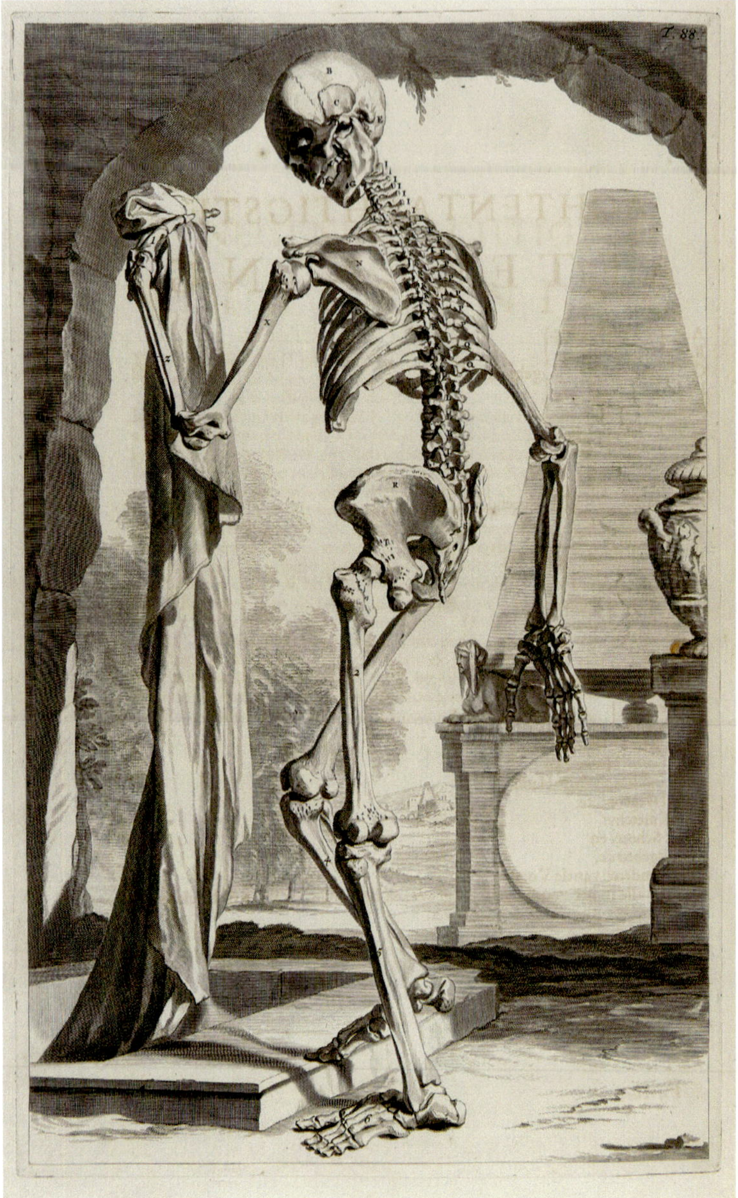

2

Sebastiaen Egbertszn[2] 1619

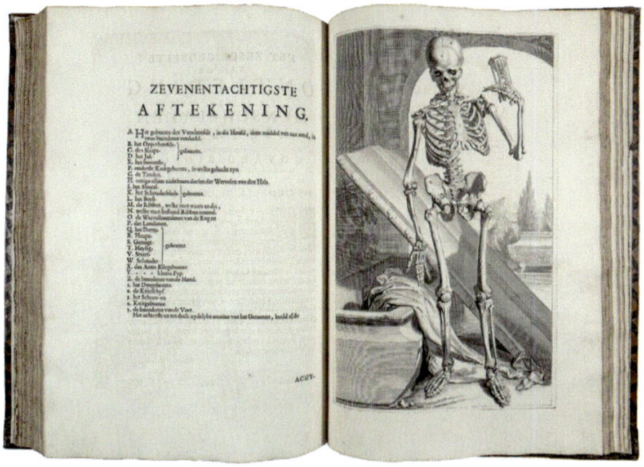

Left and right
Anatomical drawings of skeletons by Gerard de Lairesse in Govard Bidloo's *Ontleding des Menschelijken Lichaams* (Dissection of the Human Body) (1690). The bones of the skeleton are numbered and correspond to the legend. Library University of Groningen.

Rembrandt. Based on Bidloo's anatomical dissections, De Lairesse produced 105 anatomical illustrations for the book. This sixth chapter is entitled *The Complete Osteology* and contains sixteen osteological, annotated illustrations. The artistic license which De Lairesse allowed himself while producing the illustrations is unmistakable. He provided decorative attributes such as a shroud, a grave or an hour-glass to symbolize human mortality. Although the atlas is undoubtedly of great artistic value, its actual, practical use for the surgeons was seriously questioned. All in all, we could say that this atlas, which is now more than three centuries old, was the result of a fruitful collaboration between a physician and an artist.

William Cheselden (1688–1752), a leading English surgeon, learned about the works of Vesalius and Bidloo from his teacher William Cowper. He used the cadavers of executed criminals to teach anatomy at St Thomas' Hospital in London. As well as using the work of these two distinguished Dutch anatomists, he compiled his own anatomical atlas entitled *Osteographia, or the Anatomy of the Bones* (1733), which is considered to be 'one of the best English works with anatomical illustrations'. It deserves a prominent place among the series of early anatomical atlases on osteology. *Osteographia* contains 36 pages of illustrations of the bones, connective tissue and cartilage structures found in the human body.

Anatomical drawings in the field of osteology from William Cheselden's *Osteographia, or the Anatomy of the Bones* (1733).

[*a*] Abnormal curvature of the spine (*kyphoscoliosis*).
[*b*] Destruction of the bone, probably caused by an advanced stage of the sexually transmitted disease syphilis.
[*c*] Localized bone proliferation (*exotosis*) on the outer side of the shin bone (*tibia*) and the *fibula*.

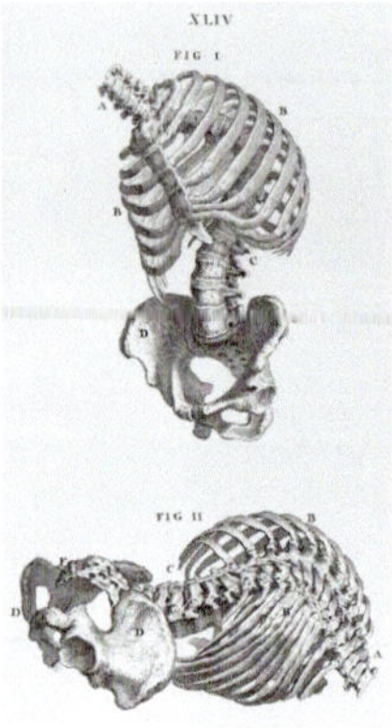

a

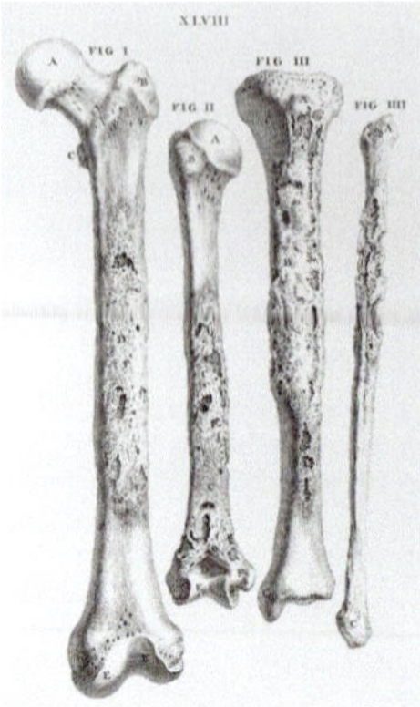

b

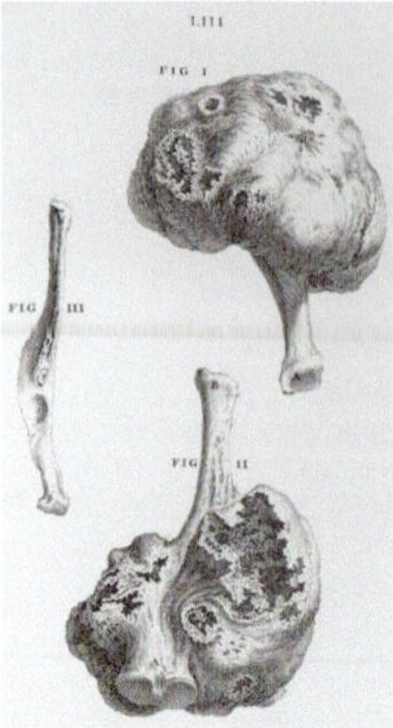

c

Cheselden was one of the first to use a *camera obscura* for the production of accurate drawings to illustrate his anatomical atlas. Using a darkened room illuminated by incoming light, he projected an image of his anatomical preparations onto a glass plate to make his drawings. He did not limit himself to studying healthy bones, as he also illustrated a number of bones affected by disease. Using this innovative technique, Cheselden succeeded in providing accurate illustrations of both healthy and diseased bones.

Bernard Siegfried Albinus (1697–1770) had the opportunity to enjoy an excellent medical education in Leiden. During his studies, he was taught anatomy by the incumbent professor, Govard Bidloo. Albinus followed in his professor's footsteps and later he also became professor in anatomy and surgery in Leiden. In 1747, he published his anatomical atlas, *Tabulae sceleti et musculorum* (Atlas of Bones and Muscles), in which he strove to produce the image of the *homo perfectus* (the perfect human). He was of the conviction that an anatomist should understand the structure of the human body the same way that an architect should understand the foundations of a building he designs. He considered the skeleton to be the basis of the body. He immersed himself in the study of bones and muscles in his quest to fathom the mechanical aspects of the body. In 1753, the professor published his anatomical atlas entitled *Tabulae ossium humanorum* (Atlas of Human Bones).

2

Sebastiaen Egbertszn[2] *1619*

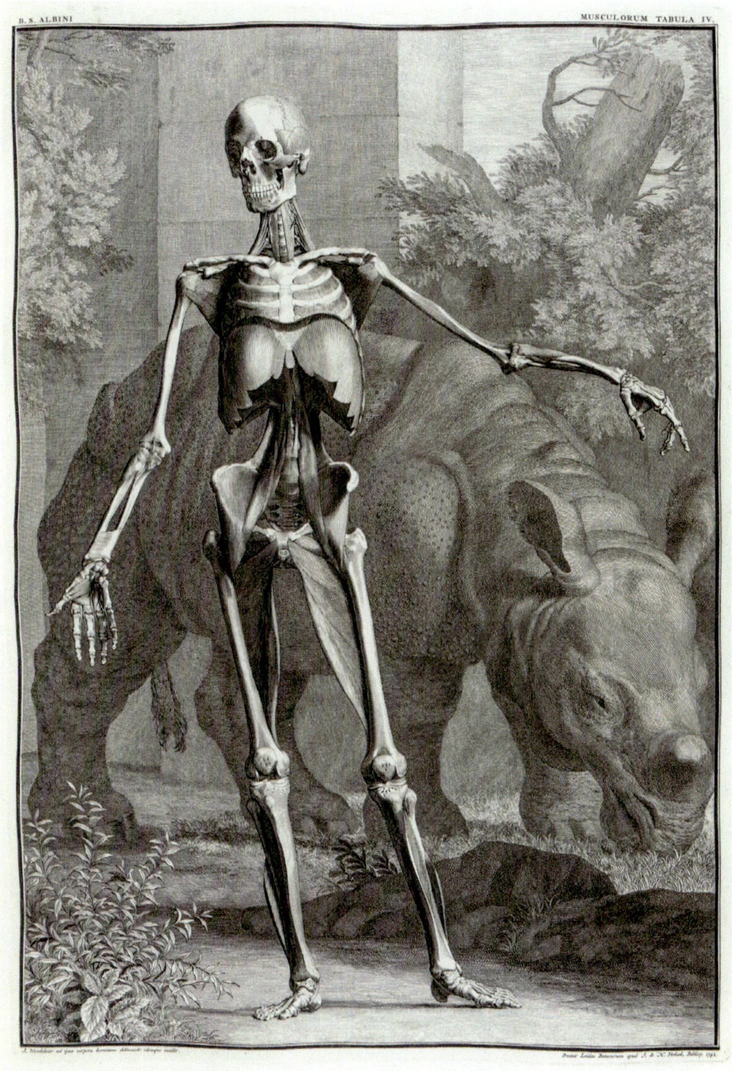

(*Also see the next page*)
Anatomical illustrations of *homo perfectus* (the perfect human being) from Albinus' *Tabulae sceleti et musculorum* (Atlas of Bones and Muscles) (1747). Albinus and Wandelaar devoted a great deal of attention to the background of the illustrations. A rhinoceros is depicted behind one of the skeletons. In 1741, a rhinoceros brought back from Bengal by Dutch sailors was exhibited in Amsterdam. Wandelaar made a drawing of the animal and used it as the background to his anatomical illustration. The rhinoceros symbolized the impetuous life force that prevailed throughout the natural world. Library University of Groningen.

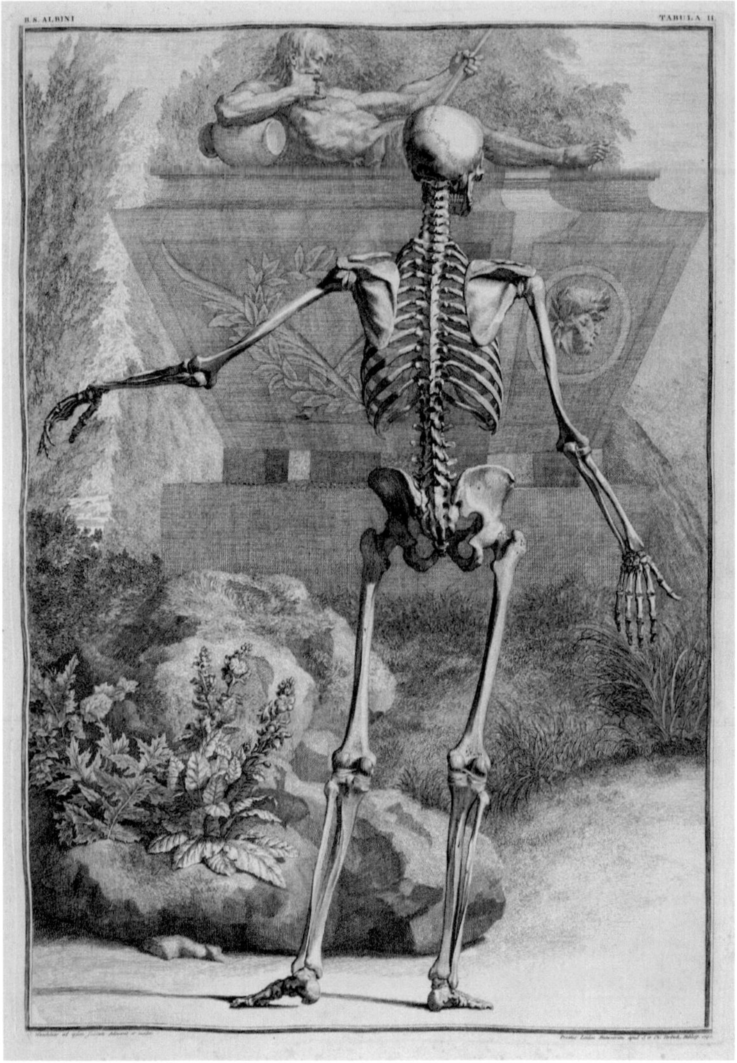

2

Sebastiaen Egbertszn[2] *1619*

> Albinus worked in close collaboration with the draughtsman and engraver Jan Wandelaar (1690–1759). In order to reproduce the image of the skeletons as objectively as possible, they used wooden frames strung with string to make grids. These grids were placed in front of the skeleton, after which the draughtsman copied the skeleton exactly onto drawing-paper from one single perspective, using the grids as reference. Albinus believed that the image of the perfect human should meet the criteria of objectivity, symmetry and vitality. The *Tabulae ossium humanorum* was published in folio (72x50 cm) and contains thirty-four illustrations relating to osteological topics. Each illustration is provided with a further explanatory illustration in which the relationship between the bones, joints, muscles and tendons is shown. By integrating his knowledge of osteology with that of muscles and joints in this way, the anatomist gained more insight into the mechanical aspects of the human body.

This series of anatomical atlases clearly shows that even three to four hundred years ago, people in the medical world had already built up a decent level of knowledge in the field of osteology. The study of bones and the construction of the human skeleton were important parts of the training and examination of surgeons. The fact that a lecture in osteology was chosen as the topic of the second group portrait of the Amsterdam Surgeons' Guild, only goes to show just how much importance the surgeons attached to these lectures.

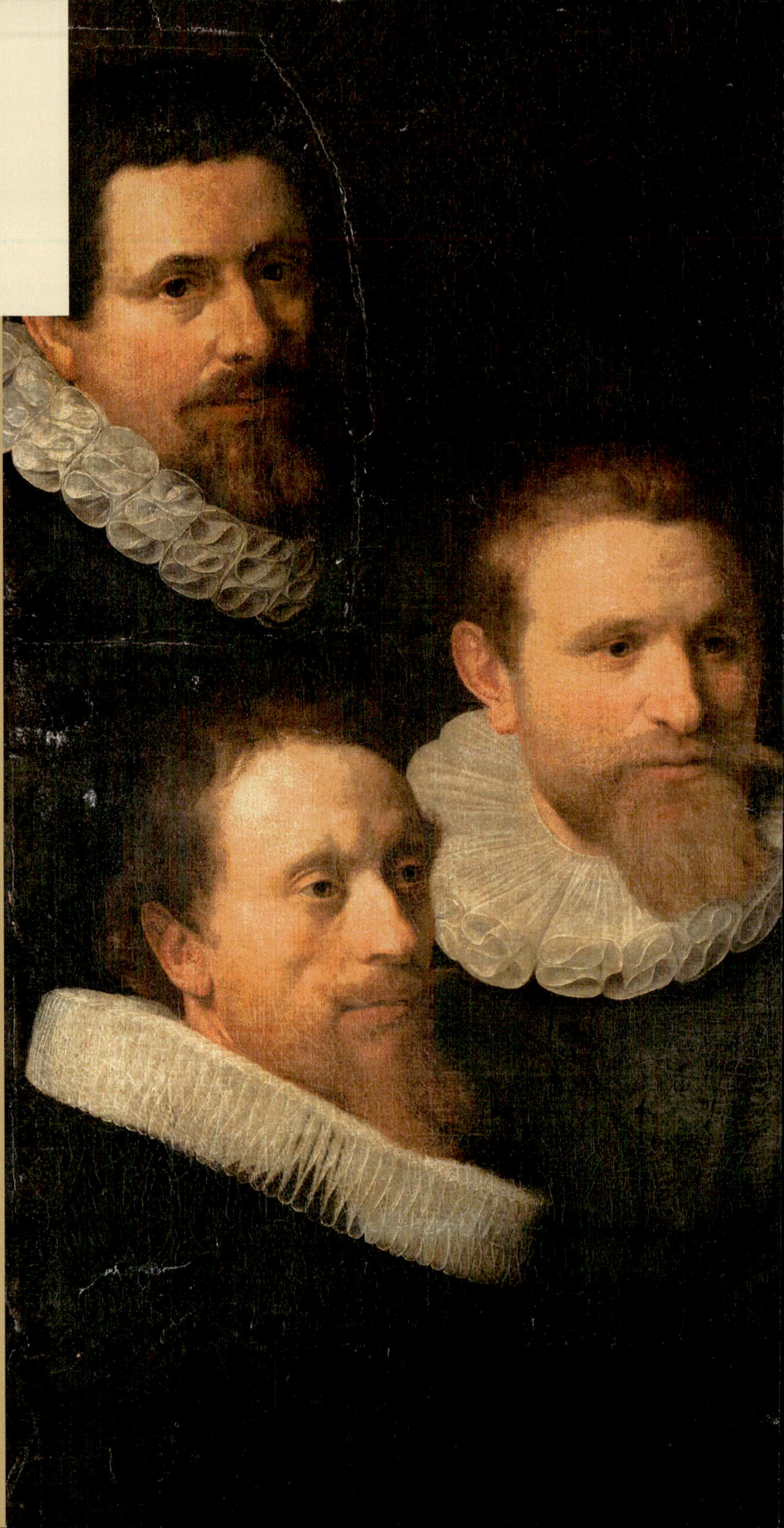

Nicolaes Eliaszn Pickenoy, *The Anatomy Lesson of Jan Fonteijn*, (1625–1626). Detail. Collection Amsterdam Museum.

3

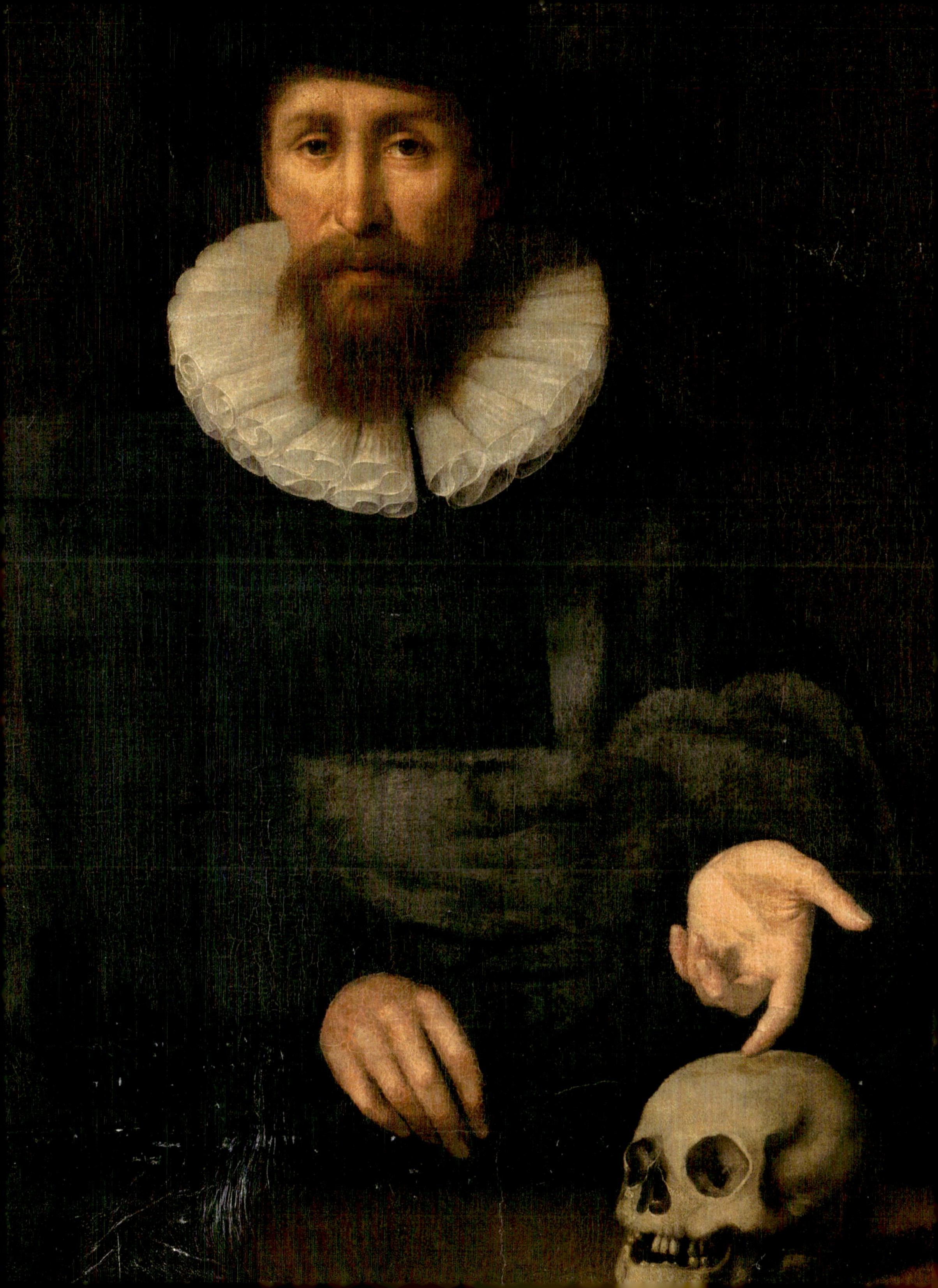

Johan Fonteijn

The Anatomy Lesson of Johan Fonteijn,
painted by Nicolaes Eliaszn Pickenoy in 1625–1626

▸ **The Painting** On September 6th, 1625, Johan Fonteijn, the *praelector anatomiae* of the surgeons' guild, commissioned the artist Nicolaes Eliaszn Pickenoy, to paint him in company of a number of other surgeons. This group portrait was delivered in October 1626 and hung in the guildhall of the Amsterdam Surgeons' Guild. This painting, *The Anatomy Lesson of Johan Fonteijn,* is the third so-called 'anatomy lesson' from the series of nine that were painted for the guild. In 1621, Johan Fonteijn was appointed *praelector anatomiae* of the guild, as successor to Sebastiaen Egbertszn. In his early years as the praelector, he continued to give his anatomy lessons on the upper floor of the former chapel of St.-Margaret's Convent on the Nes

Nicolaes Eliaszn Pickenoy, *The Anatomy Lesson of Jan Fonteijn,* (1625–1626). Collection Amsterdam Museum.

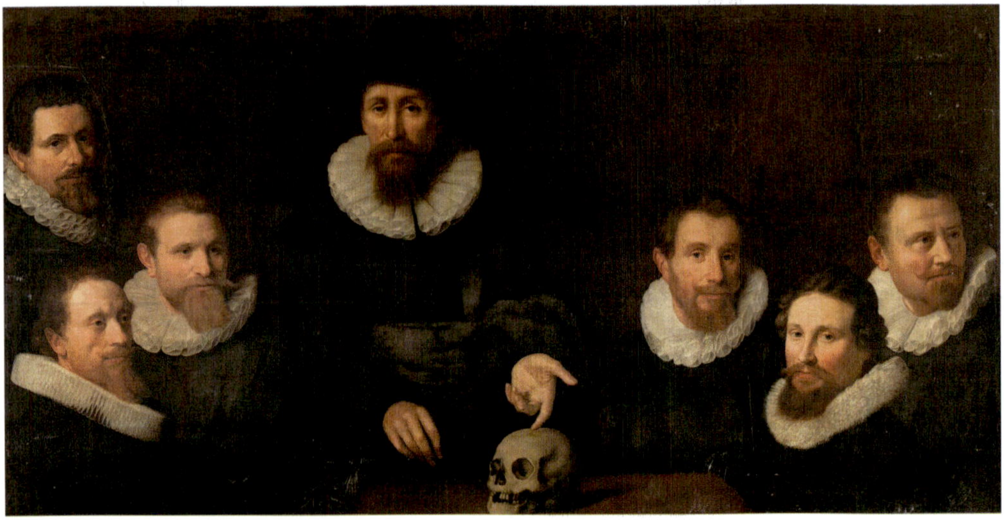

(see p. 14). In 1624 the guild's dissection-room was moved to the Weighing House on the Nieuwmarkt, after which he taught at these new premises. The commission for the group portrait could possibly have been prompted by the move, while they might also have wanted to portray the more recent members of the board who had not yet been painted in the years between 1603 and 1619.

In *The Anatomy Lesson of Johan Fonteijn,* the *praelector* is shown with six surgeons gathered around a table on which a skull has been placed. Originally, there were another four surgeons to be seen in the portrait but the fire in the guildhall in 1723 badly damaged the canvas — the same fate which befell the *Anatomy Lesson of Jan Deijman.* When the painting was restored in 1723, the parts of the canvas which were irreparably damaged were discarded, with the loss of the portraits of four of the surgeons, leaving just six of the original ten. Unfortunately, there is no way of knowing what the original painting looked like when it was still intact. It was probably originally 160 cm long, of which only 97.5 cm remains.

The surgeon shown at the upper left in the painting originally had another position in the composition. During the restoration of the partly burnt canvas, they managed to salvage the portrait and was assigned to another place. At present, the *Anatomy Lesson of Johan Fonteijn* is housed in the Amsterdam Museum.

▸ **The Painter** Nicolaes Eliaszn Pickenoy (1588–1650/56) was born in Amsterdam as the son of the Flemish seal-engraver, Elias Claeszn Pickenoy, and Heijltje Laurens s'Jonge. In 1621 the artist married Levijntje Bouwens with whom he had ten children. He learnt his craft from the portrait painter Cornelis van der Voort. In fact, Pickenoy can be considered Van der Voort's successor, as after the latter's death in 1624, Pickenoy took over his position and thereby acquired the majority of his clientele. When Pickenoy painted *The Anatomy Lesson of Johan Fonteijn* between 1625-1626 at the age of thirty-seven, he still had a successful career ahead of him, as it turned out.

Pickenoy was no stranger to Amsterdam's medical establishment. A few years after the completion of the canvas, his seriously ill young daughter came to be treated by Dr Nicolaes Tulp. The girl suffered from an osteomyelitic rib, a sickness that caused multiple abscesses which severely weakened her body and eventually led to her death. As a token of appreciation for all he had done for his child, Pickenoy painted his portrait. It depicts the doctor with a burning candle with the caption *Aliis inserviendo consumor* (I will be consumed as I serve others). Two years later, the artist painted a very fine portrait of the Tulp family (see p. 83).

Around about this time, Pickenoy also painted a large number of individual portraits of members of the Amsterdam elite. Among his works are the prestigious portrait of husband and wife, Cornelis de Graeff and Catharina Hooft, both scions of Amsterdam's leading patrician families. Between 1630 and 1645, Pickenoy established himself as an artist specialized in painting group portraits of civil militia. In this period, he produced no fewer than five large-scale paintings of musketeers. Besides this genre, he also painted various portraits of boards of directors, including the directors of the Female House of Correction (*Spinhuis*) and the French Protestant Orphanage (*Walen Weeshuis*). Nicolaes Pickenoy was an excellent portrait painter whose oeuvre consists of more than one hundred individual and group portraits.

▸ **The Dissector** Johan Fonteijn (1574-1628) came from a family of apothecaries. He was the son of the Amsterdam apothecary, Thonis Janszn, who owned the apothecary's shop 'Fountain on the Dam' (*Fonteyn op de Dam*). There was a splendid fountain right next to Thonis Janszn's house and this piece of civic architecture must have inspired his choice of his new family name 'Fonteijn' (before this time many Dutch people did not have surnames just patronymics). Thonis also owned two herb gardens on the outskirts of the city, where he cultivated herbs with healing properties, which he used in the preparation of his medicine. His other son, Rembertus Fonteijn, continued the family apothecary tradition, also cultivating his own medicinal herbs. Johan had at least three sons, two of which — Bernard and Nicolaes — also entered the medical profession.

Johan Fonteijn studied medicine, whereupon he established himself as doctor in Amsterdam. He was a highly respected medical physician who occupied a number of prominent positions. Nicolaes Tulp even went so far as to refer to him as *medicus felicissimus, college nostra* (our colleague, a very successful doctor). A fine portrait of him has survived, bearing the Latin caption *Johannus Fontanus Antoni F. Amsterodamensis, Medicinae Doctor*. Besides his medical

Jan Harmenszn Muller, *Portrait of Johan Fonteijn*, 1626 (Municipal Archive Amsterdam). The English translation of the caption runs as follows:

Christ is the source of life. Johan Fonteijn, son of Anthony, physician from Amsterdam.
An attribute to his city is depicted here in such a wonderfully lifelike way: the likes of which could not be surpassed even by the ivory of Phidias' Jupiter (Zeus).[1] This is a work by Muller. But the land of the Batavians applauds this talent, so akin to that of Apollo,[2] just as it sings the praises of its own Hippocrates. What does it benefit you, oh Citizens, to turn to the divinity at Epidaurus.[3] Even healthier shall be the water that is drunk from the Amstel-FONTEIJN.

P. Scriverius H.

1 Phidias was one of the greatest artists of Greek Antiquity. He sculpted a gigantic chryselphantine statue (gilded and inlaid with ivory) of Zeus kept at Olympia. The statue is counted among the Seven Wonders of the Ancient World.
2 Apollo was the god of 'fine art'.
3 Epidaurus was a town in Ancient Greece, famous for its sanctuary of Asclepius, the god of medicine.

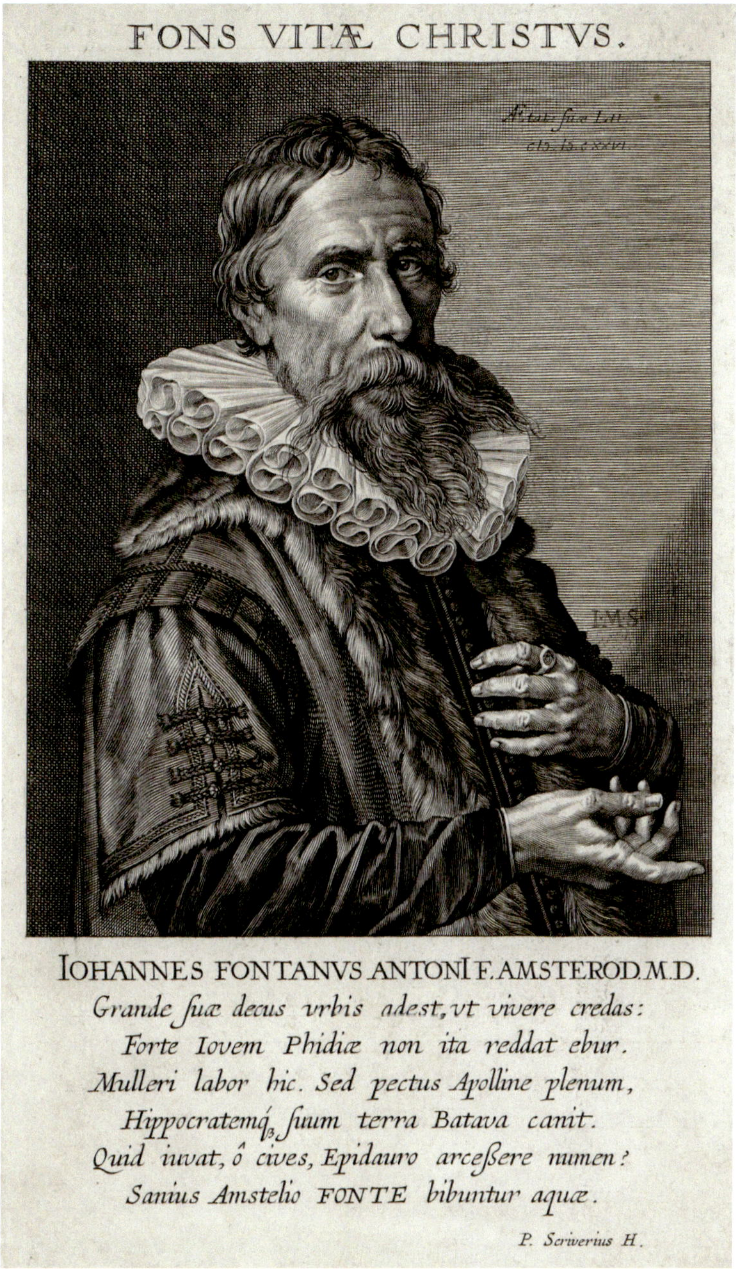

work, Fonteijn took a great interest in art and culture. Among his good friends was the famous Dutch poet and playwright, Joost van den Vondel, who described Fonteijn as 'a lover of all the fine arts, especially of the art of poetry which he embraces with charming enthusiasm and sometimes practices with a passion.'

In 1621, at the age of forty-seven, Johan Fonteijn was asked to become court physician to Prince Maurits (1567–1625), the Prince of Orange, Count of Nassau, Stadtholder and Captain-General of the Republic of the Seven United Netherlands. A year later, in 1622, the health of the ageing prince slipped into a slow decline. After a long illness during which he was attended by Fonteijn, the prince died in April 1625. His body was placed in the Orange-Nassau family vault in the New Church in Delft. Fonteijn himself passed away more than three years later. He was buried in the New Church in Amsterdam.

▸ **The Surgeons** The names of all ten surgeons whose likenesses have been perpetuated in the original painting are known. In consecutive order, they are Cornelis Kerkhem, Anthony Testament, Barend Trist, Jan Scherm, Jan Hartman, Steven Venekool, David van Meurtel, Arend Allertszn, Jacob van Leeuwen and Gerrit Hartman. Two of these ten men, Cornelis Kerkhem and Jan Hartman, had just been appointed to the guild's board of governors. Of the other eight, six had already been Assistant Tutor. This Assistant Tutor was generally appointed for a number of years, his duties were to assist the *praelector* during the anatomy lessons. He also kept the attendance roll, noting which apprentices and surgeons were present at these lessons. Apparently, *The Anatomy Lesson of Jan Fonteijn* also offered an opportunity for surgeons showing great promise to be portrayed, as most of the governors had already been included in previous group portraits. Arend Allertszn, one of the surgeons depicted, died before the portrait was completed in 1626. As four portraits were destroyed by fire, it is no longer possible to identify the six remaining men on the restored painting.

▸ **The Subjectum anatomicum** Neither the table nor the skull were part of the original composition. Perhaps these were added by the painter-restorer Jan Maurits Quinkhard (1688–1772), when he was commissioned to salvage what he could of the damaged painting. Remarkably, the skull is almost identical to the one Quinkhard

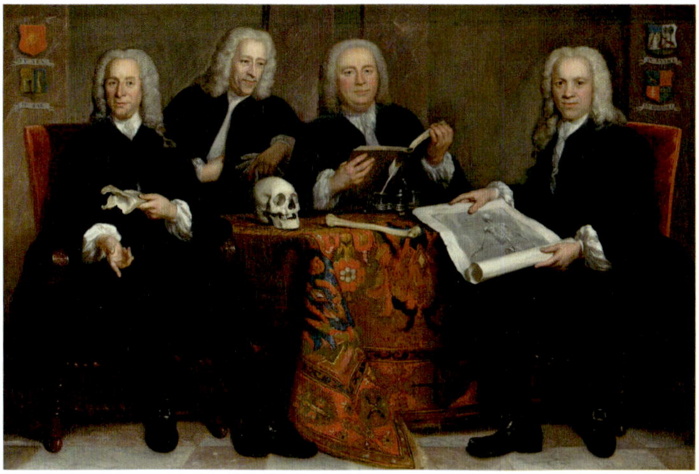

Jan Maurits Quinkhard, *Four Members of the Board of the Surgeons' Guild*, 1744. Collection Amsterdam Museum.

painted in the portrait of the members of the board which he painted in 1744. The dentition of the skulls is strikingly similar. The greatest difference is that they are reproduced as mirror images of one another.

It seems very likely that *The Anatomy Lesson of Jan Fonteijn* originally included the corpse of an executed criminal, used to give the anatomical demonstration. There should have been enough space at the bottom of the painting for it to have been displayed there. However, the question of what the subject of *The Anatomy Lesson of Jan Fonteijn* could actually have been, will always remain a matter of speculation.

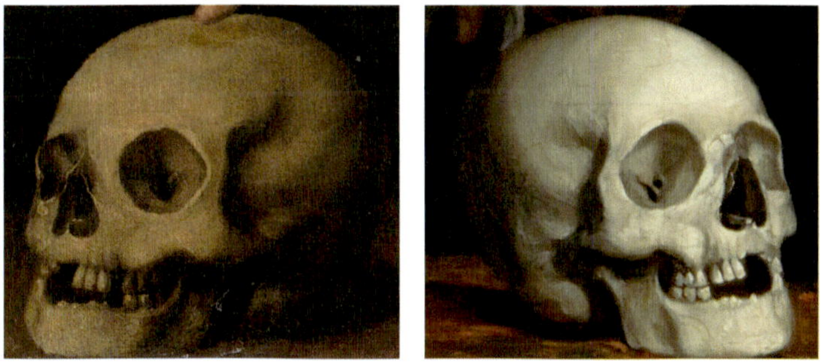

Comparison between the skulls in *The Anatomy Lesson of Johan Fonteijn* (left) and *Four Members of the Board of the Surgeons' Guild*, 1744 (right).

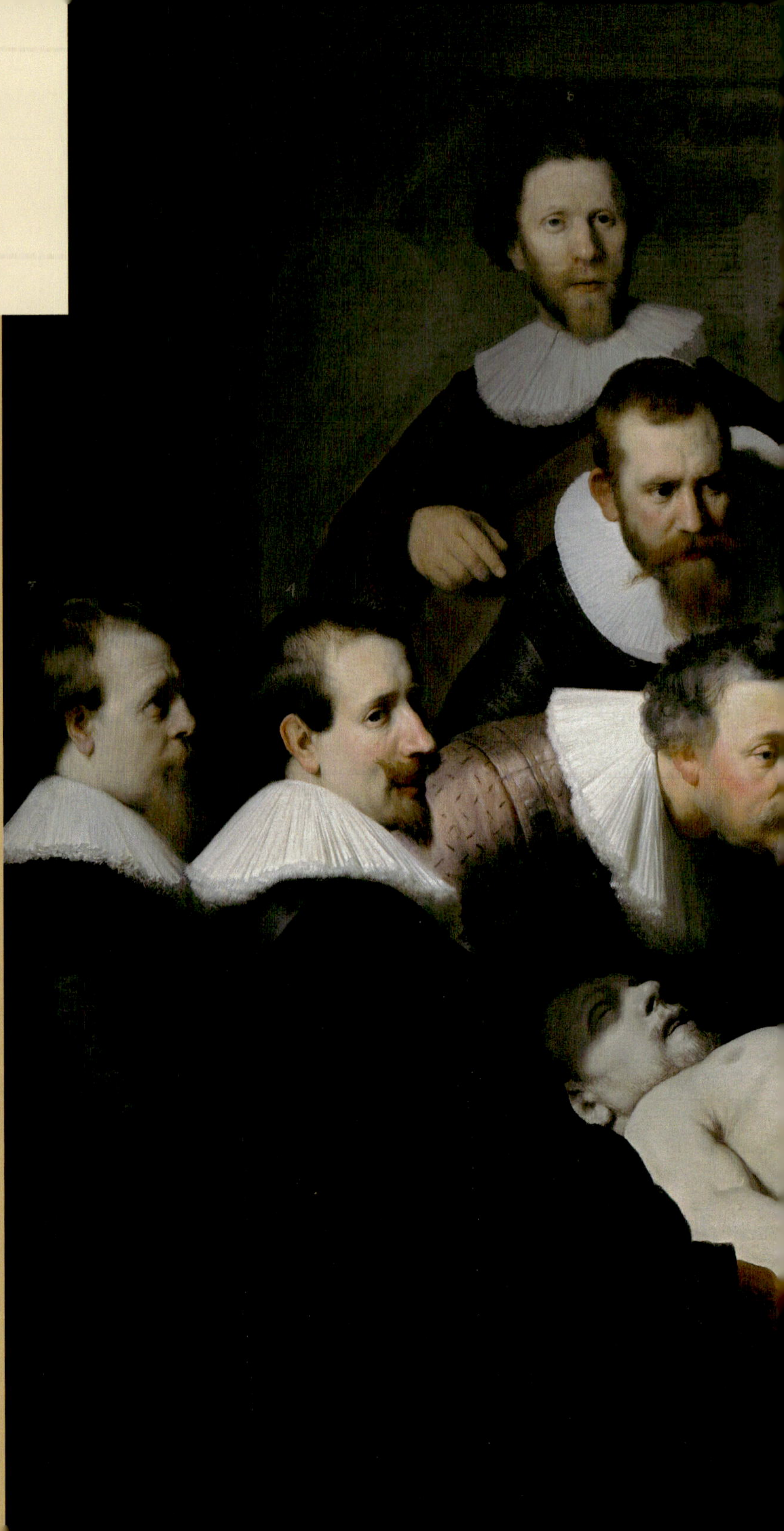

Rembrandt. *The Anatomy Lesson of Nicolaes Tulp*, 1632. Koninklijk Kabinet van Schilderijen Mauritshuis (Royal Picture Gallery Mauritshuis), The Hague.

4

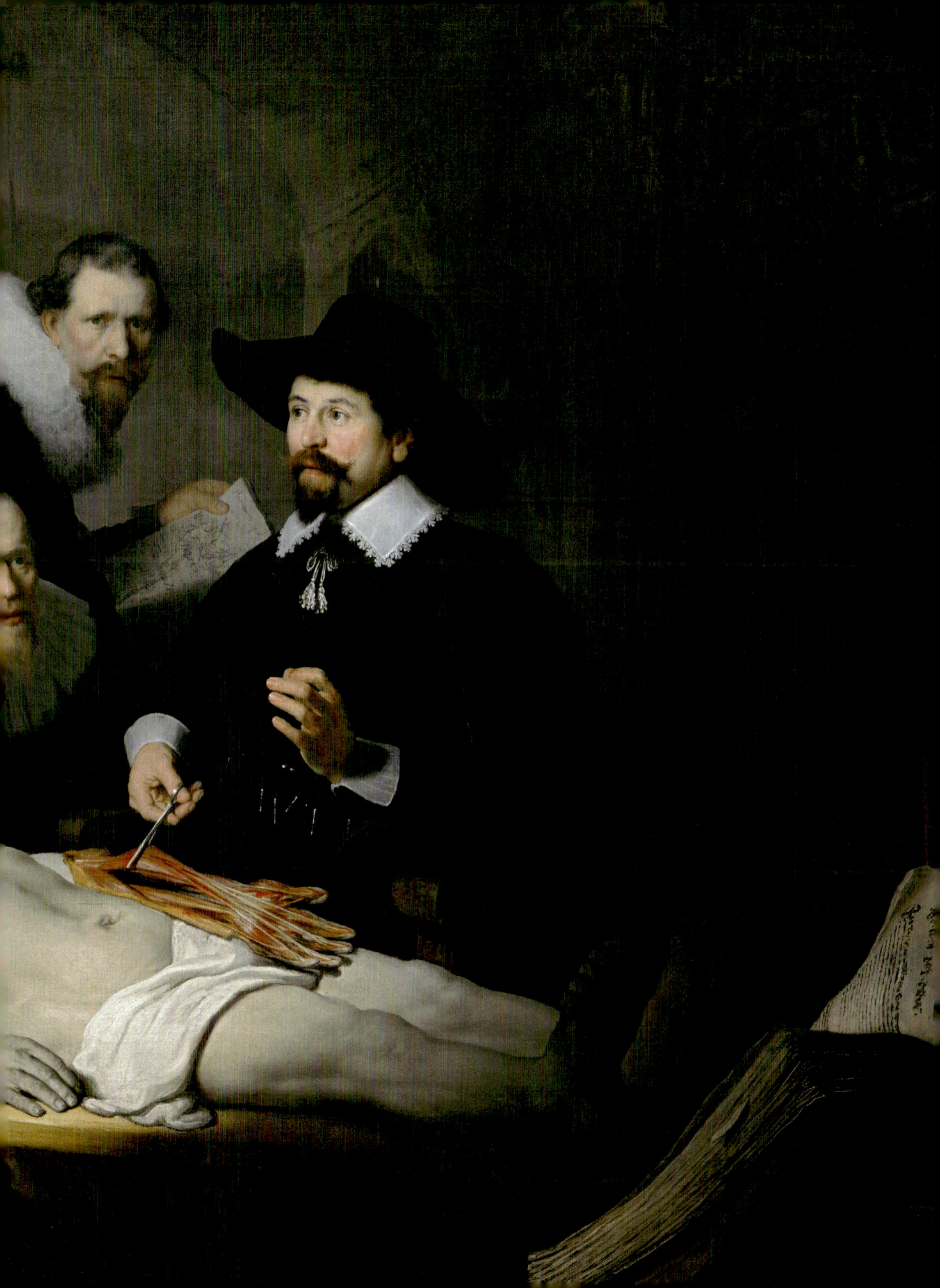

Nicolaes Tulp

The Anatomy Lesson of Nicolaes Tulp,
painted by Rembrandt in 1632

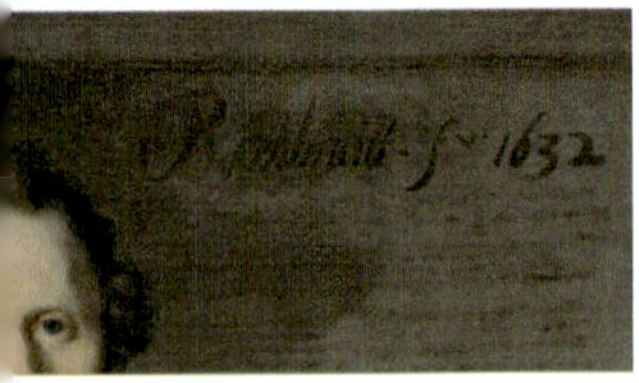

Rembrandt's signature

▸ **The Painting** Almost four hundred years ago, the twenty-six-year-old Rembrandt van Rijn painted a group portrait of the Amsterdam Surgeons' Guild during an anatomy lesson. This 1632 painting, *The Anatomy Lesson of Nicolaes Tulp,* is one in the series of anatomy pieces painted for the guild, the first dating from 1601/1603 and the last dated the end of the eighteenth century. This painting is considered a masterpiece, not least because of its refreshingly new composition, in which the traditional, formal arrangement of the subjects has been relegated a thing of the past to make way for a new configuration, showing the *praelector* and the surgeons in action. Rembrandt's signature can be seen in the background of the composition.

In the painting, Nicolaes Tulp, *praelector anatomiae* of the Amsterdam Surgeons' Guild, is dissecting the forearm of an executed criminal. Seven guild members are depicted on his left. In a masterful way, the varying facial expressions and the direction of the surgeons' gaze help to draw one's attention to Tulp's anatomical demonstration. By way of illustration, Tulp gestures with his left hand, to point out the function of the flexors in the forearm. Tulp's body language is that of a man who is giving instruction to convey his knowledge, while the surgeons listen in order to learn from him.

On the occasion of the anatomy lesson using the body of the twenty-eight-year-old condemned criminal Adriaan Adriaenszn, alias Aris 't Kint (Aris the Kid) on 31 January, 1632, Tulp probably took the initiative to have himself and a number of guild members commemorated in a group portrait by Rembrandt, following in the tradition of his predecessors. Tulp's lesson on anatomy was held in the dissection room which the surgeons had installed on the St Anthony Weighing House on the Nieuwmarkt in Amsterdam. The painting decorated the walls of the guild-hall for many years. These days, it is part of the

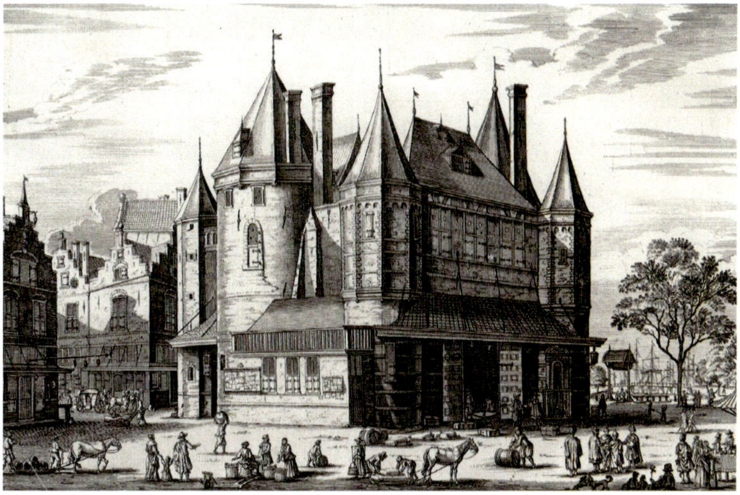

Saint Anthony's Weighing House on Nieuwmarkt (New Market) in Amsterdam. These were the official premises of the Amsterdam Surgeon's Guild where Nicolaes Tulp delivered his anatomy lesson in 1632. Municipal Archive Amsterdam.

collection at the Royal Picture Gallery at the Mauritshuis museum in The Hague.

▸ **The Artist** Rembrandt van Rijn (1606–1669) is one of the most famous painters in the history of the Netherlands. He produced more than 300 paintings, 300 etchings and 2,000 drawings. Rembrandt was born in Leiden on June 15th, 1606, as the son of a miller. While still in his teens, he was taught by the Leiden historical painter Jacob van Swanenburgh. Later, he left for Amsterdam to become the apprentice of the leading artist Pieter Lastman, and began to receive important commissions at a relatively young age. In 1632, at the age of twenty-six, the Surgeons' Guild's members of the board asked him to capture them on canvas; resulting in the fabulous masterpiece *The Anatomy Lesson of Nicolaes Tulp*.

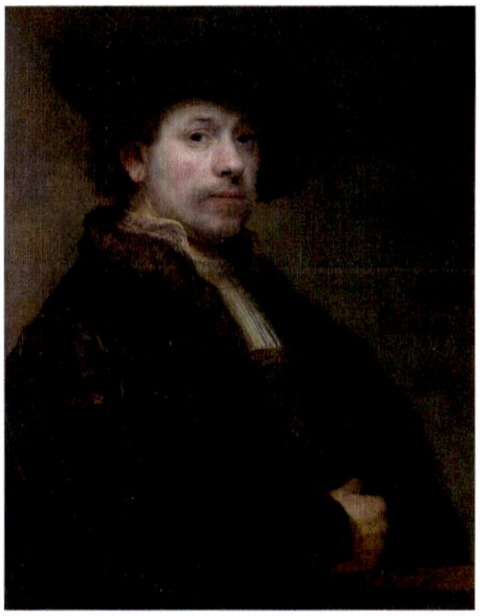

Rembrandt van Rijn, *Self Portrait*, 1640. The National Gallery, London.

Trying to discover how Rembrandt went about painting Dr Tulp, the surgeons and the corpse, is an intriguing exercise. Did he make sketches during Tulp's public lesson to use them in order to paint the scene on canvas in his studio later? There is no evidence that Rembrandt did actually witness this particular anatomy lesson given by Tulp. Nor are there any known drawings or sketches which he might have made during the public lesson. Did Rembrandt use a real dissected arm, and did he paint the portrait with or without supplementary information from atlases of anatomy? There are no known records that suggest that a corpse had been taken to his studio. And yet, the realistic details, as well as the colouring of the skin of the dead man's arm which has been laid bare, suggest that Rembrandt did have a real dissected arm at his disposal. So far, attempts at identifying the book on the desk and the anatomical illustration on the piece of paper held by one of the surgeons have proven unsuccessful. Unfortunately, it has not been possible to reconstruct the precise circumstances in which Rembrandt painted the picture.

Rembrandt collaborated with the art dealer, Hendrick van Uylenburg, who, among other things, provided him with work commissions in Amsterdam. In 1634, the artist married Hendrick's first cousin, Saskia van Uylenburg. Their son, Titus, was born in 1641, and Saskia died that same year. Following her death, the widow Geertje Dircx came to work in Rembrandt's home as a maid. Geertje and Rembrandt had an affair, but after a few years, they parted in anger. Geertje was succeeded by Hendrickje Stoffels, with whom Rembrandt had a daughter who they called Cornelia. In the years that followed, Rembrandt had to contend with major setbacks. In 1653 he found himself in great debt, and a few years later, he was declared bankrupt so that he could no longer meet his financial obligations. In 1658, his house and its contents were sold and he moved into a small rented house on the Rozengracht. Rembrandt died on October 4th, 1669.

▸ **The Dissector** Nicolaes Tulp (1593–1674) was born in Amsterdam as Claes Pieterszn. In 1611 he enrolled as a medical student at the University of Leiden. Three years later he was awarded the degree of *doctor medicinae*. When he left Leiden to return to Amsterdam, he moved into a house situated on the Herengracht. In 1617, he married Eva van der Voech (1593–1628) with whom he lived on the Prinsengracht. Four years later, the couple moved again, this time to the Keizersgracht. They had six children whom they named Pieter, Egbert, Gherytgen, Catharina, Diederick and Claes. Much to their parents' grief, four of the children died before they reached the age of thirty. However, their son Diederick prospered: he became a senior administrator of the Dutch East India Company (VOC), an alderman

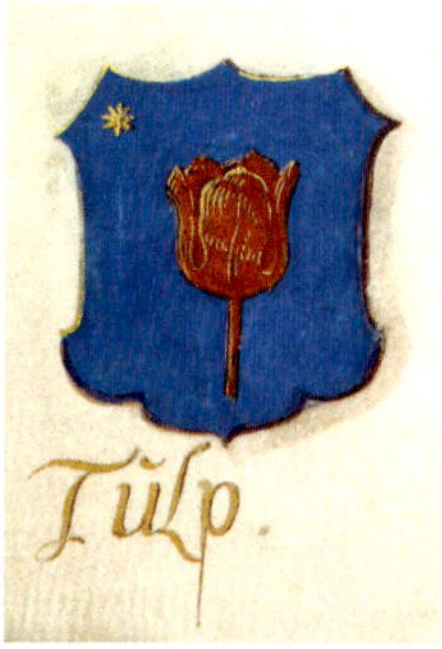

Coat-of-arms of Nicolaes Tulp. Six Collection, Amsterdam.

of Amsterdam, and he was a lieutenant-colonel with the Amsterdam civil militia corps.

From the façade of Pieterszn's family home, a signboard hung with an image of a tulip. This flower might have been chosen due to the affinity Claes had with botany, as well as the fact that, at this time, the tulip was a very exclusive, expensive flower. Claes Pieterszn, or Nicolaes Tulp, was far more than a physician: he also played an active part in public administration. In 1622, when he was appointed an alderman of Amsterdam, he had an official seal made bearing a tulip, which he could affix to official documents. Thereafter, he changed the family name to Tulp.

After the death of Tulp's first wife, he remarried in 1630, this time to Margaretha de Vlaming van Outshoorn (1598–1678). From

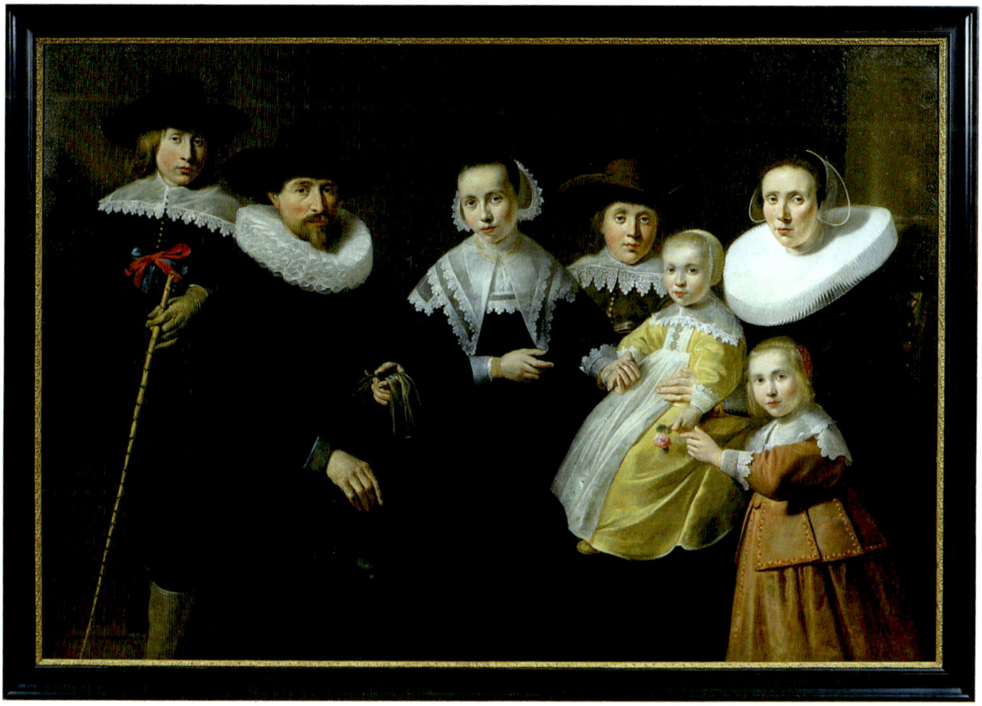

Nicolaes Eliaszn Pickenoy, *The Tulp Family*, 1635. Portraited from left to right: Diederick Tulp, Nicolaes Tulp (senior), Catharina Tulp, Nicolaas Tulp (junior), Margaretha Tulp, Eva Tulp and Margaretha de Vlaming van Outshoorn. Six Collection, Amsterdam.

this second marriage, Tulp had another three children, named Eva, Margaretha and Symon. At this point, the Tulp family was complete. In 1655 his daughter Margaretha married Jan Six (1618–1700), who occupied positions in the Amsterdam municipal administration for more than forty years, including that of burgomaster. To the present day, a large portion of Nicolaes Tulp's legacy has been preserved in the Six family archives.

Like his son-in-law, Tulp had a long record of service in the municipal administration. He served as an alderman for no less than fifty years, and four years as burgomaster of the city of Amsterdam. On top of this, he also played a major role in the improvement and organization of the city's health care. Under his leadership, the first *Pharmacopoea Amstelredamensis* — a handbook for the preparation of medicines — was compiled. Its purpose was to raise the standard of the quality of medicinal preparations. The book appeared in 1636, its publication no doubt spurred on by the 1635 plague epidemic in which more than 17,000 people died in Amsterdam alone. It was a very critical period when there was a great need for standardized prescriptions for the preparation of medicine. Up to that time, an enormously diverse range of medications had been compounded, often composed of no fewer than twenty-to forty different medicinal ingredients. In 1636, Amsterdam counted fifty-eight medical doctors (*doctores medicinae*) and sixty-six apothecaries. The medical doctors were prohibited from compounding their own medicine and had to write out a prescription to be prepared by the apothecary.

Tulp did Amsterdam's suppliers of medicine a great service when he took the initiative to compile a prescription book. The same year the book was published in 1636, medical doctors and apothecaries were legally obliged to work in accordance with the requirements it set. A new governing body composed of physicians and apothecaries — the Collegium Medicum — was established to ensure that the rules were followed. The duties of this governing body went far beyond keeping an eye on regulations affecting medicine, as it also had the task of supervising the examination of physicians, apothecaries, surgeons and — later — midwives, as well as the awarding of degrees. As far as we know, there were twenty-six editions of *Pharmacopoea Amstelredamensis* between 1636 and 1795, a telling indication of Tulp's enormous contribution to health care.

Tulp worked as a doctor in Amsterdam for more than forty years. His daily duties were actually comparable to those of a modern

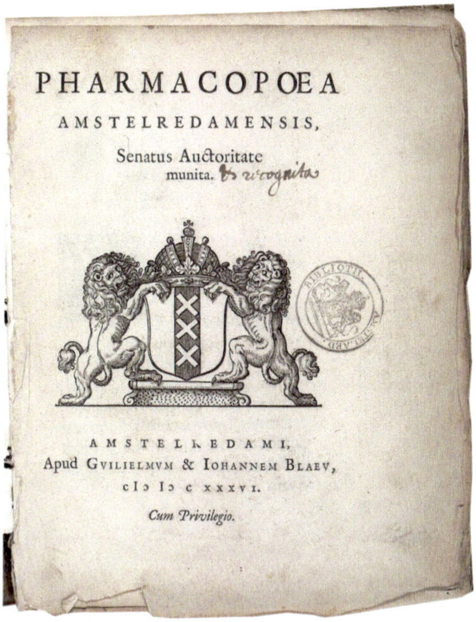
PHARMACOPŒA
AMSTELREDAMENSIS,
Senatus Auctoritate
munita.
AMSTELREDAMI,
Apud GVILIELMVM & IOHANNEM BLAEV,
cIↄ Iↄ c xxxvi.
Cum Privilegio.

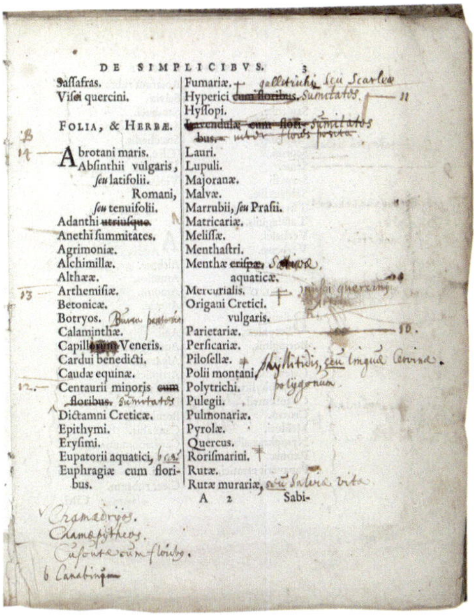
DE SIMPLICIBVS. 3

Saſſafras.
Viſci quercini.
FOLIA, & HERBÆ.
Abrotani maris.
Abſinthii vulgaris, *ſeu* latifolii.
Romani, *ſeu* tenuifolii.
Adanthi utriuſque.
Anethi ſummitates.
Agrimoniæ.
Alchimillæ.
Althææ.
Arthemiſiæ.
Betonicæ.
Botryos.
Calaminthæ.
Capillorum Veneris.
Cardui benedicti.
Caudæ equinæ.
Centaurii minoris cum floribus.
Dictamni Creticæ.
Epithymi.
Eryſimi.
Eupatorii aquatici.
Euphragiæ cum floribus.

Fumariæ.
Hyperici cum floribus.
Hyſſopi.
Lavendulæ cum floribus.
Lauri.
Lupuli.
Majoranæ.
Malvæ.
Marrubii, *ſeu* Praſii.
Matricariæ.
Meliſſæ.
Menthaſtri.
Menthæ criſpæ.
aquaticæ.
Mercurialis.
Origani Cretici.
vulgaris.
Parietariæ.
Perſicariæ.
Piloſellæ.
Polii montani.
Polytrichi.
Pulegii.
Pulmonariæ.
Pyrolæ.
Quercus.
Roriſmarini.
Rutæ.
Rutæ murariæ.
A 2 Sabi-

Title page and a page with notes on the medicine prepared by Nicolaes Tulp, from *Pharmacopoea Amstelredamensis* (Pharmacopœia of Amsterdam), Amsterdam, Joh. and Willem Blaeu, 1636. Special Collections, University of Amsterdam.

general practitioner. He had a practice in his own home and made several house calls to seriously ill patients every day. For his house calls, he used a carriage so that he could use his time as efficiently as possible. Tulp wrote prescriptions and advised on diet and lifestyle. When he deemed it necessary, he consulted a surgeon for the treatment of external ailments.

Tulp's patients came from every level of society. Sometimes they were suffering from very interesting complaints. He noted remarkable cases of more than 200 patients. In 1641 these observations were published in Latin under the title *Observationes Medicae.* This book was republished three times during the author's lifetime and, after his death, another three Latin versions appeared. Dutch translations of the *Observationes* were published, but they were not much to Tulp's satisfaction. Perhaps this is why he translated the book into Dutch himself at the end of his life. His handwritten manuscript is still preserved in the collection of the Six family. Tulp's fascinating descriptions give a good insight into the way doctors thought and worked in the seventeenth century. He describes a truly diverse variety of symptoms. These descriptions are illustrated with various images related to the medical history and his observations.

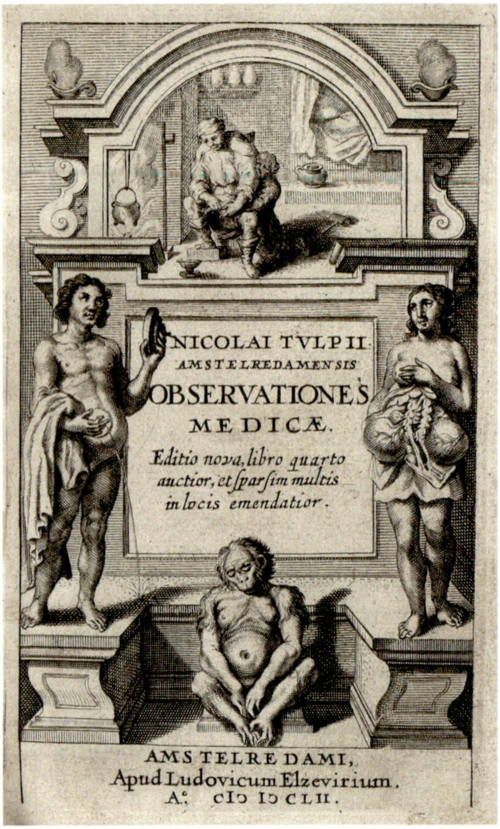

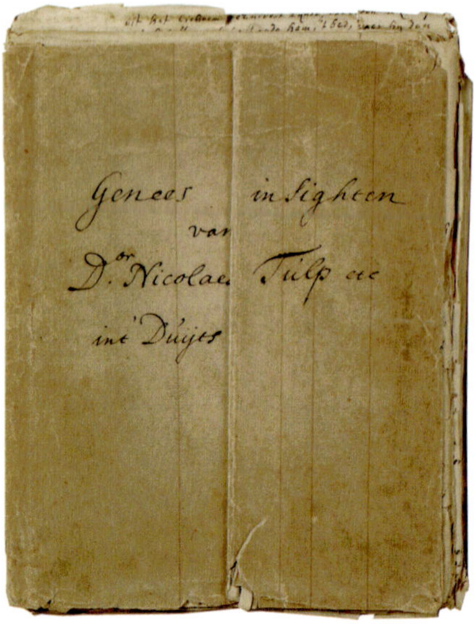

Title page of *Genees-insigten van Nicolaes Tulp* (Medical Insights of Nicolaes Tulp). This 462-page long manuscript, written by Tulp's own hand, is a Dutch translation of *Observationes Medicae*. Six Collection, Amsterdam.

←

Title page of Nicolaes Tulp's, *Observationes Medicae*, Amsterdam, 1652, second edition. Six Collection, Amsterdam.

In 1628, Tulp was appointed *praelector anatomiae* of the Amsterdam Surgeons' Guild. It was in this capacity that he was painted by Rembrandt in *The Anatomy Lesson of Nicolaes Tulp* in 1632. As a teacher he made an enormous contribution to the quality of education in dissection. In the guild's Anatomy Book, in which all its anatomy demonstrations were documented, it is recorded that, between his appointment in 1628 and his retirement in 1650, Tulp gave a total of nine lessons. He gave the first in 1631, followed by those in 1632, 1633, 1634, 1637, 1639, 1640, 1647 and 1650.

Tulp's anatomy lessons were combined with meticulous anatomical observations. A good example is his accurate description of the ileo-cæcal valve (*valvula ileocoecalis*), a sphincter muscle that

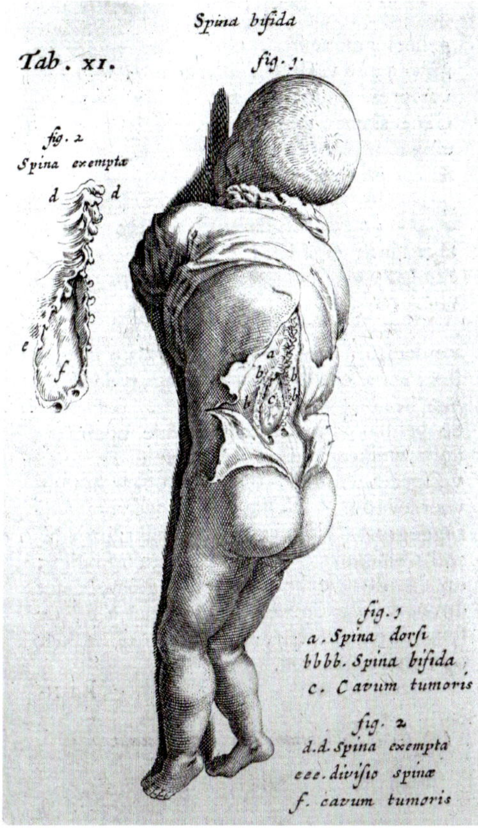

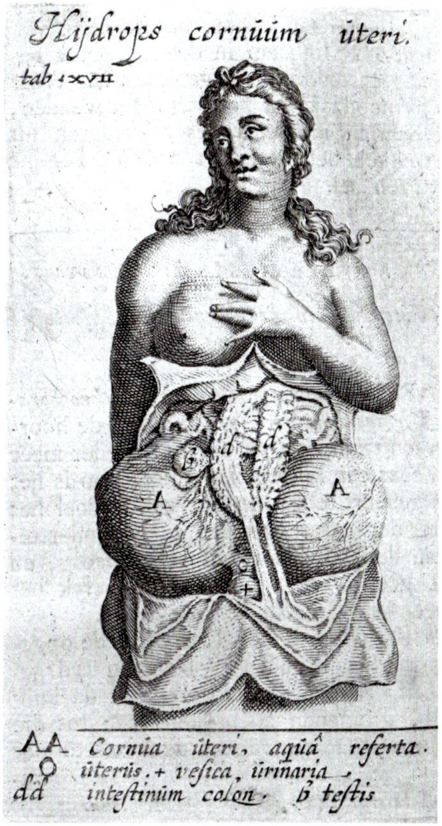

Illustration of a young child that died prematurely of *spina bifida*, from the *Observationes Medicae* of Nicolaes Tulp. The surgeons conducted an autopsy in Tulp's presence during which 'we saw that the spinal cord had completely ruptured, and the tumour caused the branches of the nerves to spread out in so many directions, that it would have been beyond the power of Medicine to remove this growth.'

Illustration of a woman with a growth in the uterus from the *Observationes Medicae* of Nicolaes Tulp. The woman had a painful abdomen that steadily distended. After nine years of enduring pain and misery, she died from what would later turn out to be a severely damaged uterus. An autopsy was carried out on her body 'during which could be seen: a putrid apron of fat in the abdomen, a pallid liver, a small spleen, a displaced large bowel enveloping both the two projecting uterine horns (*cornua uteri*), containing around nine pounds of water and pus, held within innumerable vesicles.'

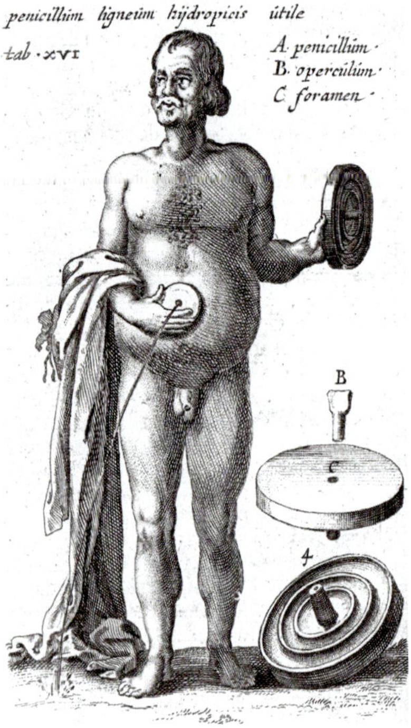

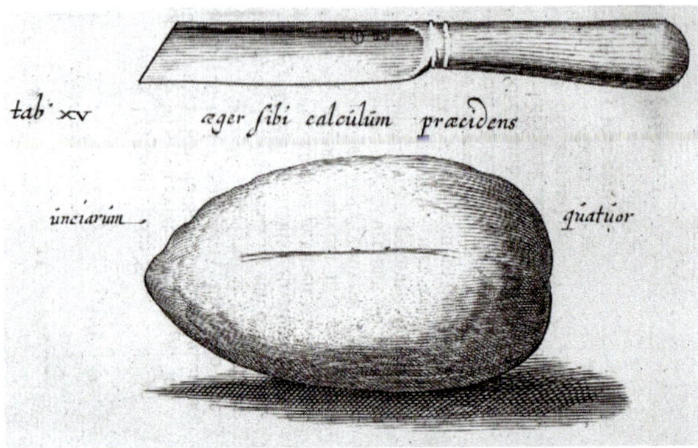

Illustration from the *Observationes Medicae* of Nicolaes Tulp of the bladder stone and knife of the Amsterdam blacksmith 'Jan de Doot' (Jan the Deadman), a patient of Tulp's, whose despair had let him to rid himself of this stone. Although he had twice been treated by a surgeon who specialized in 'cutting the stone', he continued to suffer terrible pain. Reaching a point of desperation, he decided to take matters into his own hands and extracted the stone from his bladder with a knife. He used his fingers to stretch the wound and took the stone, which was larger than a hen's egg and weighed four ounces, out of the wound.

Illustration of a man suffering from an abnormal retention of fluid in the abdomen (*ascites*) from the *Observationes Medicae* of Nicolaes Tulp. In order to tap the fluid from Tulp's dropsical patient, the surgeons fitted a wooden tap to his abdominal wall.

separates the small from the large intestine. Tulp observed this valve during one of his anatomical dissections and introduced the valve with the words: 'but this frequent talk about the intestines brings me to this intestinal valve, which has made several public appearances in the dissection scene, but may now be made more generally known.' Tulp describes this intestinal valve (*ileo-cæcal valve*) as a 'velvety ring forming a complete circle [...], from which hangs a membrane, the width of two fingers [...], which can close off the ileum, from which it hangs like a curtain or a limp sail.' Turning to the working mechanism of the valve, Tulp says that it opens in one direction and closes on the other, 'because, if any sort of unclean matter (stool) floats into the ileum from the large intestine, it resists this, forcefully preventing any matter from the large intestine or appendix from flowing back to the ileum'. Tulp thought that the mechanical forces of excrement inside the intestines determined the closing mechanism of the valve: 'the stronger this ileo-cæcal valve presses, the more force-

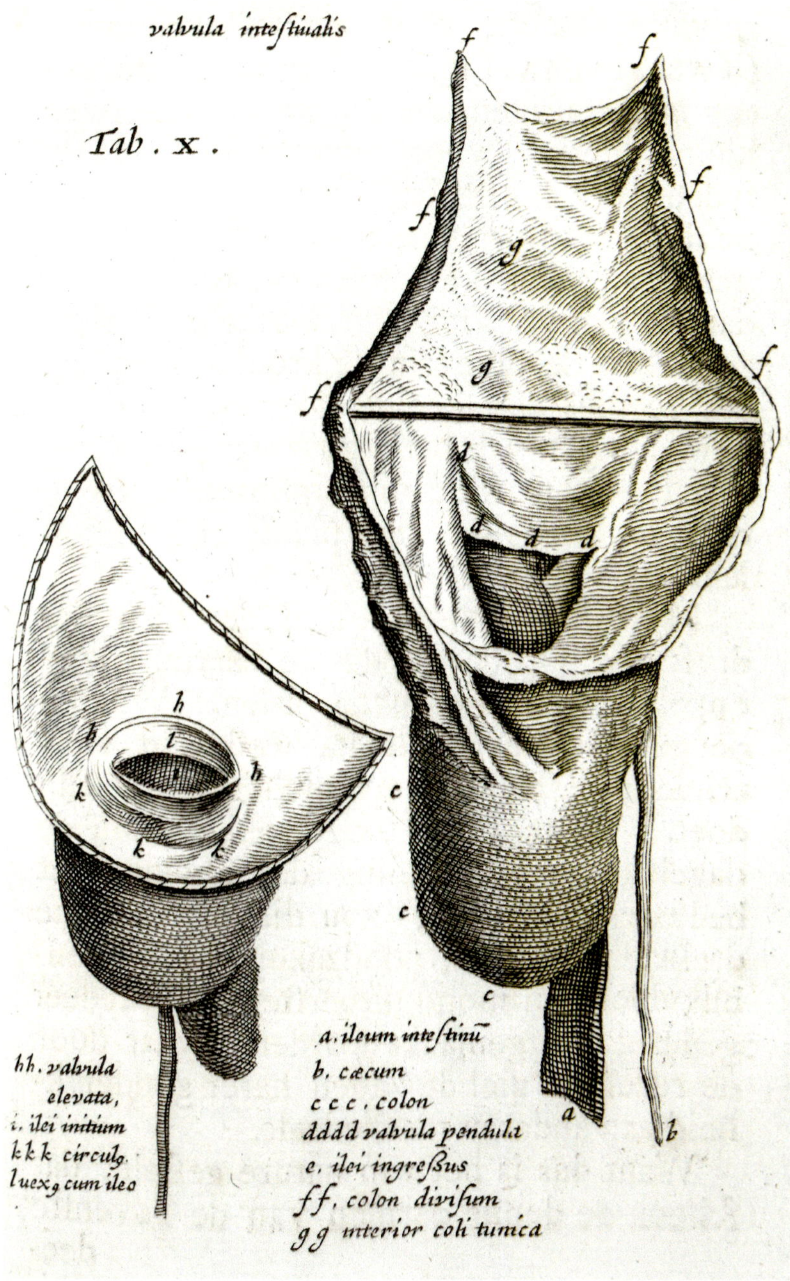

Illustration of the valve which separates the small from the large intestine (*ileocaecal valve*) from the *Observationes Medicae* of Nicolaes Tulp. Tulp observed the valve during one of his anatomy lessons.

fully it pushes, sometimes closing so tightly that even the smallest wind is not able to pass through.' He reasoned that, if the valve did not work properly, the consequence could be a dysfunction or weakening of the valve. Keeping to the age-old theory of Galen, he reasoned that 'food is brought through the intestines' because 'the intestines contract around it'. The discharge of the fæcal material through the intestine in the right direction is guaranteed by a combination of factors, namely: the presence of the diaphragm, the abdominal muscles and the ileo-cæcal valve.

Today, the functioning of the ileo-cæcal valve still has a clinical significance in the surgical treatment of obstructions of the colon. If there is an obstruction of the colon and the valve continues to function normally, the colon distends to such an extent that it can cause a perforation of the intestinal wall (cœcum blow-out), which requires surgery.

An anatomical lesson was usually spread out over several days. The report of Tulp's anatomy lesson in 1647 in the Anatomy Book gives an insight as to how it was conducted.

> *On October 19th, 1647, Levie Abrahamszn from Rotterdam was hung from the neck until he was dead. The first dissection was performed on Saturday, being the day designated by the Honourable Councilor and Alderman, Dr Nicolaes Tulpius, Anatomicus and* Praelector *of the Surgeons' Guild of this city Amsterdam, who has given five lessons using the above-mentioned* subjectum, *which has earned, on some days more than on others, the sum of two hundred and twenty-nine guilders and nine stuyvers, as shown in the account of revenue and expenditure* [...].

The following persons were present in their capacity as *proefmeesters* (Chief Tutors) and governors of the Surgeons' Guild:

Examiners	*Governors*
Mr. Jan Gerritszn Indies	*Mr. Jacob Janszn Cruys*
Mr. Dirck Janszn Wysingh	*Mr. Cornelis Kerchem*
	Mr. Jacob Janszn Colevelt
	Mr. Isaak Lambertszn Barrevoet

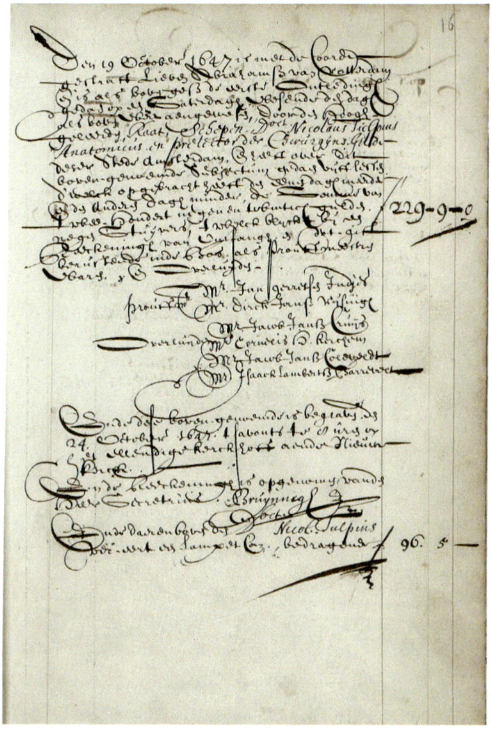

Report of Nicolaes Tulp's 1647 anatomy lesson from the Anatomy Book of the Surgeons' Guild. Municipal Archive Amsterdam.

> *And the above-mentioned was buried on October 24th, 1647, at 8 o'clock in the evening, at the paupers' cemetery of the New Church. The bill was paid by the Secretary, Bruynings.*
>
> *And the [services of] above-said Doctor Nicolaes Tulp were honoured with an ewer to the value of 96.5 guilders.*

The Anatomy Book of 1647 reveals that Tulp's anatomy lesson raised more than 200 guilders. The income from the lesson left enough money to provide the *praelector* with compensation: Tulp received an expensive silver ewer worth 96.5 guilders. Assuming that the average entry fee was 5 *stuyvers*, one can conclude that, based on the number of consecutive days, the lessons must have attracted hundreds of spectators. It would be safe to say that Tulp's 1632 anatomy lesson drew a similar number.

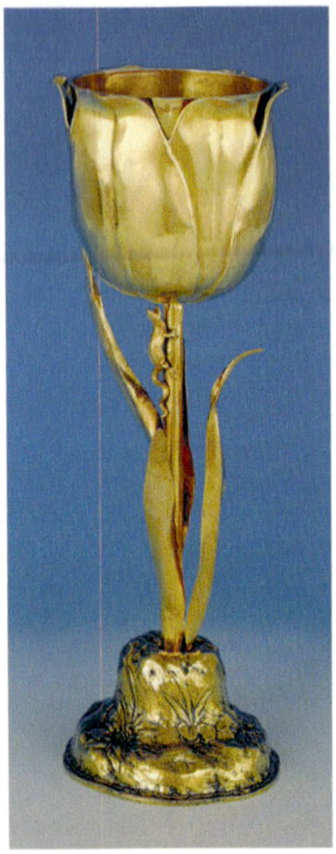

Tulip-shaped cup presented by Nicolaes Tulp to the Guild on the occasion of his retirement in 1652. Six Collection, Amsterdam.

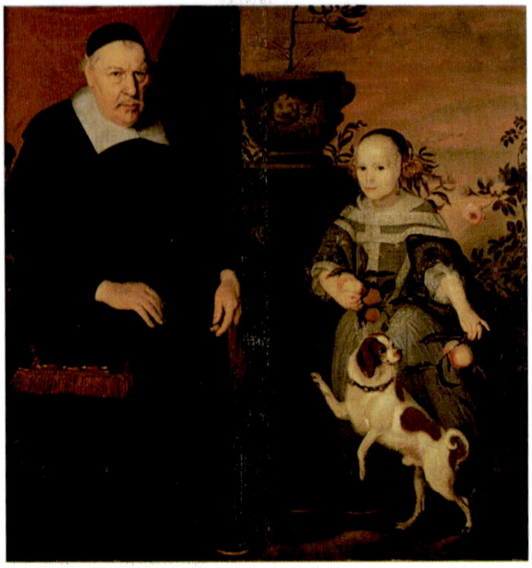

A.C. Beeldenmaker, *Nicolaes Tulp with his granddaughter Margaretha Tholincx*, 1666. Six Collection Amsterdam.

Tulp delivered his last public anatomy lesson in 1650. Two years later, he took his leave of the guild and, as a token of his appreciation, he presented the Amsterdam Surgeons' Guild with a silver cup in the form of a tulip. Having relinquished his duties as *praelector anatomiae* of the Amsterdam Surgeons' Guild, he devoted himself to civic affairs. In 1654 he was first appointed burgomaster of Amsterdam, and thereafter in 1656, 1666 and 1671. In 1666, the aged Tulp had a portrait painted of himself and his granddaughter. He died in 1674 and was buried in the Nieuwe Kerk (New Church) in Amsterdam.

▸ **The Surgeons** All the surgeons shown on this group portrait by Rembrandt have been identified. Their names are written down on a piece of paper held by one of them. Rembrandt had initially made an anatomical drawing of an arm on the paper. This was later painted over when this list of the names of surgeons was added, something which was probably done during a restoration in the eighteenth century. During the last restoration of the canvas in 1996–1998, most of the list of names was removed, so that the original layer of paint showing the anatomical sketch of the arm was visible once more.

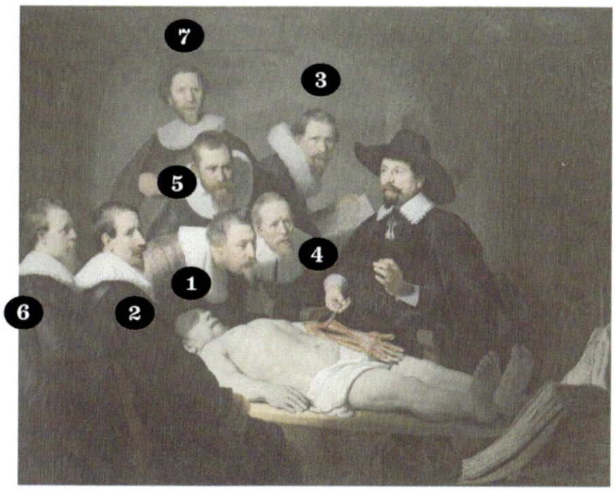

The members of the Amsterdam Surgeons' Guild depicted on *The Anatomy Lesson of Nicolaes Tulp:* 1 Jacob de Wit; 2 Adriaen Slabberaen; 3 Hartman Hartmanszn; 4 Matthijs Calkoen; 5 Jacob Block; 6 Jacob Colevelt; 7 Frans van Loenen.

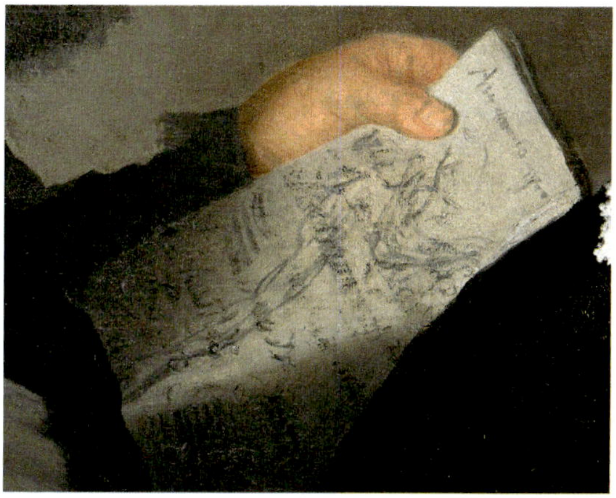

The piece of paper held by one of the surgeons in the painting. It shows the original anatomical sketch of an arm which is partially obscured by a list of names of the surgeons whose portraits are included in the painting.

In the seventeenth century, it was customary for every person depicted in a group portrait to pay the artist individually. By way of example, there is a record that, the artist Thomas de Keyser was paid 61 guilders by one of those depicted in the group portrait of the civil militia guild in 1632 (see p. 49). It is plausible that Tulp paid Rembrandt a similar sum.

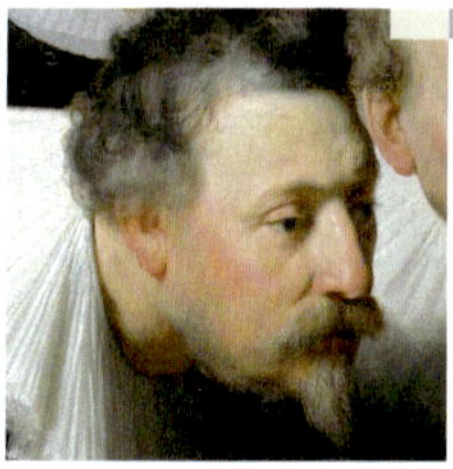

Jacob Janszn de Wit The surgeon who is leaning over the head of the corpse, staring attentively at the dissected arm, is Jacob Janszn de Wit (1582–1654). De Wit was born in Nyköping in Sweden and had come to Amsterdam at the age of fifteen. In 1611, when he was twenty-nine, he became a member of the Amsterdam Surgeons' Guild. His surgical practice, the *Vergulde Cruys* (Golden Cross), was located on the Nieuwendijk, where a sign-board bearing a golden cross hung from the façade of the house. For many years, Jacob de Wit served the Surgeons' Guild as both director and examiner. In that capacity he played a role in the guild's administration and he conducted the surgical examinations.

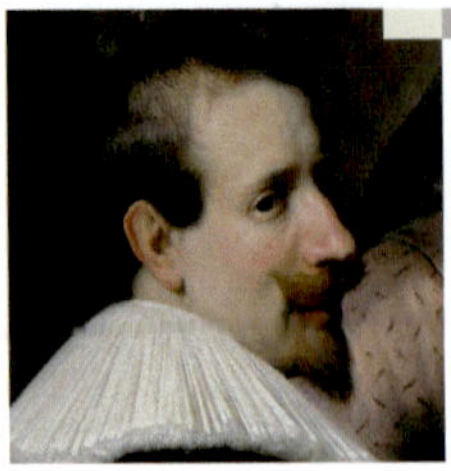

Adriaen Corneliszn Slabberaen Adriaen Corneliszn Slabberaen (1599–1661), the second on the left, was born and raised in Amsterdam. In 1614 he enrolled as an apprentice in the Surgeons' Guild. Eleven years later, he successfully submitted his masterpiece and subsequently became a guild member. He lived in the Sint Jorishof, a building on the Kalverstraat used as a house of residence for men of means who could buy a lifetime's lease and where they were provided with simple meals (*proveniershuis*). At the age of thirty-three, in 1632, his portrait was painted by Rembrandt on the occasion of his appointment as a member of the guild's board.

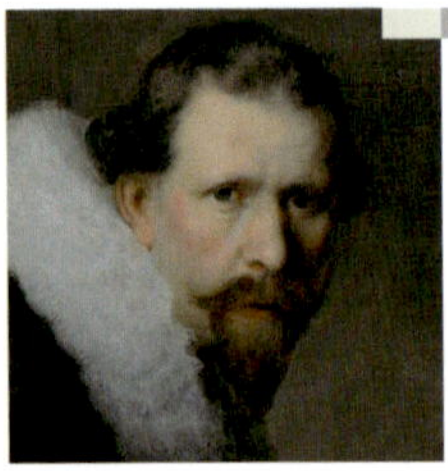

Hartman Hartmanszn The surgeon holding the piece of paper on which the names of the portrayed surgeons are listed and on which the anatomical illustration of the arm is reproduced, is Hartman Hartmanszn (1591–1659). Born in Leiden, he moved to Amsterdam at the age of seventeen. At that time, he was living in the Nes, one of the narrow streets between Dam Square and the Grimburgwal. Two years after Tulp's anatomy lesson was painted in 1632, he was appointed Head of the guild for the first time.

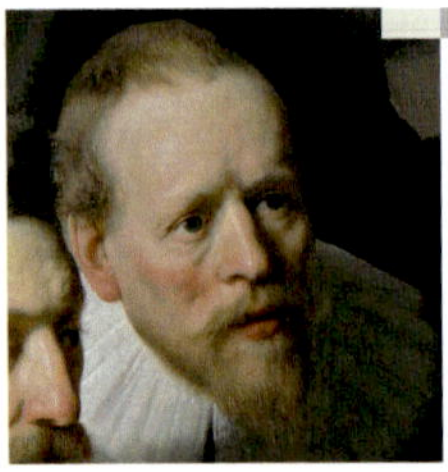

Matthijs Evertszn Calkoen The surgeon standing closest to the dissected arm is Matthijs Calkoen (1591–1653). Matthijs was born in Oldenmarkt in the province of Overijssel. He successfully passed his master's examination at the Amsterdam Surgeons' Guild at the age of twenty-four. In Amsterdam, he lived on the corner of the Haarlemmersluis and the Haarlemmerstraat. The signboard outside his house was emblazoned with a blue turkey (*kalkoen* in Dutch), a reference to his surname. The notes made by the master surgeon Job van Meekeren, who was a contemporary in the surgeons' guild, clearly indicate that Tulp collaborated with Matthijs Calkoen on the dissection of the forearm. Van Meekeren left an interesting description of the way in which Tulp and Calkoen dissected the superficial flexor muscles and tendons of the forearm:

> *The first flexor is the palmaris longus, which is woven together by a sinew-like membrane, and is so firmly attached to the skin that often, no matter how hard one rummages, it cannot be*

> *found (we let it be), let alone that it could be detached. However, we can truthfully say that Matthijs Calkoen, in life a Master Surgeon, did extract the muscle in question and peeled it back, albeit fairly roughly, from the skin and surrounding parts during a certain dissection conducted by Mr. Nicolaes Tulp, devoting himself diligently to the task for more than eight hours. The palmaris longus begins from the innermost protrusion of the arm and runs along the ulna, ending at the outermost joints of the four fingers.*

Van Meekeren reported that Calkoen and Tulp had spent hours in meticulously laying bare the flexors of the forearm. These are the same muscles shown in Rembrandt's painting. It is very likely that in this short passage from his *Heel- en geneeskonstige aenmerkingen* (Surgical and Medical Remarks) he refers to a section of Rembrandt's "Tulp's anatomy lesson of January 31st, 1632", in which it is also the subject. Calkoen was Head of the guild in 1639–1640, 1643–1645 and 1648–1649, and Chief Tutor in 1641 and 1650. His youngest son, Gijsbert, also became a surgeon and is depicted in Rembrandt's *Anatomy Lesson of Deijman* in 1656 (see p. 113).

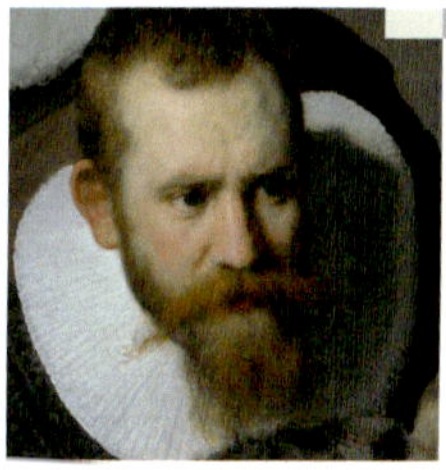

Jacob Dielofse Block Jacob Block (1600/01–1664/66) is the surgeon shown at the centre of the group, above Jacob de Wit. Jacob Block was born in Amsterdam. In 1638 he enrolled as an apprentice in the Surgeons' Guild and, five years later, he successfully submitted his masterpiece. In 1638, he was appointed Head of the guild for the first time, an office to which he was re-elected on a number of occasions. He lived on the Hartenstraat in Amsterdam. In 1649, Jacob Block was one of the two surgeons employed at the *Sint-Pietersgasthuis* (St Peter's Hospital, later the *Binnengasthuis*). A decade later, in 1659, he was summarily dismissed by the hospital's board of directors after a failed amputation of a leg. This decision was supported by his colleagues and the Amsterdam Surgeons' Guild's governors. However, Block was likely to have had good connections among Amsterdam's administrators, as they succeeded in having him re-instated at *Sint-Pietersgasthuis* in that same year. He continued to work there until his death in 1664/1666. He was buried in the Nieuwe Kerk (New Church).

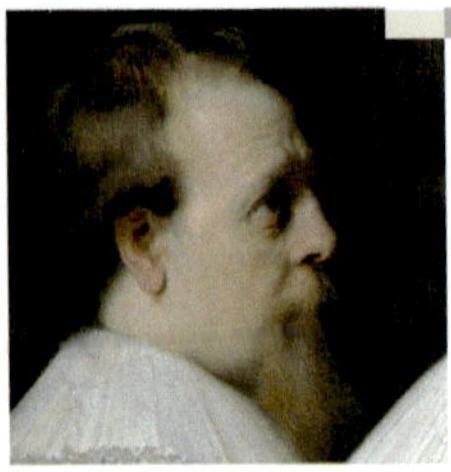

Jacob Janszn Colevelt The surgeon Jacob Colevelt (c. 1598–1649) is portrayed on the extreme left of Rembrandt's painting. At a young age, he went to work as an apprentice at the surgeon's shop of his uncle, Master Henrick Claeszn Colevelt. In 1620, he passed his masterpiece and became a member of the guild. Colevelt was elected Head of the guild in 1635, a position which, like that of chief examiner, he occupied several times after that. Besides his work as a surgeon, he had a keen interest in the theatrical arts. He wrote a number of plays, including tragedies: *Lusthofien ofte vermaeckelykheit der maechden* (1619) (Pleasure Gardens or the Amusement of Maidens), a *Droef-eyndend-spel, tusschen Graef Floris, en Gerrit van Velsen* (1628) (A Tragedy Count Floris [of Holland] and Gerrit van Velsen) and *Hartoginne van Savoyen: treur-blyd-endend-spel* (1634) (Duchess of Savoy: A Sad Story with a Happy Ending). Colevelt died in 1649 and was carried from his house in the Hoogstraat to his grave in the Nieuwe Kerk (New Church).

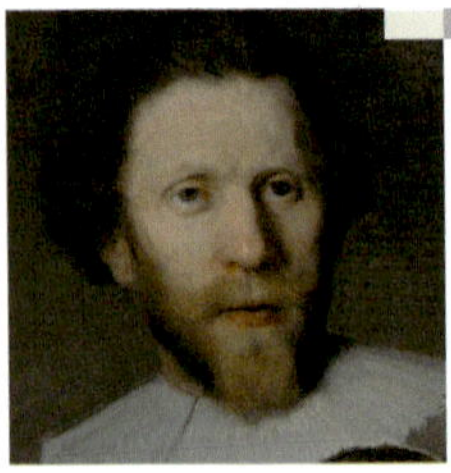

Frans Jacobszn van Loenen Frans van Loenen (1591–1662) is the surgeon seen towering above the rest of the group. He was born in Amsterdam and, in 1613, he passed the Surgeons' Guild's masterpiece, upon which he set up a practice on the Rokin. Shortly afterwards, he married Sara Jans, whose brother Anthony Jans headed the guild at the time. He married twice more after that. He is the only one in Rembrandt's portrait who never became Head of the guild.

While he painted the portrait, Rembrandt made a few alterations. When the painting was X-rayed, for instance, it was discovered

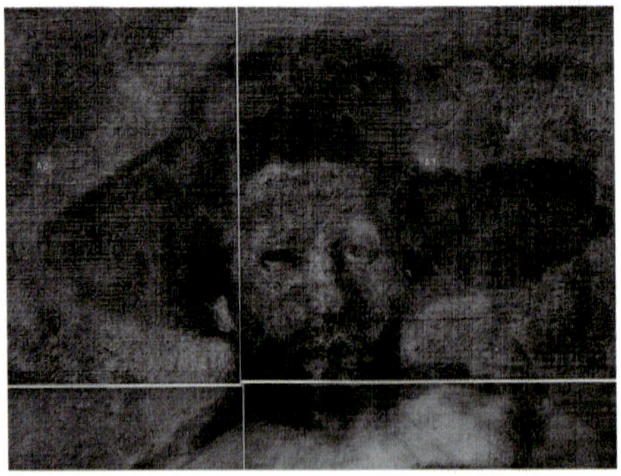

An X-ray photo of the painting shows that the surgeon Frans van Loenen was originally wearing a hat (detail of the X-ray photo on p. 103). At a later stage of the work, Rembrandt painted over the hat.

that Frans van Loenen originally wore a black hat. At a later stage, Rembrandt painted over the hat, removing it. One possible reason for this change could be that the *doctores medicinae* objected to a surgeon being depicted wearing a hat, as this was considered the exclusive privilege of physicians within the medical profession.

▸ **The Corpse** The record in the Anatomy Book of the Amsterdam Surgeons' Guild reveals that the corpse shown in Rembrandt's painting is that of the twenty-eight-year-old Adriaan Adriaenszn, also known as 'Aris 't Kint' (Aris the kid). A report of his conviction has been preserved among the deposition records at the Amsterdam judicial archives, making it possible to trace his criminal career.

Adriaan was born in Leiden and was a *kokermaker* (tube-maker) by profession. This meant that he made clay cylinders to protect earthenware from smoke and flames whilst it was fired in a kiln. In the winter of 1631, Adriaan happened to cross the Herensluis (one of the sluices on the Amsterdam canals) with two of his mates. Before long, they spotted a well-dressed gentleman wearing a cloak. They decided to rob him of this cloak, and stormed towards him, wrenching it from his shoulders. The man put up a fight, however, whereupon Adriaan began to assault the man. He would no doubt have beaten his victim to death if the night watchman had not intervened.

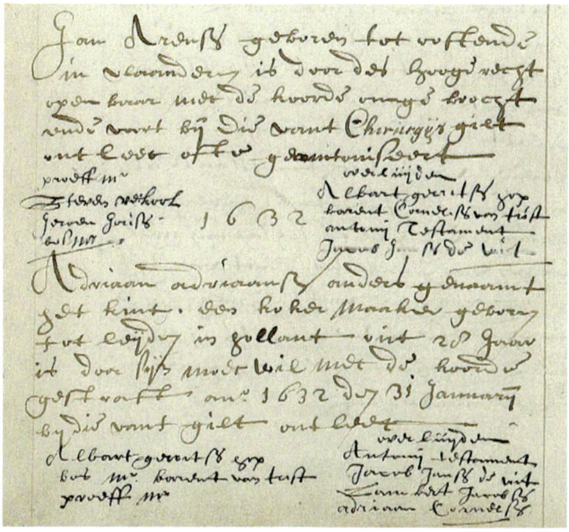

Handwritten note from the Anatomy Book of the Surgeons' Guild reporting on the anatomy lesson given by Nicolaes Tulp on 31 January, 1632. Municipal Archive Amsterdam.

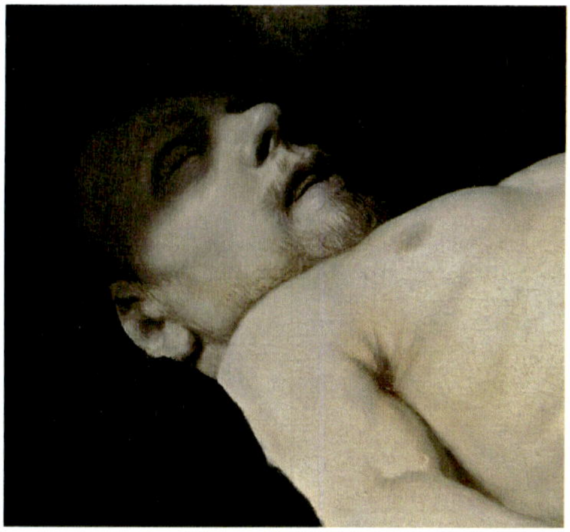

Adriaan Adriaenszn, alias Aris 't Kint (Aris the kid), the executed criminal whose body features in *The Anatomy Lesson of Nicolaes Tulp*.

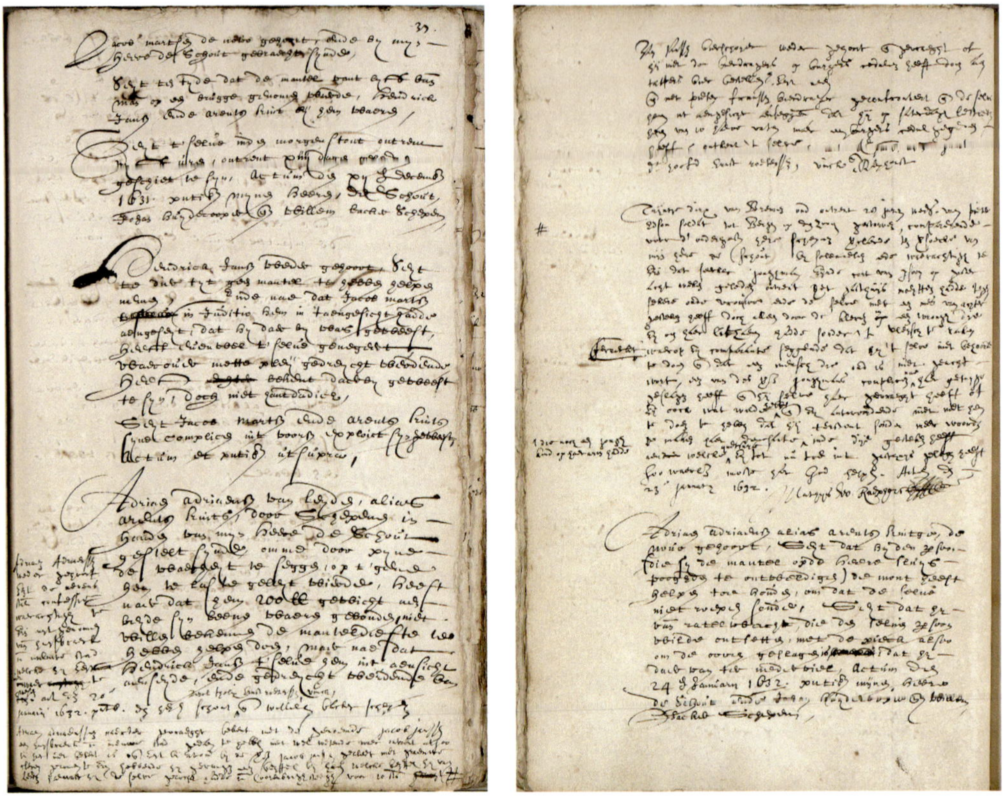

'The record of deposition from the Municipality of Amsterdam', dated 1631–1632, containing the interrogation report of Adriaan Adriaenszn. Municipal Archive Amsterdam.

The latter struck Adriaan on the head with a pike, a blow which felled him to the ground. Adriaan and his mates were arrested, thrown into prison and interrogated.

The two accomplices were sentenced to a public flogging and two years of penal servitude, either in the galleys or in a house of correction. However, Adriaan was another matter: he already had an extensive criminal record, and was therefore judged to be a habitual criminal. During a long series of interrogations and torture sessions, they managed to extract a number of confessions about his previous crimes. The first time he was arrested in 1623 for stealing a purse. For this, he was banned from Amsterdam. After this, he frequently came into contact with the officers of justice for theft and burglary. This resulted in a long list of convictions and punishments, ranging from public flogging, branding, confinement to a house of correction, to working in ships' galleys and banishment. On one occasion, Adriaan had attacked a warden in the house of correction in Utrecht with a saw, about which he made the following confession: he announced that, when committing this act, he had been 'absolutely determined to kill someone from the house of correction, even though this would entail the death penalty, and that he would far sooner die than remain confined to the house of correction any longer.' It seems that he already realized even then that he was to be condemned to death.

On January 27th, 1632, Adriaan was sentenced to death by hanging for his crimes. The death penalty was executed on January 31st and his body was put at the disposal of the Amsterdam Surgeons' Guild to be used as the *subjectum anatomicum* in the anatomy lesson of Dr Nicolaes Tulp. The reports in the deposition records reveal that during his interrogation, Adriaan had undergone considerable physical abuse. In order to elicit a speedy confession, every so often the criminal was lifted off the ground with 200 kg weights tied to his legs. He was also flogged and branded. Remarkably, the corpse in Rembrandt's painting shows no traces at all of the acts of cruelty Adriaan had to endure before he was executed. Likewise, there are no welts from the noose, and there is no sign of scars, brand-marks or welts and bruising on his legs. It is possible that Rembrandt refrained from showing a mutilated corpse in his painting for aesthetic reasons. However, it was important that the surgeons and the anatomical structures, formed the painting's focal point of attention, not the corpse of the executed criminal Adriaan Adriaenszn.

▸ **Anatomy** The question is: to what extent is the dissected forearm as painted by Rembrandt in his *The Anatomy Lesson of Nicolaes Tulp* true to life? For decades, this has been a hotly debated topic in professional literature for both medics and art historians. Until very recently, no consensus was reached and it was assumed that mistakes in the anatomy had found their way onto the painting. However, such assumptions were mostly based on comparisons with illustrations in anatomical atlases, and not on the actual anatomical dissection of a forearm.

Recently, the degree of accuracy has been tested by comparing the left forearm of the corpse in the painting with that of a deceased man. In Rembrandt's painting, the forearm is stretched out and turned outwards (supinated), with the wrist resting on the groin. The inner

The dissected forearm on Rembrandt's painting

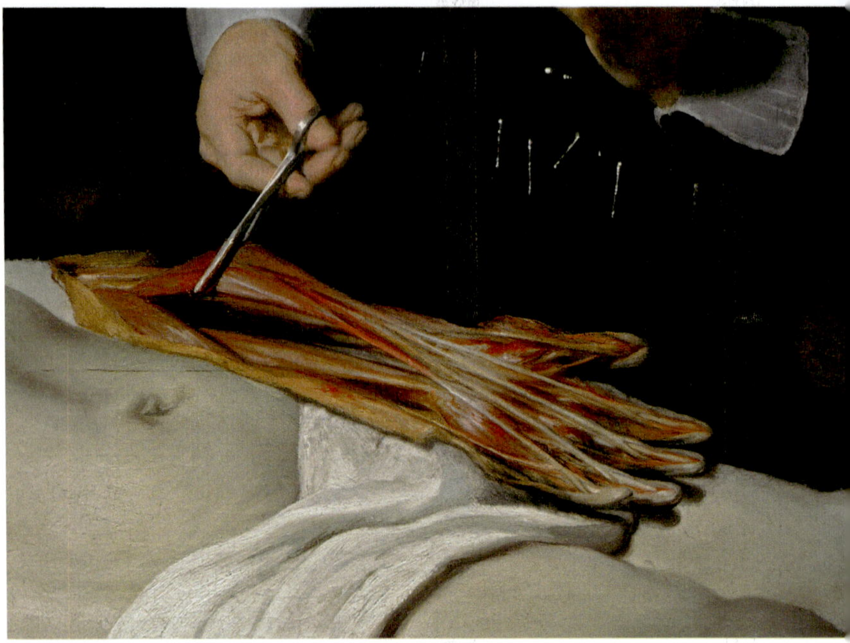

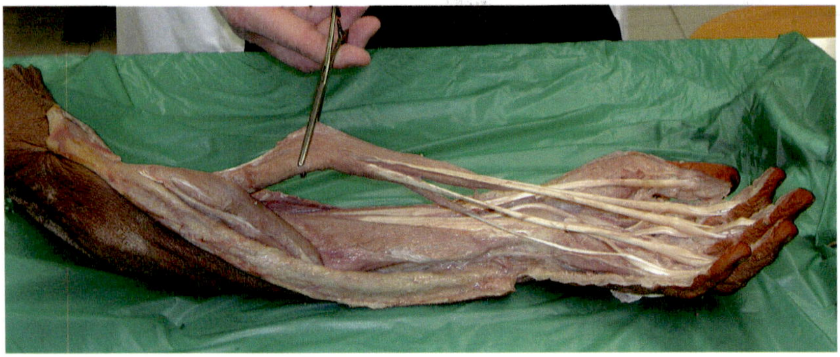

During an anatomical dissection of a left forearm, an attempt was made to imitate the anatomy of the dissected forearm as shown in Rembrandt's painting. In the first instance, the anatomical dissection revealed no oblique muscle on the inside of the forearm. The oblique muscle formed after several muscles of the forearm (*musculus flexor carpi radialis* and *palmaris longus*) had been detached and set aside. This allowed the superficial flexor muscle of the forearm (*musculus flexor digitorum superficialis*) to be lifted with the dissecting clamp. Compared to the real situation, the superficial flexor muscle in Tulp's clamp has a greater muscle volume and the muscles bellies have changed position. During the anatomical dissection, initially no white structure was observed on the side of the little finger of the hand. Therefore, one of the nerves of the forearm (*nervus ulnaris*) was moved in attempt to see if the white structure visible in the painting could be reproduced.

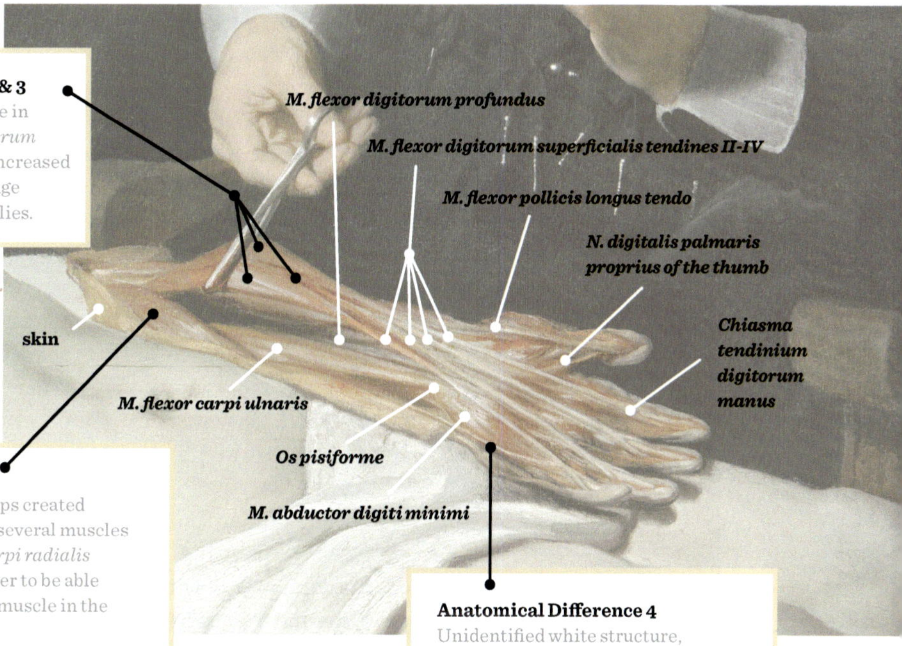

The dissected forearm on Rembrandt's painting with the identifications of the anatomical structures on which the differences established between the painting and the dissection of the forearm are indicated.

side of the elbow (*medial epicondyle*) of the humerus lies on the trunk. The outer side of the elbow (*lateral epicondyle*) is turned away from the body and hence not visible in the painting.

Tulp points to the flexor muscles of the forearm which extend from the inner side of the elbow (*medial epicondyle*). The tendons run in the direction of the hand, causing both the superficial and deep flexor tendons to cross each other at the fingers.

Comparison between the painting and an actual anatomical dissection of the forearm revealed several discrepancies. The oblique muscle shown on the inside of the forearm in the painting was not revealed in the present-day anatomical dissection. It is possible that, in order to be able to raise the superficial flexor muscles of the forearm, Tulp had detached these and laid them aside, leaving the oblique muscle on the inner-side of the forearm exposed in the painting. Tulp only lifts the superficial flexor of the forearm (*musculus flexor digitorum superficialis*), but on the painting, this muscle has greater volume than has been ascertained in the present-day dissection. On the painting,

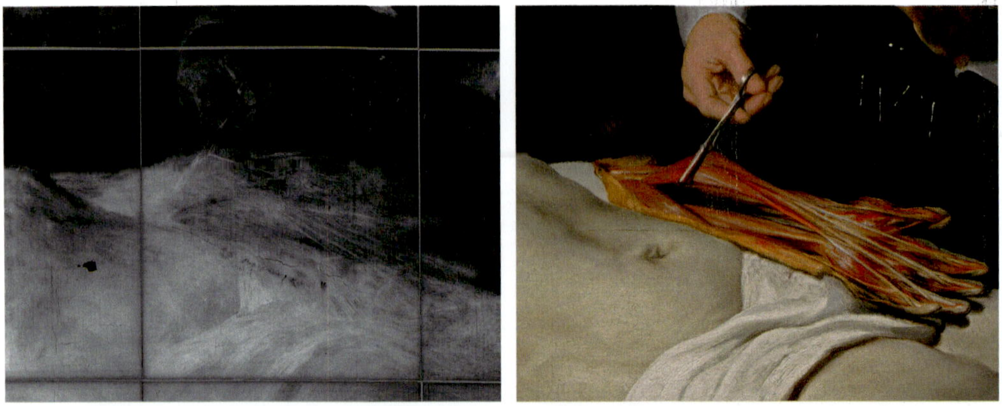

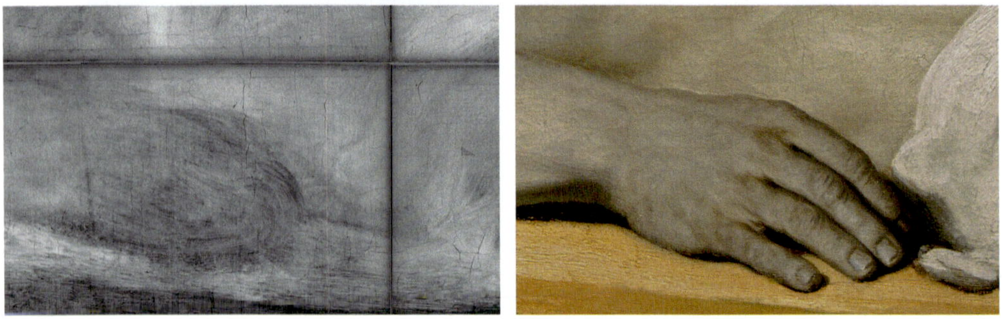

Upper
Rembrandt lowered the position of the dissected left forearm on the painting.

Lower
Detailed X-ray image of the right arm of the cadaver which Rembrandt had initially painted as an amputated stump. At a later stage of the work, he carefully reworked the stump into a meticulously painted hand.

it is the forearm that is being dissected while the rest of the corpse is still intact. This deviation from the normal procedure supports the idea that Rembrandt's painting is not a true representation of what actually took place during Tulp's anatomy lesson, but that it has a more symbolic meaning instead.

It is assumed that when Tulp chose to be portrayed with a dissected forearm, he was inspired by Andreas Vesalius (Van Wesel) (1514–1564). This famous anatomist, who was born in Brussels, had himself portrayed conducting a comparable anatomical dissection: the demonstration of the flexor muscles of the forearm in his famous anatomy textbook, *De Humani Corporis Fabrica Libra Septum* (On the Fabric of the Human Body in Seven Volumes), first published in 1543. In the sixteenth century, Vesalius revolutionised the study of human anatomy by investigating anatomical structures on the basis of his own empirical observations, thereby abandoning the traditional

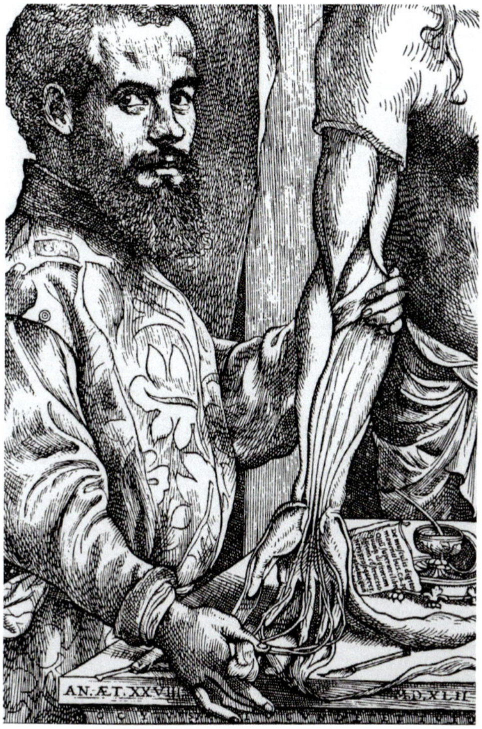

Portrait of the anatomist Andreas Vesalius who is demonstrating the flexor muscles of the lower arm in an illustration from his famous work *De Humani Corporis Fabrica Libri Septem* (1555) (On the Fabric of the Human Body Book Seven).

Greek and Roman writings of Hippocrates (470 – 400 BC) and Galen (AD 130–200). Instead of relying on ancient texts, Vesalius emphasized the importance of personal observation during anatomy lessons in which a human body was used. He considered the hand to be the physical counterpart of the psyche, and the doctor's most important instrument, the *primarium medicinae instrumentum*. He saw it as a tool which enabled the use of other tools.

Through Pieter Pauw, Tulp's own teacher in Leiden who had once been a student of Vesalius, Tulp had become quite knowledgeable on the physician-anatomist's theories. While writing on the subject, he says: 'Anatomy is the eye of medicine and unveils the truth'. The dissection of the forearm in Rembrandt's painting immortalized Tulp as the new Vesalius of his time — a 'Vesalius redivivus' — and ushered in a new era in both practical and functional anatomy.

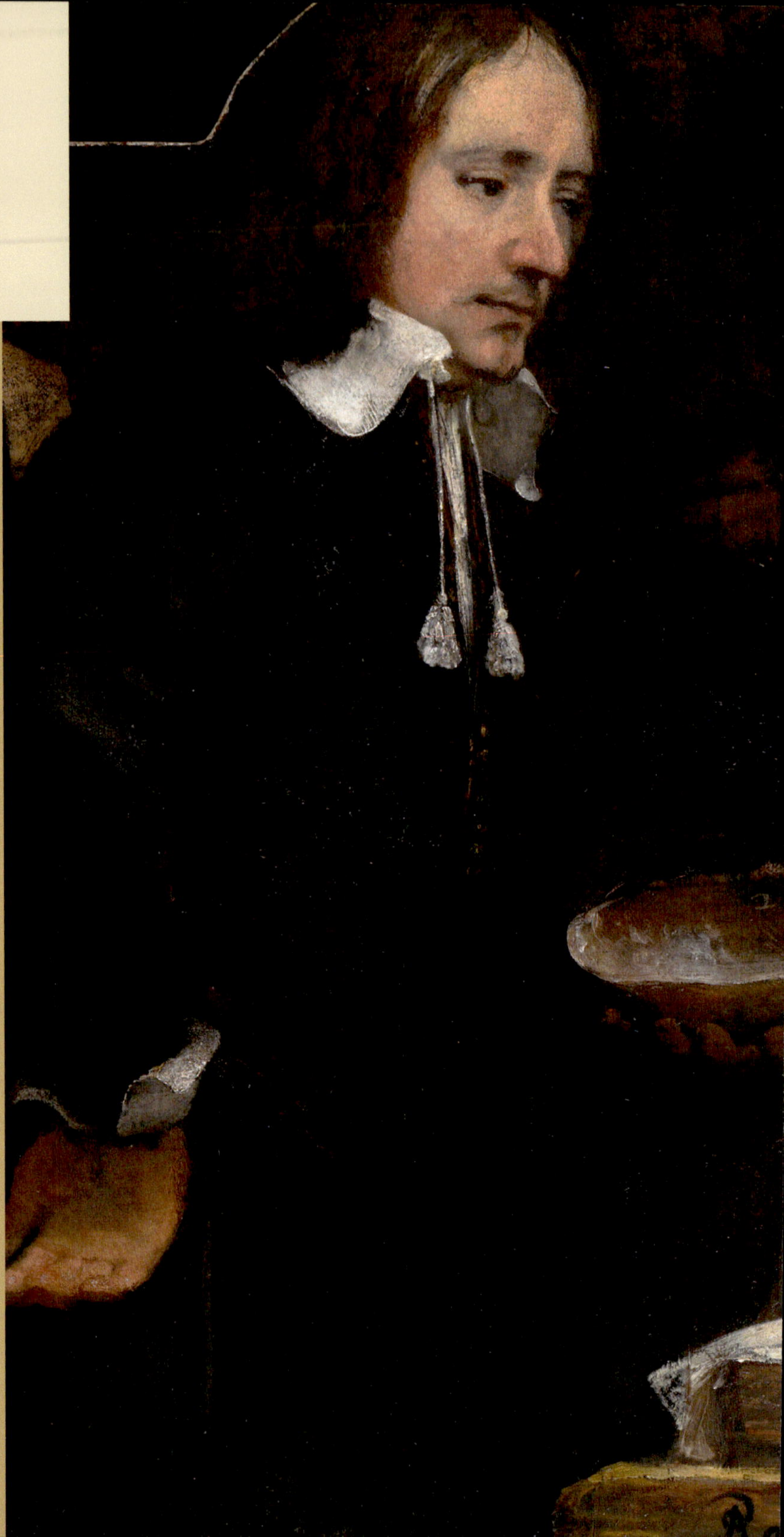

Rembrandt, *The Anatomy Lesson of Jan Deijman*, 1656. Collection Amsterdam Museum.

5

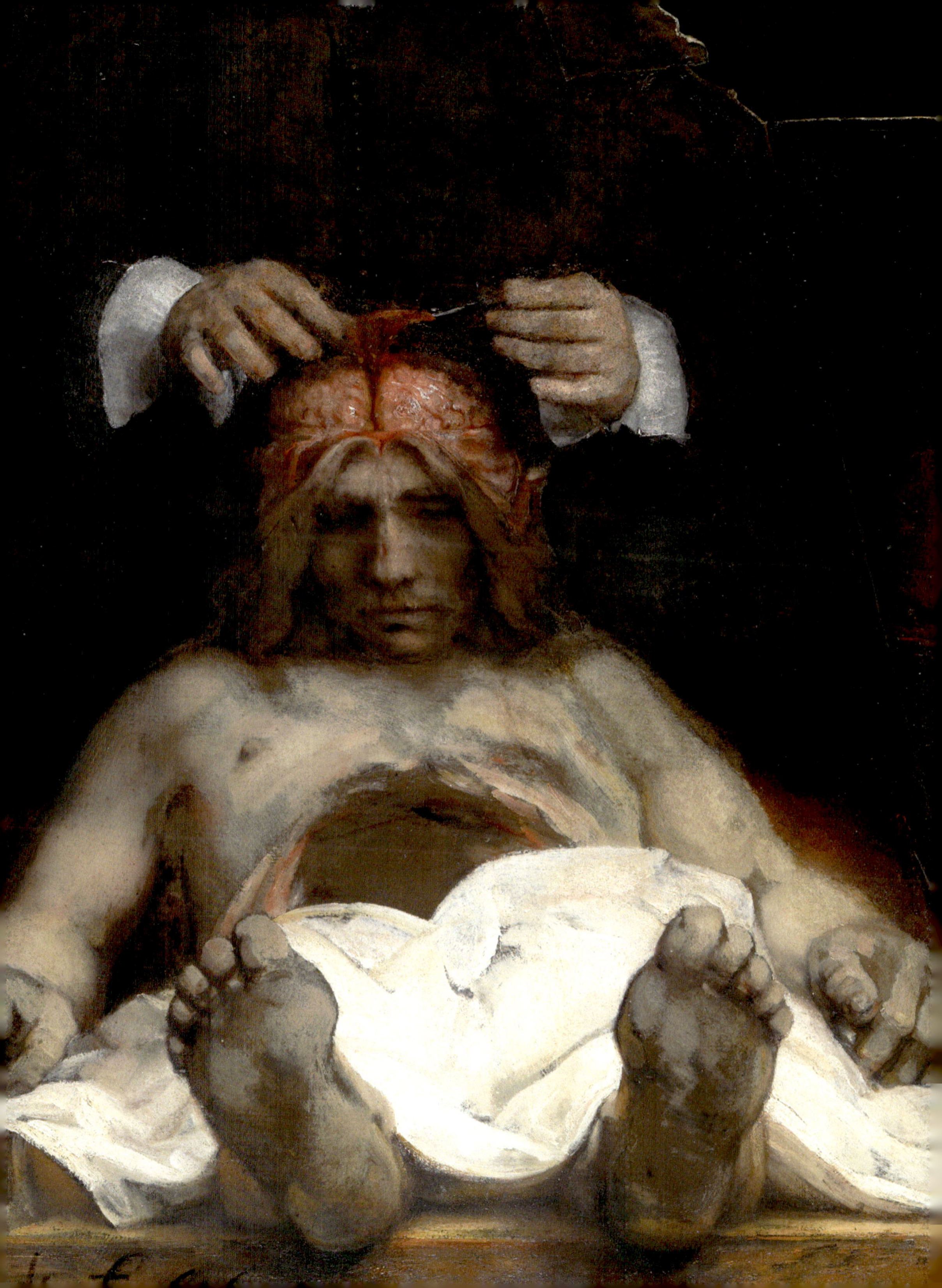

Jan Deijman

The Anatomy Lesson of Jan Deijman,
painted by Rembrandt in 1656

▸ **The Painting** Twenty-four years after he had painted *The Anatomy Lesson of Nicolaes Tulp* in 1632, Rembrandt completed his second group portrait for the Amsterdam Surgeons' Guild, *The Anatomy Lesson of Jan Deijman,* in 1656. This painting has always been overshadowed by its predecessor. This can be explained by the fact that the work was badly damaged in a fire at the Guildhall in 1732: only a small section survived. When the heavily damaged canvas was restored only the central part could be salvaged.

In 1653, Jan Deijman became *praelector anatomiae* of the Amsterdam Surgeons' Guild as successor to Nicolaes Tulp. The painting shows how, taking up his position behind the corpse of an executed criminal, he carried out an anatomical dissection of the brain and meninges of the dead man. The person standing on his right, left on the canvas, is his assistant Gijsbert Calkoen. A preliminary sketch — also by Rembrandt — gives us an idea of what the original picture must have looked like. Besides Deijman and his assistant, the drawing depicts seven other surgeons. A digital reconstruction has been made using Rembrandt's sketch, giving us an impression of what the painting must have looked like before most of it was damaged in the fire. The original painting must have measured 245 × 300 cm, of which only 113 × 135cm survived. *The Anatomy Lesson of Jan Deijman* is unquestionably one of the best-known historical representations of an anatomical dissection of the brain and meninges. The painting is now on exhibition at the Amsterdam Museum.

▸ **The Artist** At the time he painted Deijman's anatomical lesson, Rembrandt, by then fifty, was an established and experienced portrait painter. The artist included a number of interesting elements in his depiction of the anatomy lesson.

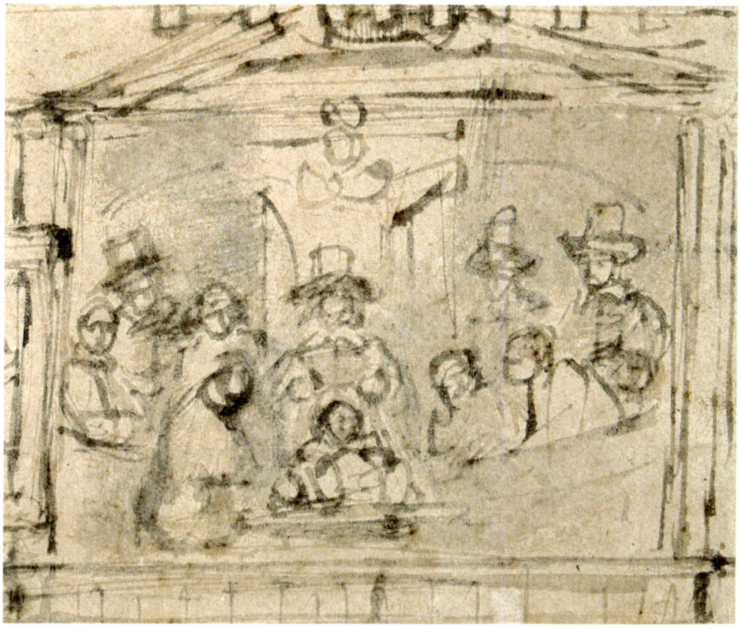

Rembrandt's preparatory sketch for *The Anatomy Lesson of Jan Deijman*, 1656. Collection Amsterdam Museum.

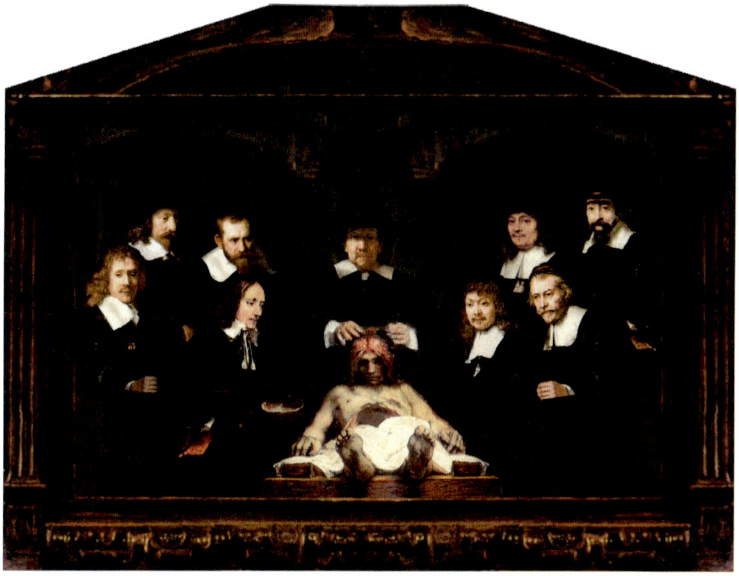

Thijs Wolzak and Norbert Middelkoop attempted to create a digital reconstruction of *The Anatomy Lesson of Jan Deijman*. A large section of the painting was destroyed during a fire at the Guildhall. Only the central section of the composition survived. Collection Amsterdam Museum.

Most seventeenth-century anatomy lessons began with the dissection of the organs of the abdominal and thoracic cavities, which were subject to rapid decomposition. The open belly is an indication that Deijman had already dissected the abdominal organs at the beginning of his anatomy lesson. In the first instance, it seems that he followed the order of stages correctly. Nevertheless, on closer inspection it appears as if Deijman did deviate from the usual sequence, because the thoracic cavity is still intact, even though he has already begun with the dissection of the brain. Of course, it is possible that Deijman had already dissected the organs of the thoracic cavity but, prompted by artistic motives, Rembrandt chose to reproduce the body with its rib-cage intact.

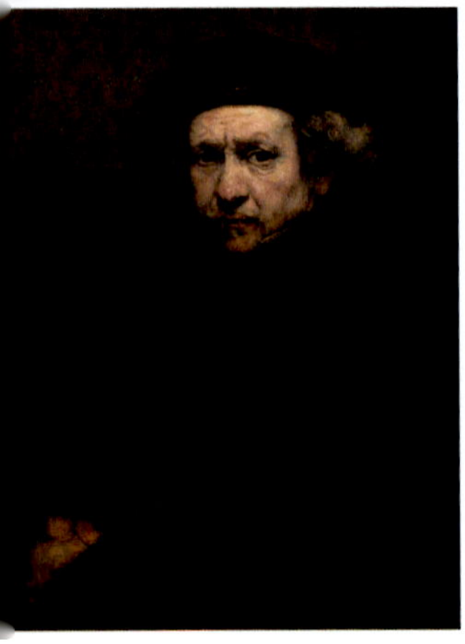

Rembrandt van Rijn, *Self Portrait*, 1659. National Gallery of Art, Andrew W. Mellon Collection, Washington.

Rembrandt's sketch and the reconstruction that is based on it, reveal that the anatomy lesson was held in an anatomy theatre. The way Rembrandt has arranged the tiers of seats around the dissection table truly involves the onlookers in the lesson. Moreover, he shows the body from the foot-end's perspective, and has placed the edge of the dissection table parallel to the lower edge of the canvas, giving the illusion that it is protruding from the painting. Under normal circumstances, the brain would have been barely visible from this angle. By portraying the body in this compact way, he has managed to combine visual depth with close-ups. The neck of the corpse has been tilted forward to an extreme degree. In reality, such a bent position for a corpse would be impossible, unless the neck had been broken after being hanged. The brain is fairly voluminous and is prominently displayed. Rembrandt obviously did his utmost to draw the spectators' attention to the *praelector's* actions.

▸ **The Dissector** Jan Deijman (1619–1666) was born the son of a sea captain. He studied medicine at the University of Leiden and obtained his doctorate in medicine at the University of Angers in France. After completing his studies, he set himself up as a physician in Amsterdam. He married Maria Bas, with whom he had four children. Deijman was appointed inspector of the Medical Supervisory Board (*Collegium Medicum*), the body responsible for supervising the quality of health care in Amsterdam. He worked as a physician in the former city hospital, Sint-Pietersgasthuis (St Peter's Hospital) in the centre of Amsterdam. When first employed there, his job was to be assistant to the well-known doctor Samuel Coster (1579–1665).

A few years later, he succeeded Coster and became physician in charge of the hospital.

Sint-Pietersgasthuis was situated between the Oudezijdse Achterburgwal and the New Doelenstraat in the center of Amsterdam. Its function was not limited to caring for the sick, it also offered a shelter for the poor and the homeless. People died there on a regular basis and if no-one came forward to claim the body or cover the cost of a funeral, the body was placed at the disposal of the infirmary's physician. A small dissection room in which postmortems could be performed on patients who had died there was set up within the infirmary itself. These 'medical' postmortems were solely accessible to the hospital's doctors, and were not open to the public. A report of one of these postmortems carried out in Deijman's presence was written by the surgeon Job van Meekeren:

> *In the year 1655,* [...] *in the Infirmary in this city,* [...] *in the presence of the Physicians Samuël Koster and Johan Deiman* [Jan Deijman], *and of that of the Infirmary Surgeon, Daniël Florianus, taking into account certain wounds, the mortal remains of Jan Roelofszoon were opened, in whose left thoracic cavity we observed a mixture of thin and pungent water; in many places this had scorched the pericardium and the endocardium, so that it resembled a roasted pear.*

As a result of this postmortem, Deijman and his colleagues established that the patient had died as a consequence of a wound to his thoracic cavity. They observed that the heart and the pericardium had been so badly damaged by the injury that this must have been the cause of death.

Alongside his work at the infirmary, Deijman was responsible for the education of surgeons in Amsterdam. In 1653 he succeeded Nicolaes Tulp as *praelector anatomiae* of the Amsterdam Surgeons' Guild. He was to occupy this position for a total of thirteen years, until his death in 1666. According to the Anatomy Book of the Surgeons' Guild, Deijman gave a public anatomy lesson in the dissection room on the upper floor of the St.-Margaret's Convent on the Nes on two occasions. (see p. 14) He gave his first lesson on January 26th 1656, and the second one three years later. The report of Deijman's first lesson in 1656 in the Anatomy Book reads as follows:

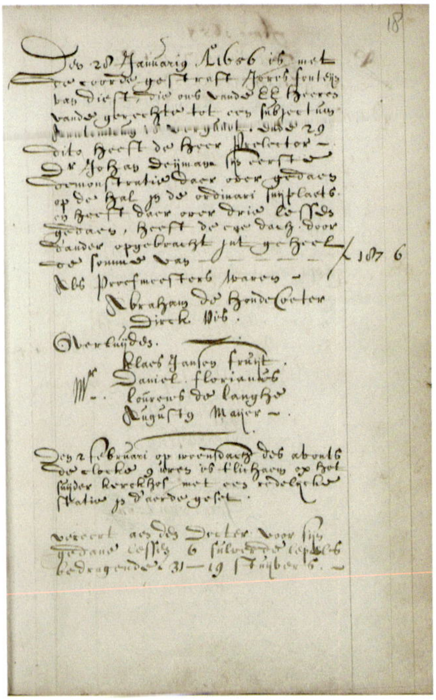

January 28th in the year 1656, Joris Fonteijn van Diest, who had been hanged, was handed over to us by Their Excellencies at the law court to serve as a subjectum anatomicum. *And on the 29th of the same month and year, the* Praelector *Dr Johan Deijman gave his first demonstration using the body in the hall of the usual dissecting place and, in all, he dedicated three lessons to it, the one and the others raising in total the sum of f 187/6.-*

[Present] as Chief Tutors were Abraham de Hondecoeter / Dirck Vis

Members of the Board of Governors — Klaes Jansen Fruijt, Daniel Florianus, Lourens de Langhe, Augustus Maijer.

On February 2nd at nine o'clock on a Wednesday evening, the body was laid to rest with all due respect in the southern churchyard.

The remuneration to the Doctor for the lessons he gave was six silver spoons valued at f 31 — 19 stuivers.

Notes in the Anatomy Book of the Surgeons' Guild pertaining to the anatomical lesson given by Deijman in 1656. Municipal Archive Amsterdam.

The lesson lasted three days in total, and according to the record, raised about 177 guilders. At the average price of 5 *stuivers* per entry ticket, the three-day spectacle must have attracted hundreds of visitors. At the end of the lesson, as a token of appreciation, Deijman was presented with six silver spoons. Deijman's first anatomy lesson was given on January 28th, 1656, coinciding with his appointment as *praelector* of the Surgeons' Guild. This provided a good opportunity to have his likeness painted by Rembrandt, following the tradition of his predecessors Egbertszn, Fonteijn and Tulp. Rembrandt's masterpiece, *The Anatomy Lesson of Jan Deijman* is the tangible reminder of this. Unfortunately, the image of Deijman's face was lost when the canvas was damaged in a fire: only his torso and his hands are still visible on what was left of the painting. And thus, we can only speculate what his facial expression might have been during this anatomical lesson.

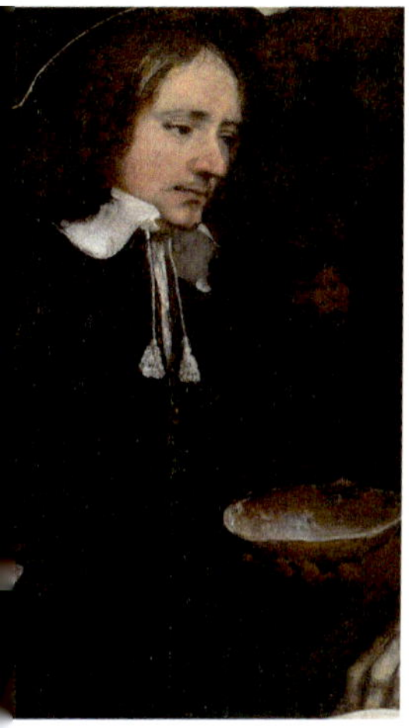
Gijsbert Calkoen, Jan Deijman's assistant.

▸ **The Surgeons** The man who is standing to the left of the dissection table is the thirty-four year old Gijsbert Calkoen (1621–1664). Gijsbert was the youngest son of Matthijs Calkoen, who is depicted in the earlier *Anatomy Lesson of Nicolaes Tulp*. He was, as the saying goes, following in his father's footsteps. In 1645 Gijsbert successfully passed his qualifying examination which allowed him to become a member of the Amsterdam Surgeons' Guild. At the time of Deijman's anatomical lesson in January 1656, he was Assistant Tutor. One of his duties in this capacity was to assist the *praelector* during anatomy lessons. He carried out his duties seriously: in the painting he is shown holding the cranial vault in his hand. A black shroud which he could drape over the corpse at the end of the lesson is seen folded on his left arm. A few months after the anatomy lesson, Gijsbert Calkoen was elected chairman of the Board of Governors.

Only one anecdote is known about Calkoen's surgical activities. From the notes made by Job van Meekeren, who was also a practising surgeon and member of the guild, it is clear that the former was involved in the treatment of the housewife Diever Jans. She suffered from goitre, an enlarged thyroid which is visible as a swelling in the throat on the level of the larynx. Before Calkoen could do anything to help her, she died while eating a chestnut which had become stuck, caught on the obstruction caused by the swelling. After her death, Calkoen and his colleagues performed an autopsy on her body, and they reported the following findings:

> [...] *having peeled back the skin of the throat, the swelling was revealed, which one* [...] *found on the windpipe,* [*and*] *which was impossible to move either backwards or forwards, in order to give her room to breathe, and for food to pass beyond the swelling* [...], *it would have been impossible to have relieved* [*the situation*] *and to have kept the patient alive by either medical or surgical procedures.*

In 1658 Gijsbert Calkoen was appointed Chief Tutor for the period of one year. His chief responsibility was the setting and supervision of the exams for trainee surgeons. He died in 1664 and was buried in the Westerkerk (Western Church) on October 23rd of the same year.

On Calkoen's right and left, the hands of the other surgeons present are partly visible, the rest was lost in the fire. Their names can be traced from the list of names which has been preserved: Dirck Vis, Klaes Fruijt, Daniel Florianus, Lourens de Langhe, Augustus Maijer, Jacob Hernij and Barend Heems.

▸ **The Corpse** On the dissection table lies the lifeless body of the twenty-two-year-old Joris Fonteijn (1633/34–1656). Joris had originally been a tailor. Besides pursuing this trade, he had also spent three-and-a-half years in the service of the West India Company (*West-Indische Compagnie*). In 1653 he came home from the coastal regions of North Africa. Upon his return, he inherited the sum of 150 guilders and, with that sum of money in his hand, he ended up in Dordrecht. After he had splurged his money, he got on the wrong path. At first, Joris tried to scrape some money together by begging. However, he had progressed to theft and burglary in no time, with a preference for stealing clothes and silverware. In Dordrecht he kept the company of a certain Elsje Otte, also known as the 'thunder whore'. Her nickname suggests that she was perhaps not the best possible company for Joris.

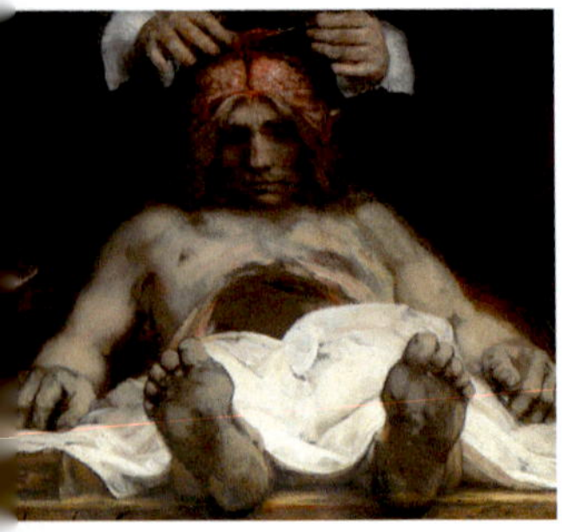

Joris Fonteijn, alias 'Black John', the executed criminal in *The Anatomy Lesson of Jan Deijman*.

Joris then continued to pursue his criminal career in Amsterdam. In broad daylight, he burgled the house of a cloth merchant on the Nieuwendijk unseen, fully intent on helping himself to a piece of broadcloth. He was caught red-handed whereupon he quickly took to his heels. However, a group of boys who had seen the incident took chase and tried to overpower him. When he reached the Oude Brug, Joris pulled a knife and wounded one of his pursuers when the latter tried to grab hold of him. His struggle was in vain, for he was soon overpowered and arrested.

In the previous year-and-a-half, Joris had been imprisoned no fewer than five times for theft. So far, he had been released after being subjected to physical punishment in the form of a flogging or a caning, before being banished from the town in which he had committed the crime and thereby losing his citizen's rights. Taking all his other offences into account, he was sentenced 'to be hung by the neck until he was dead on the scaffold on January 27th, 1656, a pistol suspended above his head as a warning and example to others'. After his death by hanging, his body was placed at the disposal of the Amsterdam Surgeon's Guild, where it was dissected during Deijman's lesson.

▸ **Anatomy** This painting shows the point at which, after having peeled off the scalp, Deijman removed the cranial vault and part of the meninges, providing us with a glimpse of the brain of the executed criminal Joris Fonteijn. Using his hand and a pair of tweezers he lifts part of the meninges. Recently, we researched these anatomical structures by comparing them to an actual anatomical dissection of the brain. This was a routine anatomical dissection during which the brain of a deceased person was removed and preserved for scientific purposes. During the dissection, the scalp was cut into and removed from the cranial vault. The cranial vault was sawn through and, once it had been taken away, the *dura mater* became visible.

Anatomical dissection of the brain and meninges of the body of Joris Fonteijn.

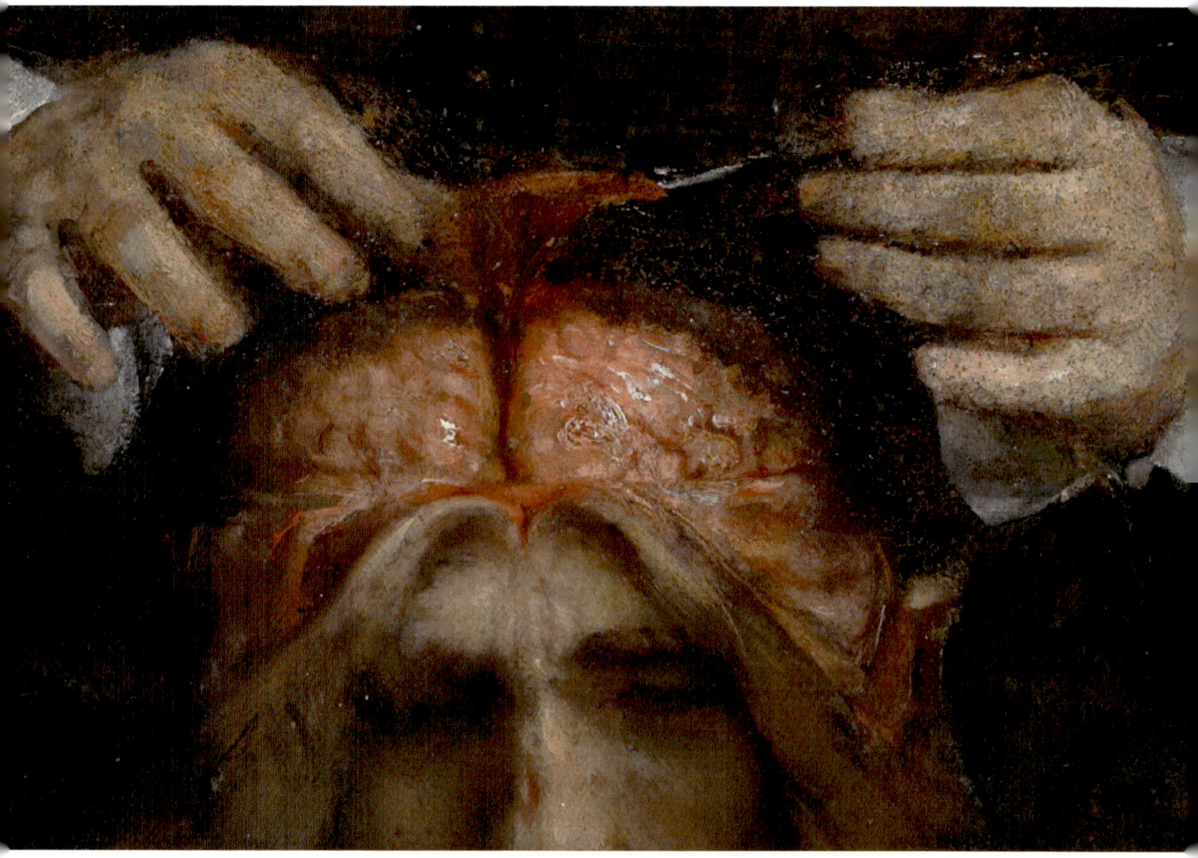

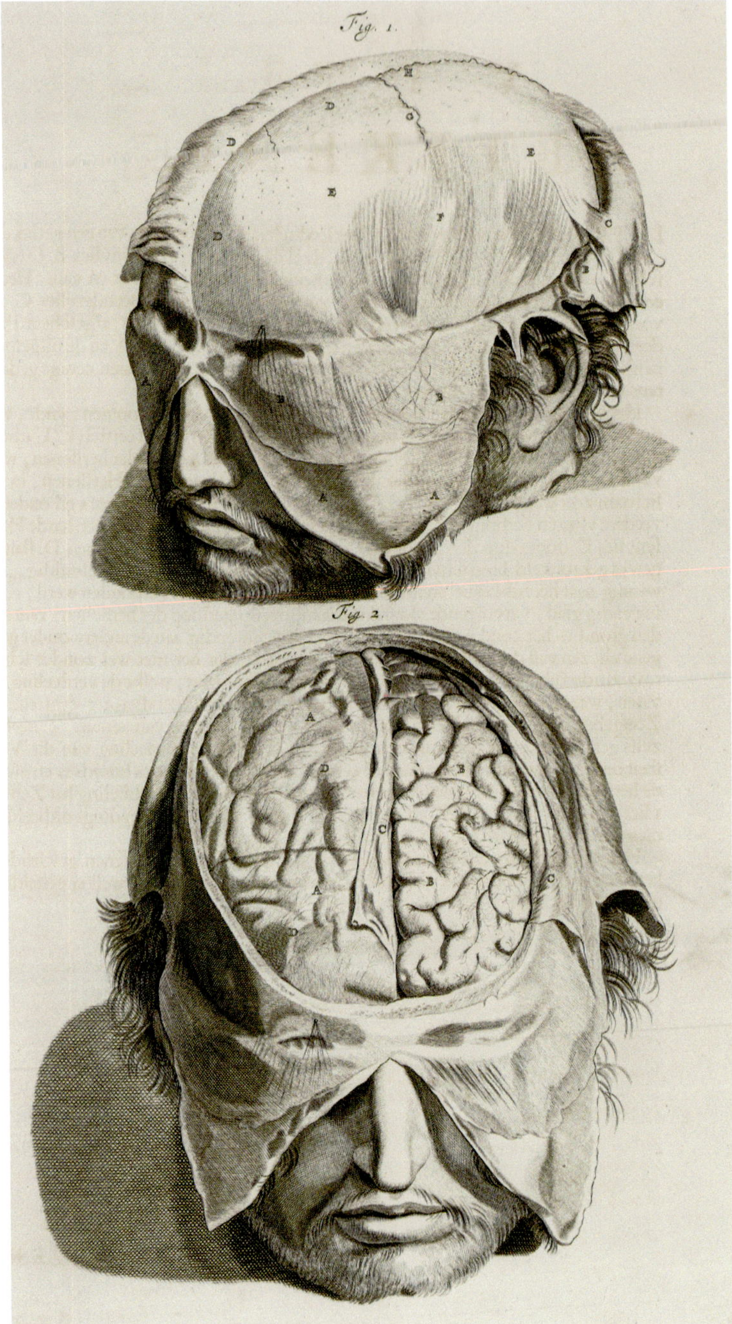

5

Jan Deijman 1656

An illustration from the anatomical atlas *Ontleding des Menschelijken Lichaams* (1690) by Govard Bidloo (1649–1713) gives an impression of the appearance of the *dura mater*, just as we also observed it during the recent dissection. In 1670, Bidloo qualified as a surgeon with the Amsterdam Surgeon's Guild. Although he would not have been present at Deijman's lesson in 1656, he did attend the lessons given by the latter's successor, Frederik Ruysch. Later in his career, Bidloo was appointed chair of anatomy in Leiden (1694), where he personally involved himself in anatomical dissections. The illustrations in his anatomical atlas are based on his observations from this period.

During our present-day dissection, it was possible to observe the way in which the *dura mater* deflects inside the groove between the left and right sides of the brain where it forms the *falx cerebri*. This is the Latin name for 'the crescent or scythe of the brain'. As the name suggests, this part of the *dura mater,* situated between the two halves of the brain, resembles the shape of a sickle or scythe. Bidloo's anatomical atlas contains a very fine illustration of the *falx cerebri*. In the accompanying caption, Bidloo calls this structure the sickle membrane (*zeissenvlies*).

In the painting, Rembrandt shows Deijman lifting up the *falx* with his hand and a pair of tweezers. In order to lift it, he had to cut away the *dura mater* along the edge of the *falx*. He would have then cut the *dura mater* into quadrants and laid these aside so as to expose the brain. The impressive reproduction of the colour of the brain in Rembrandt's painting corresponds closely to the actual appearance of the brain. This is irrefutable proof that, before he began painting, Rembrandt had seen the brain with his own eyes. In the painting Deijman not only raises the *falx*, he also turns it 90 degrees on its axis, giving a better view of the *falx*. In reality, it is impossible to lift the *falx* so far above the brain and then rotate it in the way Deijman did. During our anatomical dissection, in order to reveal the shape of the *falx*, we had to free it from the base of the skull. The front of the *falx* is firmly attached to the skull, the rear section merges into that part of the *dura mater* which separates the brains from the cerebellum (*tentorium cerebelli*). Only after both structures had been cut through and the brain removed from the skull, the sickle- or scythe-shape of the *falx* became properly visible.

←
Illustration of an anatomical dissection of the scalp, skull, meninges and the brain.

Figure 1
The scalp [A]; bone membrane (*periosteum*) [B&C]; skull [D&E]; the temporal muscle (*musculus temporalis*) [F]; coronal and sagittal sutures [F&G].

Figure 2
In the next stage of the dissection, the vault of the skull has been removed. The *dura mater* on the right side of the brain is still intact but it has been removed from the left side. The central part where the two thick membranes meet forms the cerebral falx (*falx cerebri*).

From: Govard Bidloo *Ontleding des Menschelijken Lichaams* (Dissection of the Human Body), 1690. Library University of Groningen.

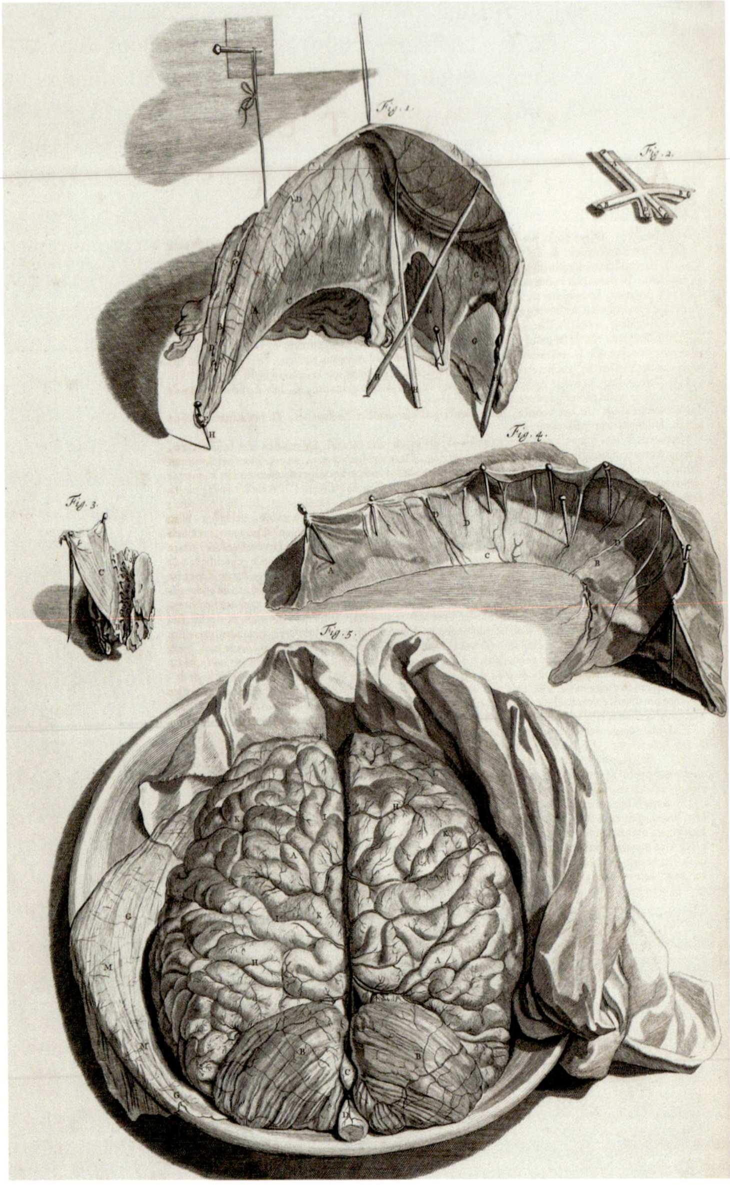

Illustration of the anatomical dissection of the brain and meninges. Above centre and to the right in the centre of the page, the *falx cerebri* is shown resembling the shape of a sickle or scythe (Figs 1 and 4). Under it in the skull are the brain and cerebellum with the meninges draped around them. From: Govard Bidloo *Ontleding des Menschelijken Lichaams* (Dissection of the Human Body), 1690. Library University of Groningen.

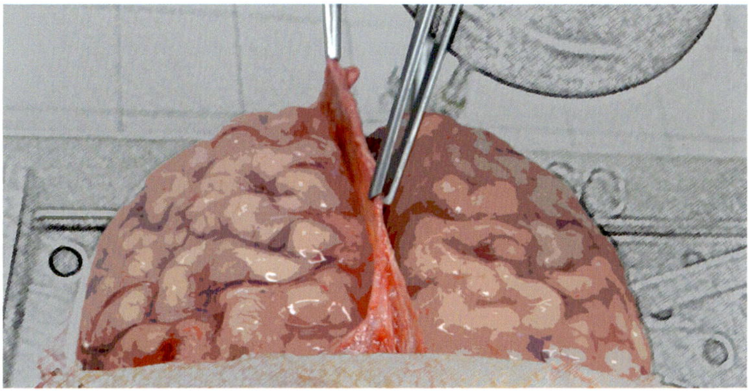

Front view of an anatomical dissection of the brain and meninges (digitally adjusted view in which the actual size of the *falx cerebri* is reproduced). The cranial vault has been removed and the *dura mater* partly removed. The *falx cerebri*, located between the two halves of the brain, has been raised with a pair of tweezers. In reality it would be impossible to lift the *falx* so far and turn it the way Deijman is shown doing in the painting. The shape of the *falx* is not easy to distinguish because it lies concealed between the two halves of the brain.

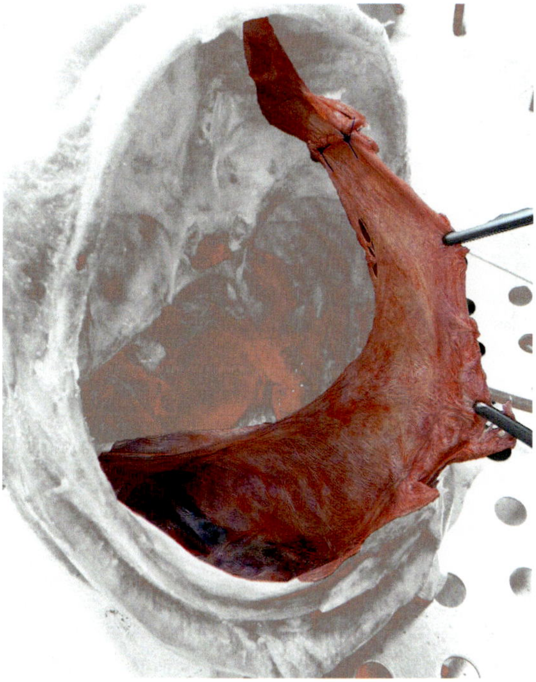

Overhead view of an anatomical dissection. The cranial vault has been removed allowing a view of the base of the skull. The crescent or scythe-shaped *falx cerebri* is indicated by two pairs of tweezers (digitally adjusted view which permits the *falx cerebri* to be reproduced in its actual size). In order to see the shape of the *falx*, it was necessary to remove the brain from the cranium. The front of the *falx* and the *dura mater*, which separate the brain from the cerebellum (*tentorium cerebelli*), had to be cut through to remove the brain. Thereafter the *falx* was repaired with two stitches making its crescent shape clearly visible.

▸ **The Anatomical Perspective** In Rembrandt's painting, Deijman is shown trying to demonstrate the 'shape' of the *falx cerebri* to his audience. In order to do this, he has raised the *falx* and tried to turn it. As said above, during the recent anatomical dissection it proved impossible to lift the *falx* up and turn it as Deijman is doing in the portrait. Therefore, *The Anatomical Lesson of Jan Deijman* is not a precise depiction of an anatomical dissection of the *falx cerebri*. This is to be expected, because the principal purpose of the painting was not to be an actual representation of an anatomical dissection, but to be a group portrait of the *praelector* and the surgeons.

An anatomical illustration of the brain from the book of the famous anatomist Andreas Vesalius (1515–1564) is generally accepted to have been Deijman's source of inspiration for his anatomy lesson. However, there is one remarkable difference: Vesalius had detached the head from the torso before he began his anatomical dissection of the brain. However, during Deijman's lesson, the head is still firmly attached to the body. Nevertheless, in seventeenth-century anatomical lessons it was regular practice to separate the head from the torso before beginning on the dissection of the brain.

Vesalius considered the brain to be the most important part of the body. In the light of this belief, the dissection of the brain will have been a suitable highlight for Deijman's anatomical lesson. However, we cannot ignore the fact that Deijman is drawing attention to the shape of the *falx cerebri*. If he had wished to stress the brain itself, it would have been more logical for him to have demonstrated a dissection of the ventricles (sinuses in the brain which contain the cerebrospinal fluid). Why was Deijman so determined to show the falx?

The sickle or scythe could symbolize death. Therefore, given its shape, the falx was principally shown as the instrument of death. Death was usually portrayed as a skeleton holding a scythe with which he could cut short the life of mortals. From this point of view, the scythe symbolized human mortality. A skeleton, whether or not holding a scythe, also features on the coat-of-arms of the Surgeons' Guild. By placing the emphasis on the 'human scythe' in the form of the *falx cerebri*, perhaps Rembrandt and Deijman wanted to underline the transient nature of existence. This sort of *memento mori* message suited the philosophy of the surgeons, who were regularly confronted with human frailty and the transient nature of human life.

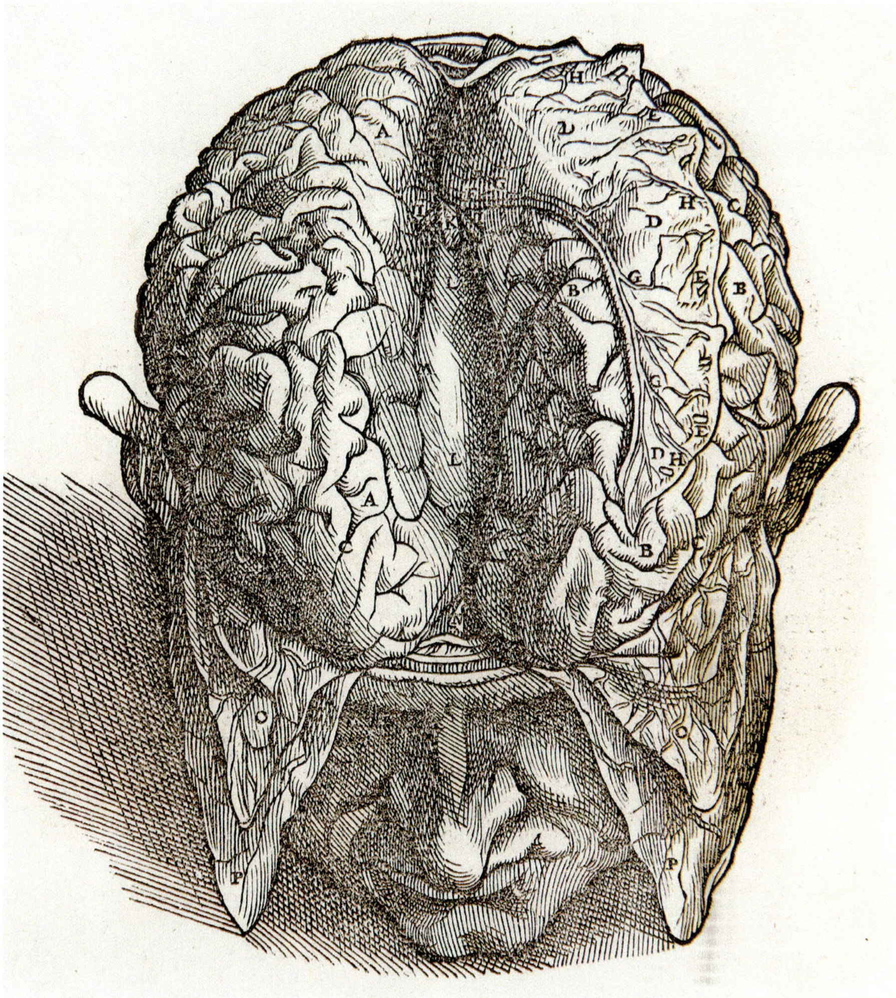

Illustration of an anatomical dissection for the brain from the book of Vesalius.
It is an overhead view of the fossa or groove between the two halves of the brain.
The *falx cerebri* has been taken out and lies on the left side of the brain.
From: Andreas Vesalius, *De Humani Corporis Fabrica Libri Septum*, 1555.
Library University of Groningen.

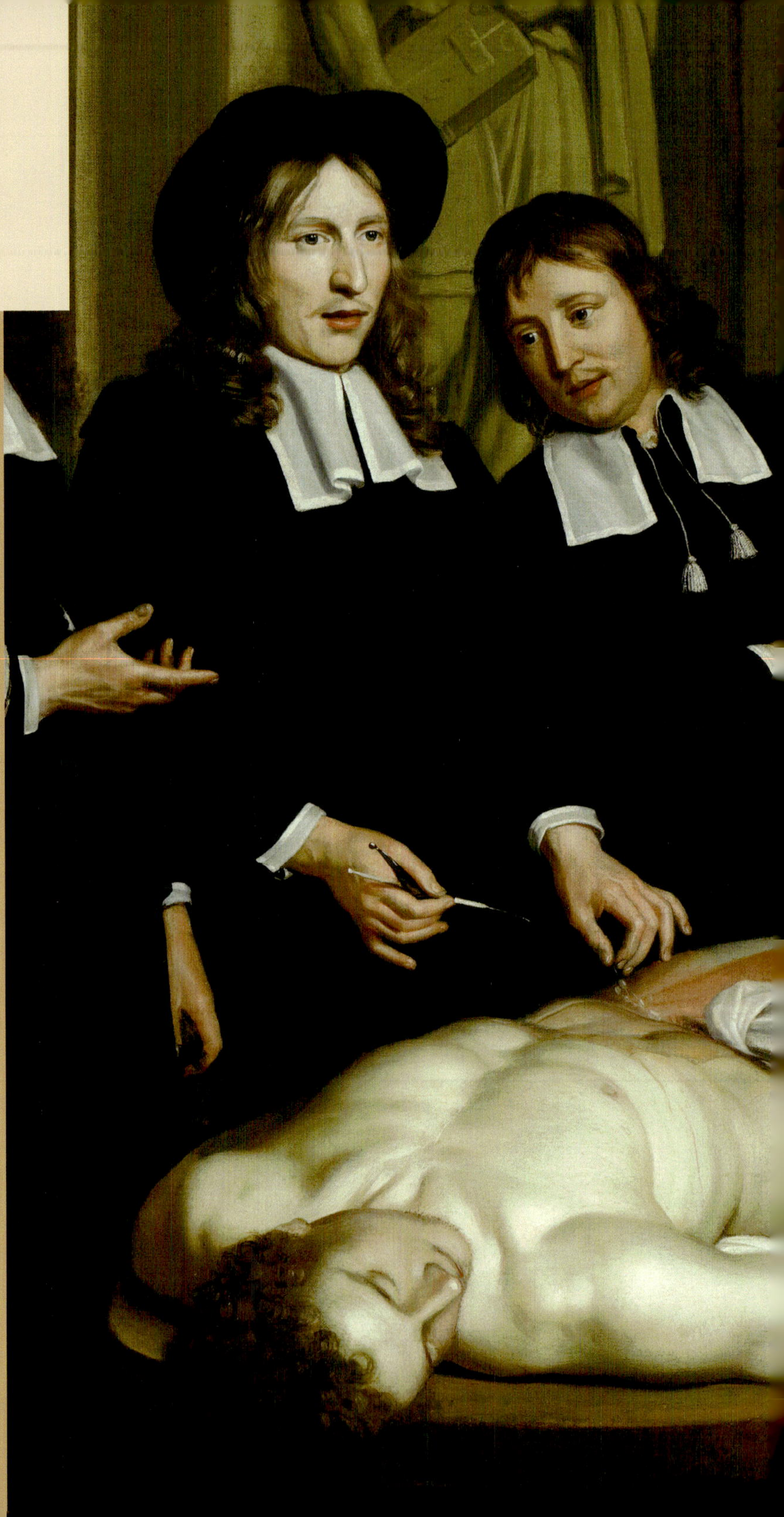

Adriaen Backer, *The Anatomy Lesson of Frederik Ruysch*, 1670. Detail. Collection Amsterdam Museum.

6

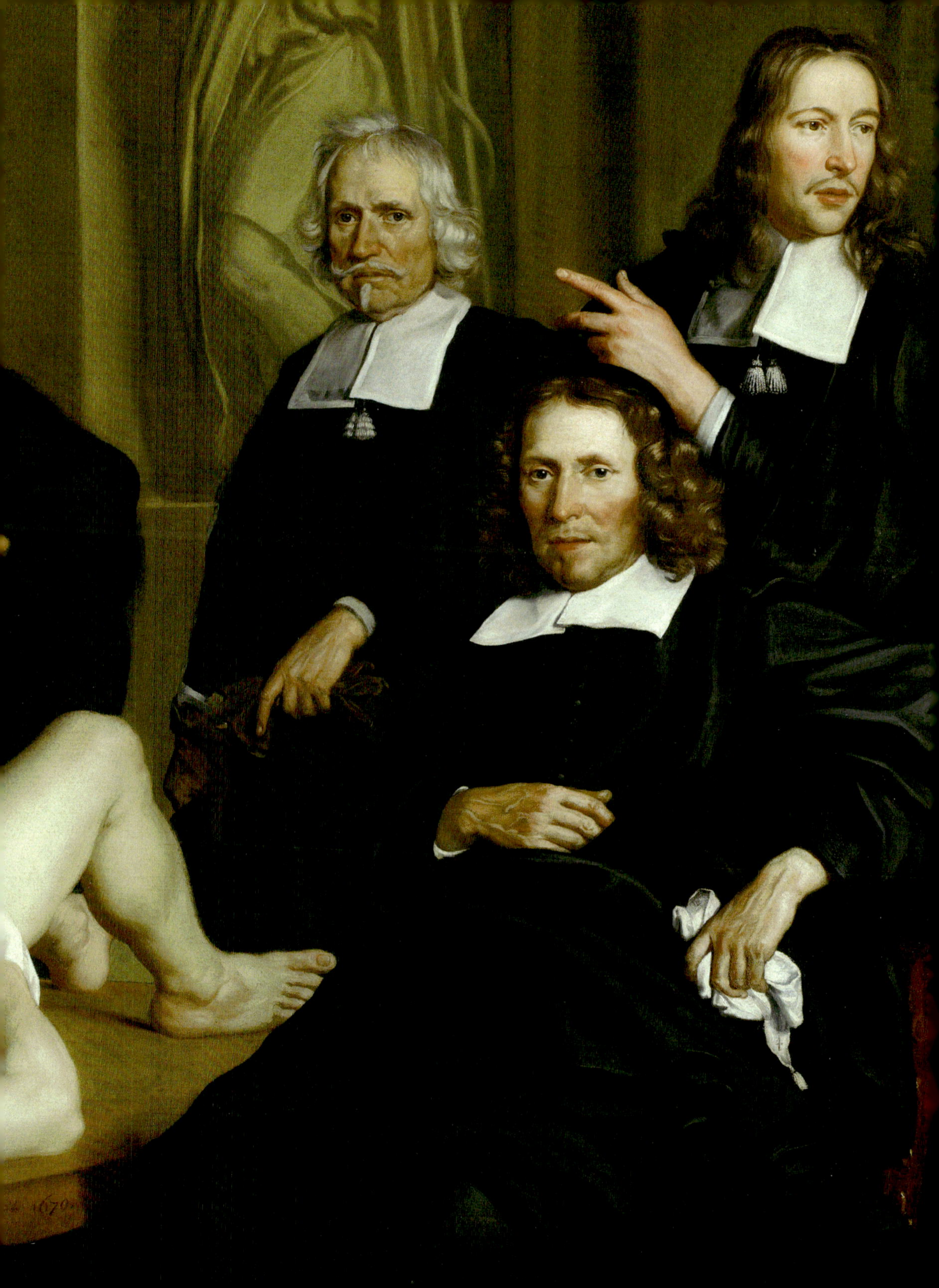
1679

Frederik Ruysch [1]

The Anatomy Lesson of Frederik Ruysch,
painted by Adriaen Backer in 1670

▸ **The Painting** In 1670, Adriaen Backer painted a group portrait of Frederik Ruysch and a few other Amsterdam surgeons posing around a corpse. It represents an anatomical lesson conducted by Ruysch, one of the most prominent, academically trained physicians in the Netherlands at that time, who was appointed *praelector anatomiae* of the Surgeons' Guild in 1667. In this anatomical lesson, he is shown dissecting the lymph nodes in the groin. This masterpiece is one of the oldest representations of the lymphatic system. Ruysch had spent years doing research into the anatomy of the lymphatic vessels. It is therefore not surprising that he chose the dissection of the lymph nodes as the main theme for a portrayal of himself. The dissection takes place in an unidentified room, the walls of which are decorated in the Classical style. In the niches in the background there are statues of (from left), the physician Galen of Pergamon (AD 130–201), and (right), Aesclepius, the god of medicine, with reference to the profession of those portrayed.

The Anatomy Book of the Amsterdam Surgeons' Guild contains a report of this public anatomy lesson, telling us a great deal about the duration of this demonstration, the profit it made, the surgeons present, and the identity of the body:

> *On March 29th, Pasquier Joris from Iperen was sentenced to death by strangulation. He was assigned to us with permission [to be used] as an anatomical subject by the Honourable Gentlemen of the Courts of Justice and, on the 30^{h}, doctor and* praelector *Fredericus Ruysch gave his first demonstration on him in the usual dissection room on the upper floor, using the body to give lessons on five consecutive days, the one and other raising a total of two hundred and fifty-five guilders and sixteen* stuivers / *sum total f 255.16–.*

The first demonstration / on Sunday 155 guilders and 16 stuivers / Monday 48.19 / Tuesday April 1st 36.18 / Wednesday 26.26 / Thursday 26.27 / sum total 255.16.

Dean (chairman) and Chief Tutor (examiner of candidate surgeons) was / Barent Heems

Governors / Gillis Hondecoeter / Leendert Fruijt / Joris van Loon / Daniel Florianus.

The anatomy lesson covered five days and was conducted in 'the usual dissection room'. This refers to the dissection room on the upper floor of the Meat Hall on the Nes, which was used by the surgeons between 1639 and 1691 (see p. 14). It should be noted that the room decorated with classical pillars and niches as shown in the painting, is not a realistic representation of the room. After Backer completed *The Anatomy Lesson of Frederik Ruysch*, the painting was hung in the Surgeons' Guildhall at the St Anthony Weighing House on Nieuwmarkt in Amsterdam. These days, it is exhibited at the Amsterdam Museum.

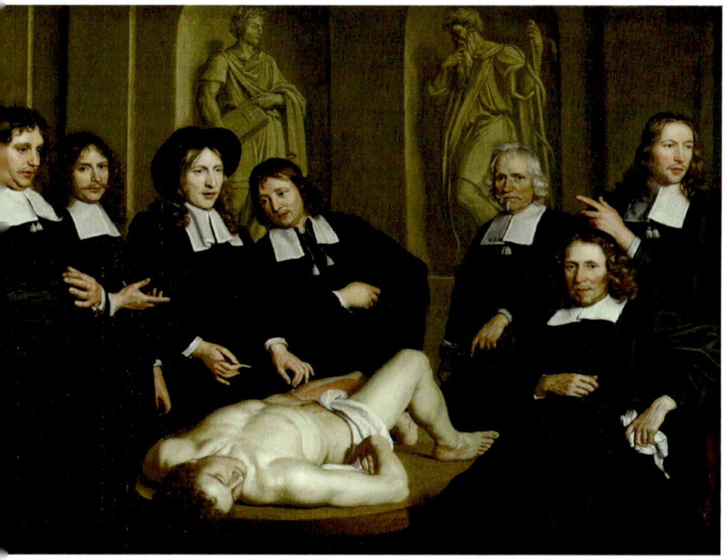

Adriaen Backer, *The Anatomy Lesson of Frederik Ruysch*, 1670. Collection Amsterdam Museum.

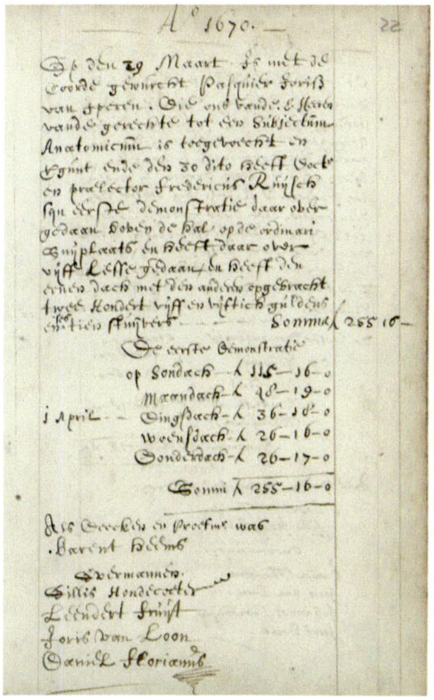

Aº 1670. 22

De eerste Demonstratie
op Sondach ƒ 155—16—0
Maendach ƒ 48—19—0
1 April Dingsdach ƒ 36—18—0
Woensdach ƒ 26—16—0
Donderdach ƒ 26—17—0
Somma ƒ 255—16—0

Als Deeken en Proefmr was
Barent Heems
Overmannen
Gillis Hondecoeter
Leendert Fruijt
Joris van Loon
Daniel Florianus

Report of the anatomy lesson given by Frederik Ruysch in 1670. From: Anatomy Book of the Amsterdam Surgeons' Guild. Municipal Archive Amsterdam.

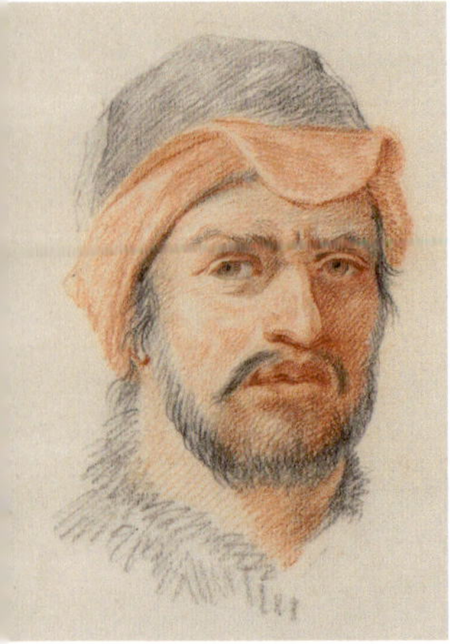

Adriaen Backer, *Self-portrait*, 1671. National Office for Art Historical Documentation.

The Painter The artist who painted the 1670 group portrait of the surgeons was Adriaen Backer (c. 1630–1684) from Amsterdam. He was the son of the Mennonite Tjerk Adriaensz and the Remonstrant Marritje Dootshooft. He was probably apprenticed to his uncle, the historical painter Jacob Adriaenszn Backer. In 1666 Adriaen Backer travelled to Italy, where he spent a year. After he returned to the Netherlands, he married Elsje Colyn in August 1669. The newly-weds moved into a house on the Spui in Amsterdam. Backer was mostly a portrait painter, his works including group portraits of the governors of the Home for Old Men and Women (1676), the City Orphanage (1683) and the *Amsterdam Collegium Medicum* (1683), which now hang in the Amsterdam Museum and the Rijksmuseum. He also painted historical pieces, among them *The Last Judgement* above the entrance of the Aldermen's Court at the Amsterdam town hall, now the Palace on the Dam.

The Dissector Frederik Ruysch (1638–1731) was born to a family of lawyers and civil servants, but he was trained as an apothecary in The Hague. He passed his final exams in 1661 and opened an apothecary's shop in that city. That same year he married Maria Post, the daughter of the renowned architect Pieter Post, who, among others, worked on commission for Frederick Hendrik, third Stadtholder of the House of Orange. Frederik Ruysch and Maria Post were blessed with a large family. The best-known among their children are their son Hendrik and daughter Rachel. Like his father, Hendrik was a doctor and was included in the second group portrait of Frederik Ruysch and the surgeons, painted by Jan van Neck in 1683 (see Chapter 7). Rachel's great artistic talent was already apparent at a young age: she was later celebrated for her flower and fruit still lifes. She married the artist Jurriaan Pool in 1695.

As soon as he was married, the twenty-three-year-old Frederik Ruysch — who also had a great interest in anatomy — was very eager to expand on his knowledge. Every day, he would make the effort to travel from The Hague to Leiden: his goal was to hone his proficiency in medicine at the University of Leiden. He would leave at the crack of dawn in order to be on time to attend the anatomy lectures given by Johannes van Horne (1621-1670), which were given at the *Academiegebouw* (now the main university building) on the Rapenburg. In the winter, Van Horne taught anatomy by conducting demonstrations

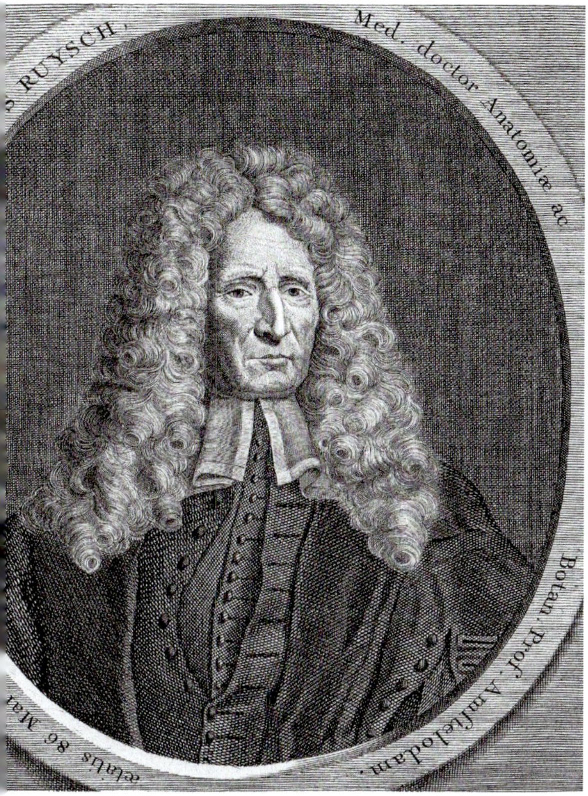

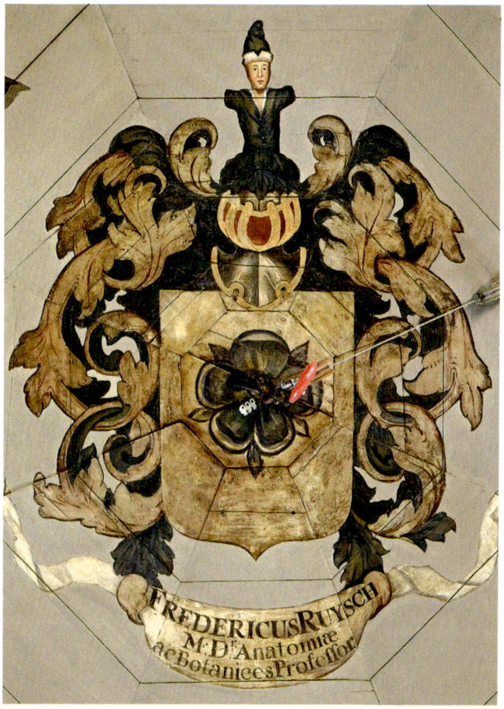

Ruysch coat of arms in the central of the vault in the *Theatrum Anatomicum* at the Weighing House in Amsterdam.

Jan Wandelaar, *Portrait of Frederik Ruysch.* From: *Alle Ontleed-, genees-, en heelkundige werken van Frederik Ruysch* (The Complete Anatomical, Medical and Surgical Works of Frederik Ruysch), 1744.

at the *Theatrum Anatomicum* on the other side of the canal, (now incorporated in Museum Boerhaave). Ruysch also studied botany, which regularly took him to the *Hortus Botanicus* (Botanical Gardens), where all sorts of exotic species with medicinal properties were grown. In 1664 Ruysch was awarded the title of doctor; Van Horne was his supervisor. The subject of his dissertation was pleurisy. A year later he published a book in which he described how, with the help of innovative preparation methods, he had proven that there are valves in the lymphatic vessels.

His discovery did not go unnoticed within scientific circles. It was therefore not surprising that the ambitious Ruysch was invited to become the *praelector anatomiae* of the Surgeons' Guild in Amsterdam, a city with a long tradition in anatomical education.

In 1667, he was appointed to this position as successor to Jan Deijman (1620–1666) and would fill this post for more than sixty years. Ruysch made enormous strides in the education of dissection, which explains the prominent position occupied by his coat of arms at the centre of the vault of the *Theatrum Anatomicum* in the St Anthony's Weighing House, surrounded by the coats of arms of the members of the Guild's Board. In his role as *praelector*, Ruysch saw to the aspiring surgeons' weekly training sessions. His public anatomy lessons were given at the *Theatrum Anatomicum (Anatomy Theater)*. In the period between 1667 and 1719, Ruysch gave a total of thirty-one anatomy lessons, all recorded in the surgeons' Anatomy Book.

Nearly thirty years later, Ruysch dissected the body of Pieter Antonius, who had been hanged to death. This particular dissection covered a record number of days: no fewer than eleven. This protracted period meant that vermin had to be kept at bay. On one occasion, one of Ruysch's anatomy lessons was interrupted by a rat. On this, he later said: '[...] a few years ago, when I was giving anatomical instruction of the muscles of the arm which I had prepared to be demonstrated for the next day, I removed the cloth from the cadaver to show the muscles, this rat had not only torn and eaten the prepared muscles, it had also bitten off a large part of the cheek.' Ruysch acted without a moment's hesitation. He chased and caught the rat which had so badly mutilated the cadaver. He then seized the opportunity to conduct a public dissection on the rat. In doing so, he made a remarkable discovery: he found a small stone in the animal's bladder. He kept the rat's skeleton in his possession for a very long time.

In 1684, Ruysch had the body of a dead pregnant woman placed at his disposal by the Sint-Pietersgasthuis (St Pieter's Hospital). The anatomy lesson on the body of the woman was spread over three days and raised the modest amount of 60 guilders. It is possible that this lesson was given as part of the training for midwives. From the year 1668 onwards, the midwives in Amsterdam were obliged to take an exam as proof of their professional skills. In 1672, Ruysch succeeded the incumbent master instructor of Amsterdam' midwives, Hendrik van Rhoonhuijsen. This position meant that he was responsible for the education and examination of the midwives. In 1674, he requested permission of the town council to use a woman's body from the hospital four times a year for the purpose of giving anatomical instruction to the midwives. A subsequent position bestowed on Ruysch in

1679 was that of forensic examiner, otherwise known as coroner. The various important positions he filled in the course of his long career made it easier for him to procure 'anatomical material'.

In 1685, Ruysch was given the chair of Professor to teach Botany at the *Athenaeum Illustre*. This school, which was founded in 1632 and regarded the forerunner of the University of Amsterdam, was located at the Agnietenkapel (St Agnes Chapel) on the Oudezijds Voorburgwal. In 1684, when the Amsterdam Botanical Gardens (Hortus Botanicus) were opened on the Plantage Middenlaan, Ruysch took on the extra task of teaching botany to apothecaries, surgeons and their assistants. Ruysch was a polymath who continued to teach anatomy, obstetrics and botany well into old age.

Surgeons still had to deal with many limitations when it came to anatomical dissections during the seventeenth century. One limitation was, that the dissector had to work fast in order to stay ahead of the decomposition process. The growing stench of decay was extremely unpleasant. The cadaver could only be kept for a few days, which did not leave enough time to examine the anatomical structures properly. Needless to say, this was a very inefficient way of working. In short, there was a pressing need for a technique to preserve body parts so that they could be studied in more depth. Ruysch's teacher, Van Horne, had already been working diligently on a method to enable him to preserve them properly. One of Ruysch's fellow-students in Leiden was Jan Swammerdam (1637–1680). He experimented with wax as a method to preserve insects. The contact between Van Horne and Swammerdam was of great importance to Ruysch's later ideas about how to preserve anatomical specimens.

Ruysch continued the pioneering work of both these men, in search of preservation techniques. He first tried to preserve the body by rinsing the vessels of all the blood and filling them with air. As time passed, he refined on technique by injecting the blood vessels full of coloured, molten wax. After this had cooled, it solidified and remained inside the specimen. He would then keep most of his specimens in glass jars which were filled with an alcoholic liquid, known as *liquor balsamicus*. This liquid preserved the consistency and lifelike colour of the body parts. Although Ruysch was only too happy to share his anatomical knowledge with others, he kept the recipe for the intravenous injections and preservatives to himself. Recent research on Ruysch's surviving anatomical specimens has shown that glycerine and mercuric sulphide (*cinnaber*) were the principal ingredients in this quickly solidifying waxy substance. Ruysch's methods of preservation led to astounding results. The most minute blood vessels in the human body, which had hitherto never been seen, were now visible. Through the addition of the dyes, the lifeless specimens regained their natural colour, imbuing them with a life-like appearance.

Ruysch lived and worked in Amsterdam for a good sixty years. Before they moved to the Bloemgracht in 1685, the Ruysch family had lived on the Nieuwezijdse Achterburgwal. Throughout his working life, Ruysch prepared and conserved more than two thousand anatomical specimens. These were put on display in large cabinets in his home. The shelves were full of jars containing specimens of all kinds of body parts, which had retained their natural colour after being injected with the wax preparation. Some of the organs had been opened to reveal their internal structure. Ruysch called a sub-collection, usually kept together in one cabinet, a 'Thesaurus'. The anatomical section formed the bulk of his collection. Alongside it, Ruysch also had various cabinets and boxes filled with natural objects of interest.

Ruysch opened his private collection to the general public. It was the first time that a collection of lifelike preserved body parts had been exhibited. Visitors were asked to pay an entry fee, but medical people, if they so wished, could be given a personal guided tour by Ruysch. To assist the visitors, he had compiled a catalogue with detailed descriptions of his specimens. Foreign visitors had a Latin version of his catalogue at their disposal. Ruysch's cabinets mainly exhibited healthy anatomical specimens. He did his best to present the specimens in such a way that they would not distress the general public. His wife and daughters assisted him in his work, adorning dismembered baby arms and legs with lace. Preserved limbs were frequently placed in glass containers together with another type of anatomical structure. For instance, by placing a lung section, intestine or meninges in the palm of a baby's hand, Ruysch managed to put the focus on the specific details of the anatomical structure. By presenting the specimens in this way, he avoided it that people looked at the anatomical specimens with revulsion or horror. Most of the specimens were intended for teaching or scientific purposes, but some were of a more decorative nature.

6

Frederik Ruysch [1] *1670*

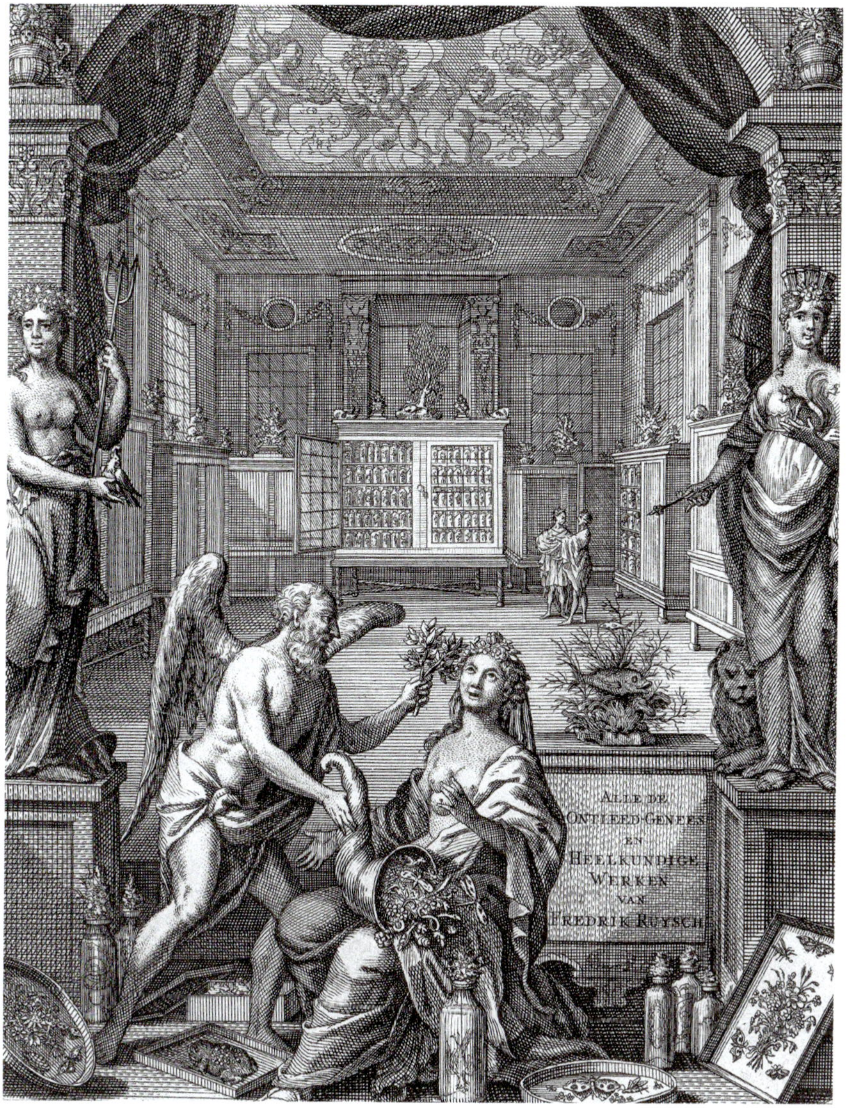

Idealized depiction of Frederik Ruysch's collection which was exhibited in the home on the Bloemgracht in Amsterdam. Against the walls, there are cabinets containing anatomical specimens in glass jars. Ruysch had placed an 'anatomical still life' on top of each cabinet. These resembled works of art, composed of various anatomical structures placed on a pedestal. The lids of the bottles in the foreground are also decorated. This illustration is the title page of the collected work of Frederik Ruysch. From: *Alle de ontleed-, genees-, en heelkundige werken van Frederik Ruysch* (The complete anatomical, medical and surgical works of Frederik Ruysch), 1744.

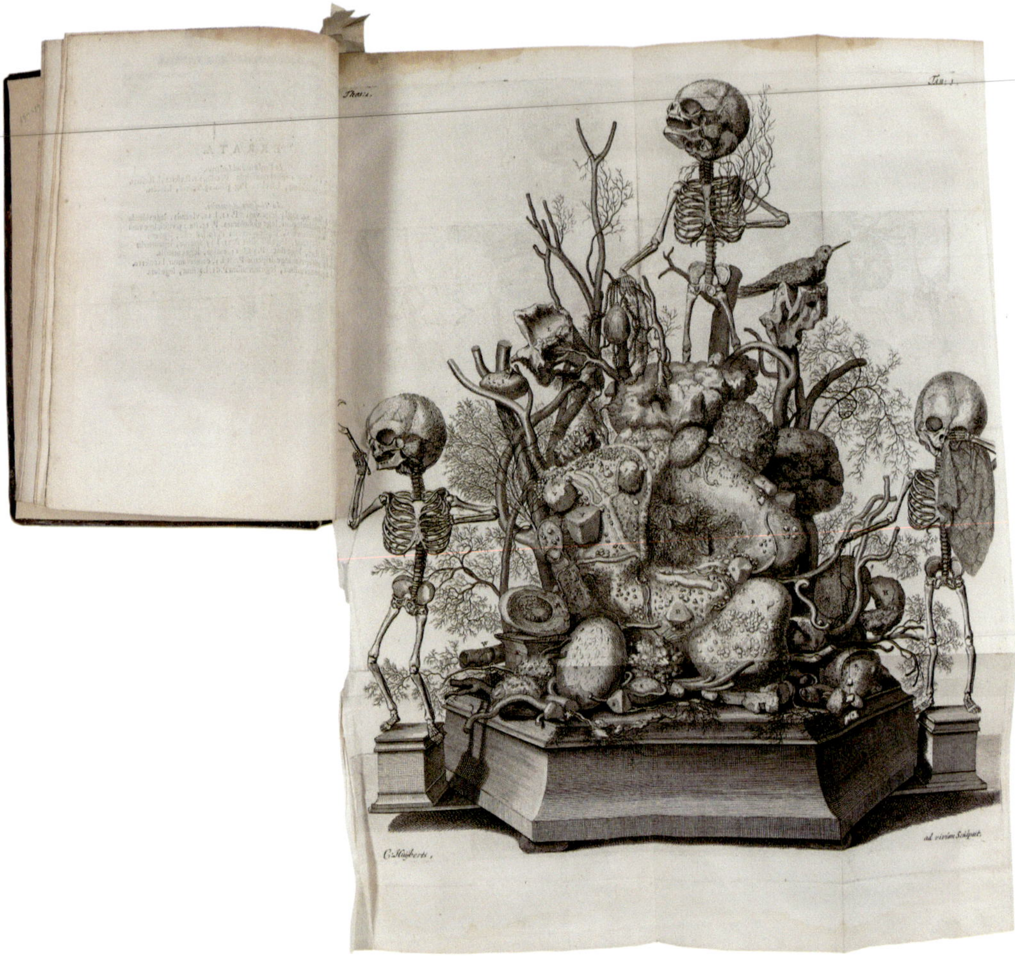

Cornelis Huijberts, Illustration of an 'Anatomical Still Life' from the first anatomical cabinet of Frederik Ruysch. From: *Alle de ontleed-, genees-, en heelkundige werken van Frederik Ruysch* (The Complete anatomical, medical and surgical works of Frederik Ruysch), 1744.

6

Frederik Ruysch [1] *1670*

The collection consisted of a considerable number of fetal skeletons and preserved body parts of newborn babies. These specimens were provided with captions showing moral proverbs to remind visitors of the temporary nature of our existence. This concept of vanitas permeated the presentation of the entire collection. The moralistic proverbs and symbols of our mortality helped to put the terror of death into perspective by emphasizing the relativity of life.

For a number of cabinets, Ruysch created special works of art appropriate for the display in the form of an 'anatomical still life'. For example, for the first cabinet containing a group of children's skeletons, he made an arrangement of gall-, kidney and bladder stones on a rock. This rock was decorated with 'trees' made out of dried blood vessels, which had been filled with red wax. Below, to its right stood the skeleton of a four-month-old fetus. In its left hand, it held a tiny handkerchief made of a delicate membrane lined with capillaries. Tearful, it expresses the misery of mankind, emphasized by Ruysch's accompanying mournful text: 'Man that is born of woman, lives but a short while, and is full of sorrow.' The baby skeleton below left held a scythe in its hand and said: 'Death does not even spare the defenceless children.' The third small skeleton, positioned on top of the rock held a necklace of pearls in its right hand. With uplifted head it gazes towards heaven and cried: 'Why should I desire worldly goods?' By creating these dioramas, Ruysch transformed the anatomical specimens into allegorical works of art.

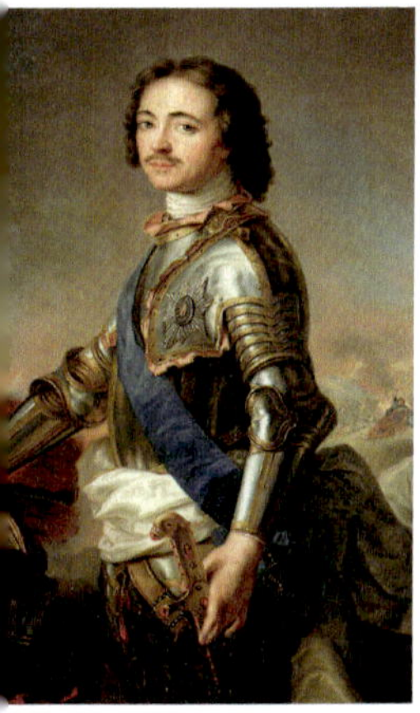

Jean-Marc Nattier: *Portrait of the Russian Tsar Peter the Great*, 1717. The State Hermitage Museum, Saint Petersburg.

Frederik Ruysch's collection attracted tremendous interest, both at home and abroad. In 1697, the Russian Tsar Peter the Great (1672–1725) made a study tour of various European countries accompanied by a retinue of 250 people. The chief purpose of his travels, was to familiarize himself with Western progress in such fields as shipbuilding and medicine. During his travels, he visited the exhibit at Ruysch's home in Amsterdam. The Tsar was greatly impressed by the lifelike appearance of the children's remains in Ruysch's collection, so much so, that he knelt down and kissed one of baby corpses. On September 17th, Peter the Great wrote the following words in Russian in the museum's guest book:

> *I, the undersigned, — while travelling through the greater part of Europe — have been here in Amsterdam, [in search of] knowledge and expertise of which I have had a need for some time, observing*

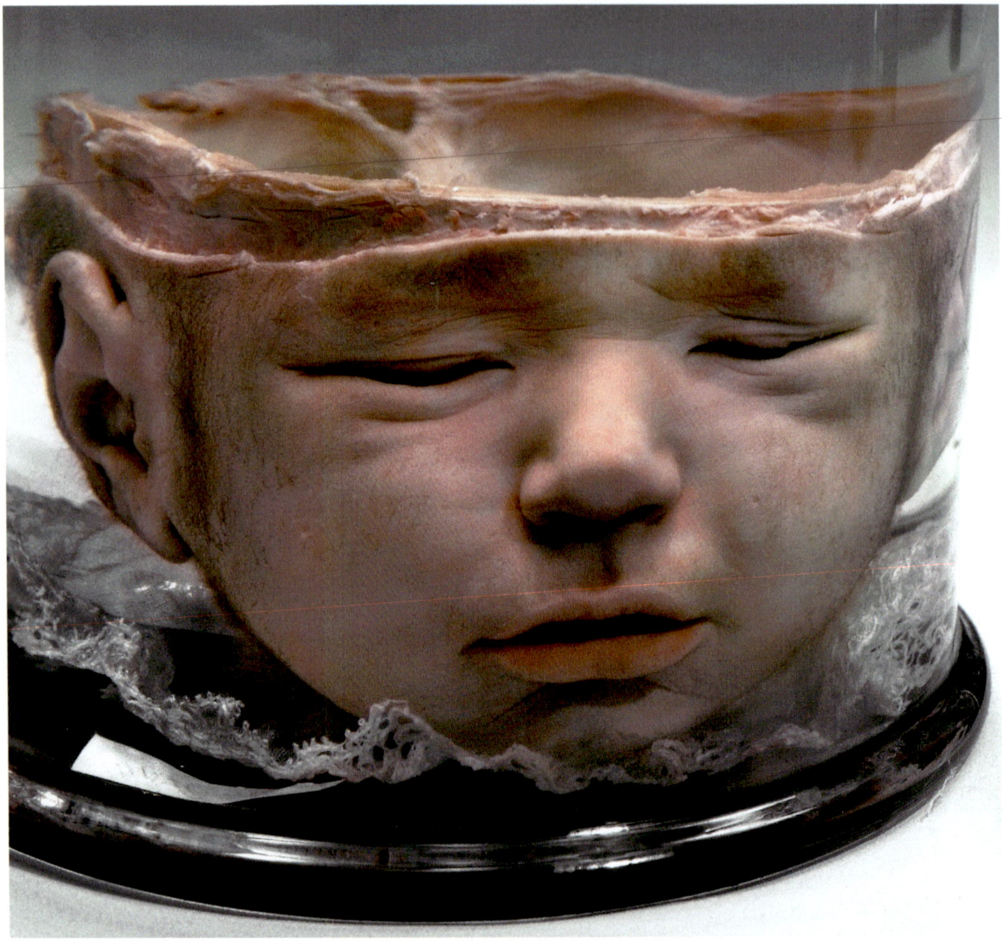

Anatomical specimen of the head of a baby from the collection of Frederik Ruysch. The collection contains several of these heads. Peter the Great was so overcome by the impression made by the preserved bodies of the children that he kissed one of them during his first visit to Ruysch's 'museum'. It is possible that this corresponds to the specimen in Cabinet X, N XVIII, the description of which (taken from *Alle de ontleed-, genees-, en heelkundige werken van Frederik Ruysch*; The Complete anatomical, medical and surgical works of Frederik Ruysch), runs as follows: 'A large glass [jar] containing liquid, and therein the head of a child whose eyes are closed, resembling that of a living child who is asleep, its tiny cheeks rounded and unwrinkled, the lips red, very neatly preserved and it has been kept by me for some years. Remarks: As the top of the head has been removed and the brain taken out, it was possible to see under the skin the natural composition of the subcutaneous tissue, the endings of the cranial nerves, auditory nerves &c.' Peter the Great Museum of Anthropology and Ethnography (*Kunstkamera*), Russian Academy of Sciences, St Petersburg.

6

Frederik Ruysch[1] *1670*

> *things, among which in particular Mr Ruysch 's skill in anatomy, and in accordance with the custom of this house, I have signed this with my own hand.*

The Tsar wanted Ruysch to inform him extensively on anatomy, he even attended several of Ruysch's lessons in anatomy at the *Theatrum Anatomicum* in Amsterdam. Twenty years after they first met, Peter the Great was to buy Ruysch's entire collection for the sum of *f* 30,000, the equivalent of € 300,000 today. The collection, comprising approximately two thousand preserved anatomical specimens, was shipped to St Petersburg. Initially it was given a temporary home in the Tsar's summer palace. However, in 1728, the Peter the Great Museum of Anthropology and Ethnography (*Kunstkamera*) was prepared in order to house Ruysch's collection. Now, almost three hundred years later, nine hundred of the original two thousand anatomical specimens are still preserved. In the course of time, some of the specimens were assigned another role, while others have been lost because of their fragility. The original descriptions of the specimens are included in Ruysch's collected work, *Alle de ontleed-, genees-, en heelkundige werken van Frederik Ruysch,* which was published posthumously in 1744. The complete work, including the accompanying illustrations, consists of nearly 1,800 pages. The book also contains a biography of Ruysch, correspondence with eminent medical men of the time, descriptions of the anatomical collection, and notes on a large number of medical histories. Ruysch was able to pursue his work on the preservation of specimens until an advanced age, and died in 1731 at the respectable age of ninety-three.

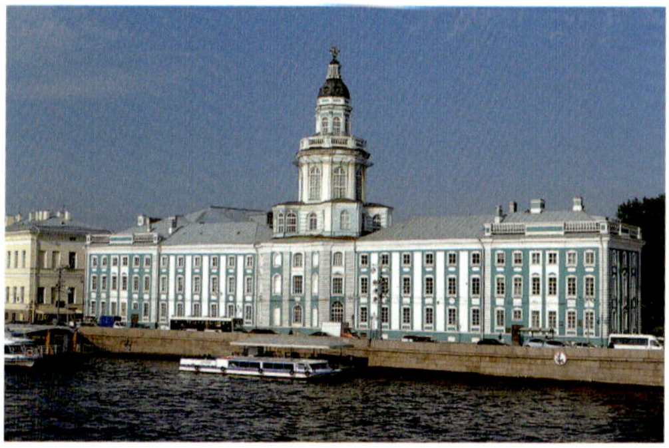

The Peter the Great Museum of Anthropology and Ethnography (*Kunstkamera*) on the banks of the Neva in St Petersburg. Frederik Ruysch's collection of anatomical specimens has been kept in this building for almost three hundred years.

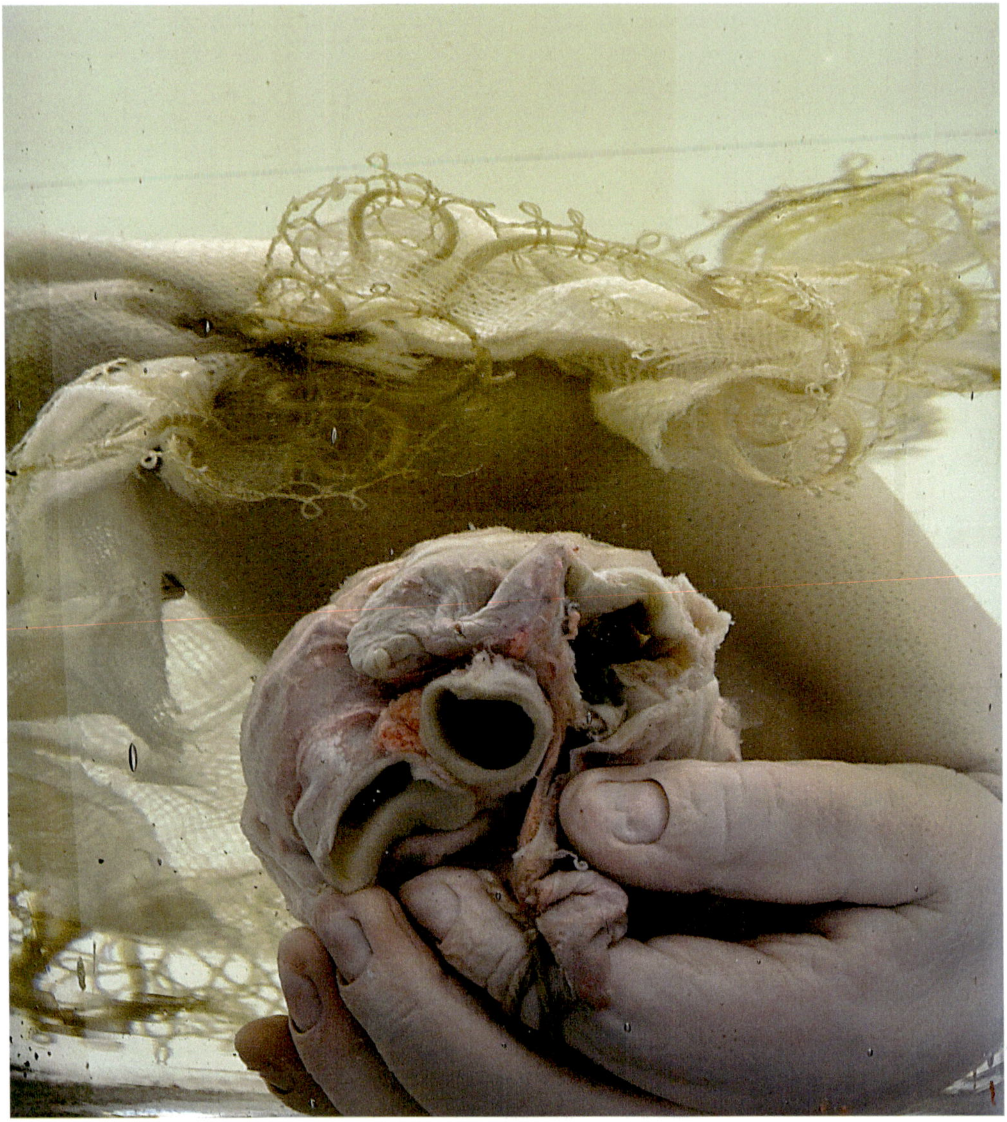

Anatomical specimen of a child's arm presenting a preserved heart from the collection of Frederik Ruysch, Peter the Great Museum of Anthropology and Ethnography (*Kunstkamera*), Russian Academy of Sciences, St Petersburg.

6

Frederik Ruysch [1] *1670*

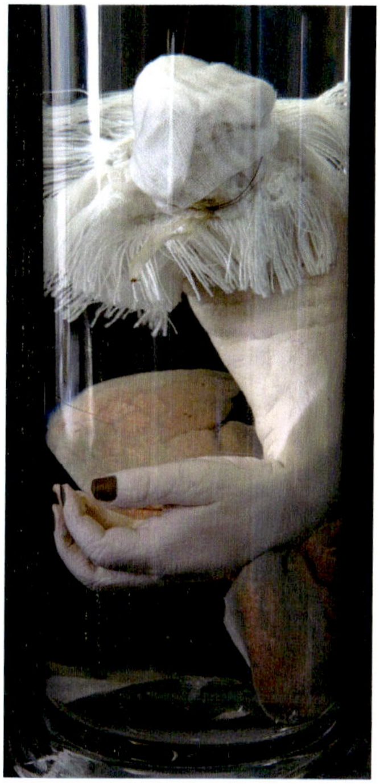

Anatomical specimen of a child's arm presenting a section of a lung, from the collection of Frederik Ruysch. It corresponds to the description of the specimen from Cabinet VI, N XXVI: 'The arm and hand of a young child, holding a small section of a lung between its fingers, cut diagonally, in which the alveoli — which make up a substantial part of the lung — open up, as they do whilst breathing, without having to be inflated by me, so that one can see its natural size and dimension.' Peter the Great Museum of Anthropology and Ethnography (*Kunstkamera*), Russian Academy of Sciences, St Petersburg.

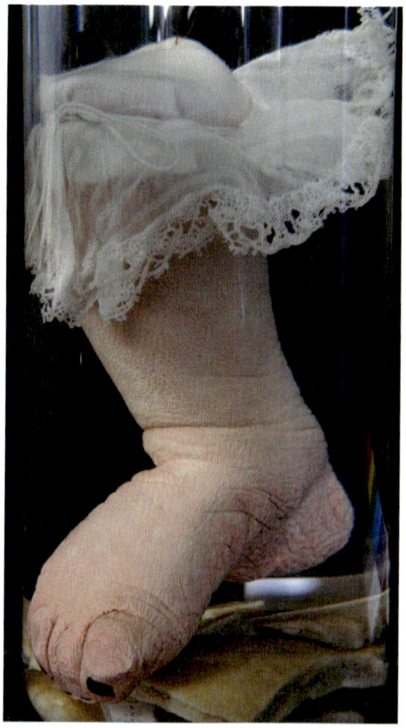

Anatomical specimen of a child's foot trampling a fragment of a skull said to have belonged to a whore, from the collection of Frederik Ruysch. Description of the specimen from Cabinet VII, N XIV: 'The naturally coloured leg of a Child, under whose foot one finds a small fragment of the decayed skull belonging to a most renowned Whore, named Anna van Hoorn, once well known by those who patronised prostitutes, of whom some are still alive, or so I am told. Why a fragment of the skull has been placed underneath the small foot is not difficult to imagine, after all this doxy would not have been felled by this hideous disease had she not pursued her abominable profession: because this is the sort of fish one catches in such waters; all is preserved in a clear liquid.' It is highly likely that this was the skull of a whore struck down by syphilis. Peter the Great Museum of Anthropology and Ethnography (*Kunstkamera*), Russian Academy of Sciences, St Petersburg.

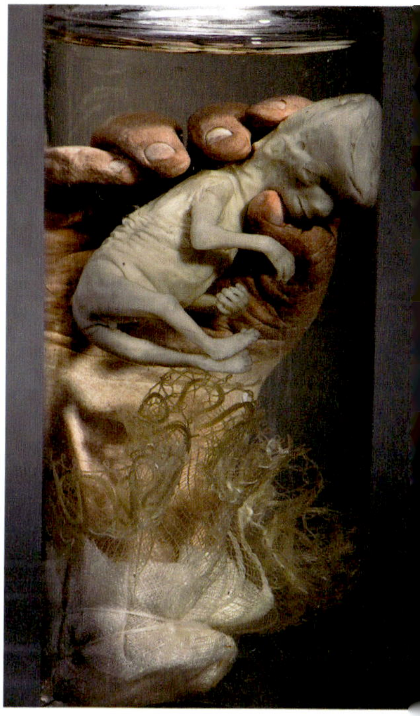

Anatomical specimen of a child's arm with a fetus from the collection of Frederik Ruysch. Peter the Great Museum of Anthropology and Ethnography (*Kunstkamera*), Russian Academy of Sciences, St Petersburg.

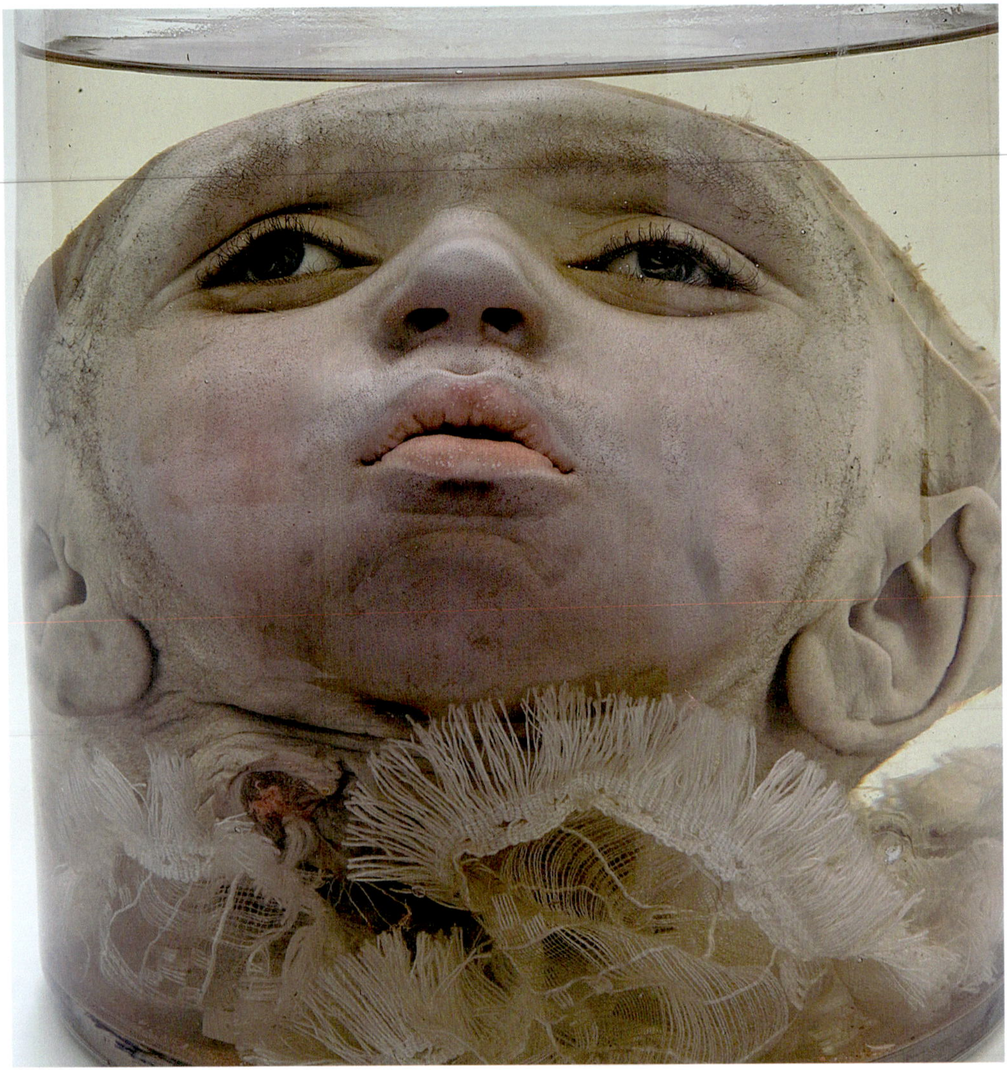

6

Frederik Ruysch [1] *1670*

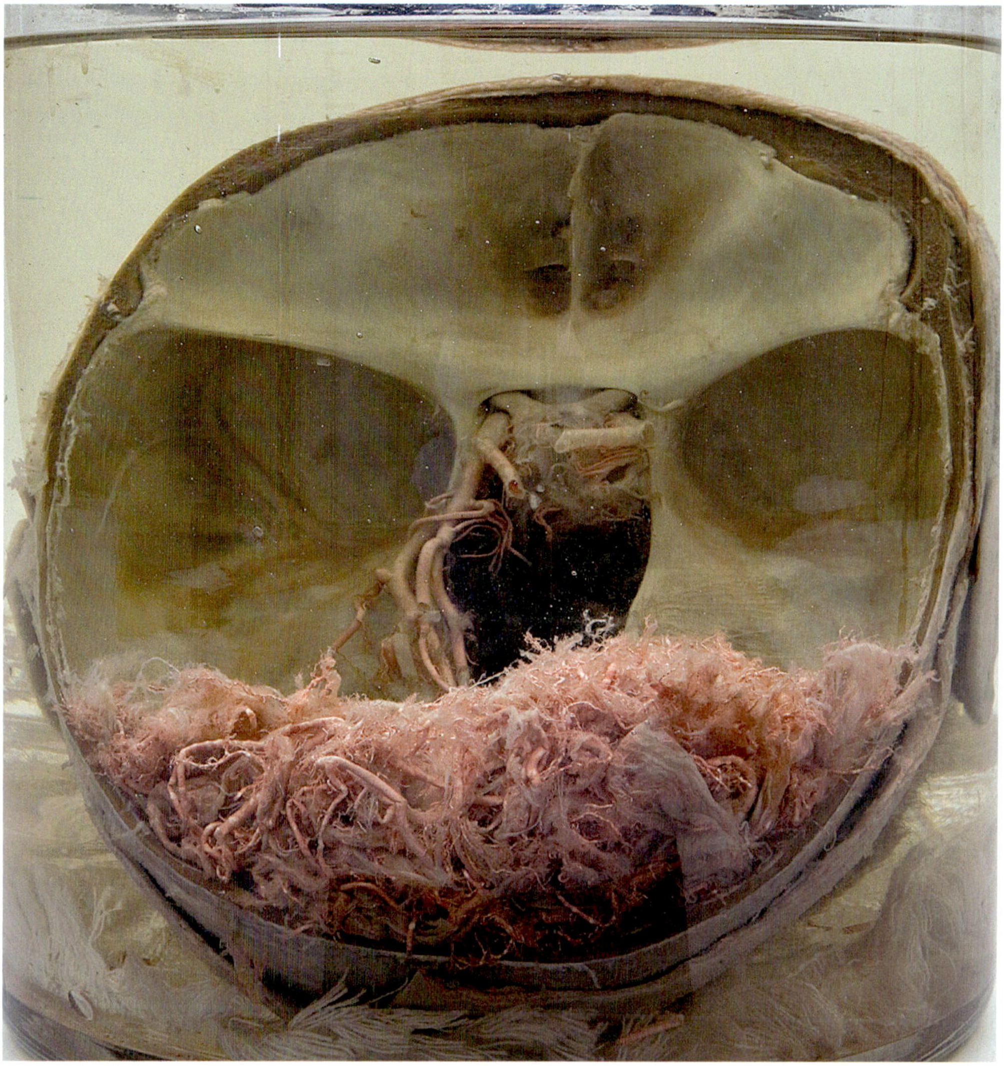

Left and right Anatomical specimen of the head of a small child with glass eyes from the collection of Frederik Ruysch. Ruysch has managed to create a lifelike appearance by using small injections of coloured wax. The child has pink lips and rosy cheeks. The cranial vault has been removed and the brain disposed of. The blood vessels of the meninges injected with pink wax lie in the base of the skull. Peter the Great Museum of Anthropology and Ethnography (*Kunstkamera*), Russian Academy of Sciences, St Petersburg.

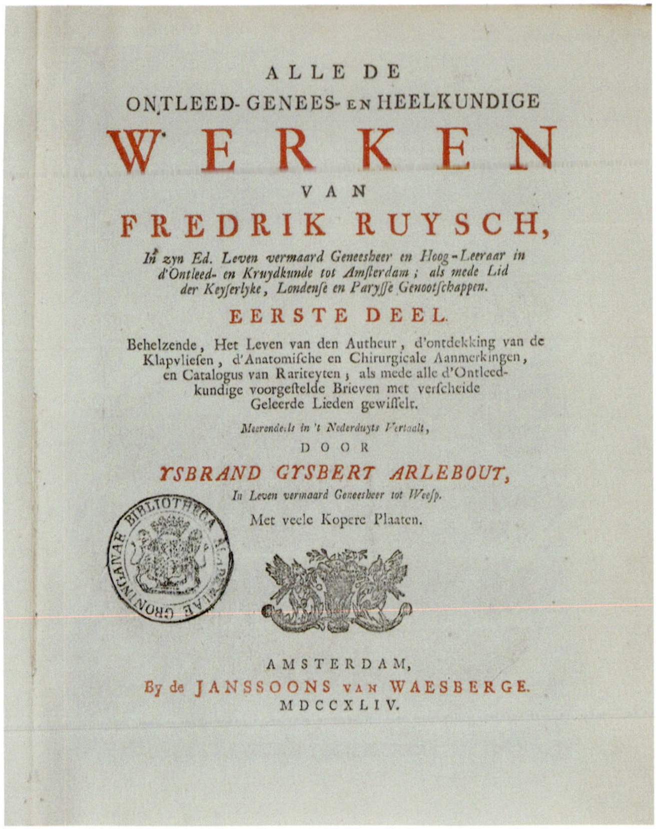

ALLE DE
ONTLEED- GENEES- EN HEELKUNDIGE
WERKEN
VAN
FREDRIK RUYSCH,
In zyn Ed. Leven vermaard Geneesheer en Hoog-Leeraar in d'Ontleed- en Kruydkunde tot Amsterdam; als mede Lid der Keyserlyke, Londense en Paryse Genootschappen.
EERSTE DEEL.
Behelzende, Het Leven van den Autheur, d'ontdekking van de Klapvliesen, d'Anatomische en Chirurgicale Aanmerkingen, en Catalogus van Rariteyten; als mede alle d'Ontleedkundige voorgestelde Brieven met verscheide Geleerde Lieden gewisselt.
Meerendeels in 't Nederduyts Vertaalt,
DOOR
YSBRAND GYSBERT ARLEBOUT,
In Leven vermaard Geneesheer tot Weesp.
Met veele Kopere Plaaten.

AMSTERDAM,
By de JANSSOONS VAN WAESBERGE.
MDCCXLIV.

Title page of the collected works of Frederik Ruysch: *Alle de ontleed-, genees-, en heelkundige werken van Frederik Ruysch* (1744). Library University of Groningen.

6

Frederik Ruysch[1] *1670*

▸ **The Surgeons** Originally, all the names of the surgeons portrayed in *The Anatomy Lesson of Frederik Ruysch* were recorded in the upper right-hand corner of the canvas. Only three of them are still vaguely legible. The rest of the names can be derived from the numbered list of names in the Minutes of the Surgeons' Guild, whose numbers correspond to those of the surgeons in the painting. Those portrayed are, from left to right: Leendert Fruijt (1620–c. 1701), Aert van Swieten (1618–1685), Frederik Ruysch (1638–1731), Gillis Hondecoeter (1635–1697), Rogier de Coen (c. 1600–1678), Joris van Loon (1607–1680) and Jacob Brandt (1628–1680).

So far, very little is known about the individual surgeons' surgical activities. The surgeons' Anatomy Book mentions that Fruijt, Hondecoeter and Van Loon were members of the Board at the time of Frederik Ruysch's anatomy lesson on March 19th, 1670 (see p. 125). In September of that same year, Van Swieten and Brandt were eligible for the position of Head of the Surgeons' Guild. Perhaps they invested in having their portraits included in the painting, in the hope of raising their chances at being appointed. The surgeon Rogier de Coen, then seventy years old, was the uncle of Aert van Swieten. De Coen never obtained the position of chairman of the Surgeon's Guild's Board. His appearance in the painting could be attributed to the fact that he financed his own portrait, and that of his ambitious nephew.

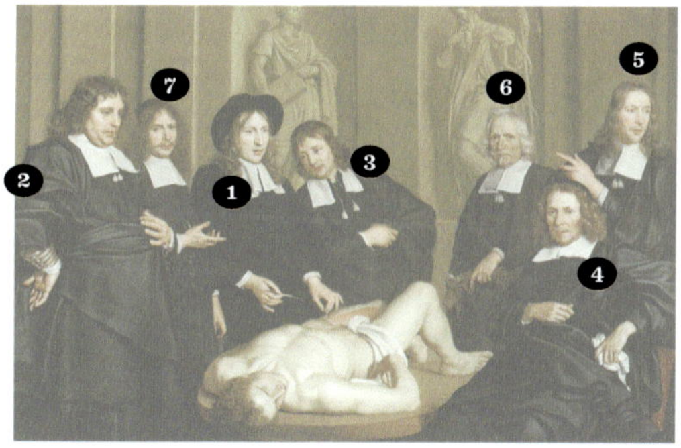

Those depicted in *The Anatomy Lesson of Frederik Ruysch*, 1670.

1 Frederik Ruysch
2 Leendert Janszn Fruijt
3 Gillis Abrahamszn Hondecoeter
4 Joris Janszn van Loon
5 Jacob Brandt
6 Rogier Janszn de Coen
7 Aert Claeszn van Swieten

▸ **The Corpse** The subject of Ruysch's anatomy lesson in the spring of 1670 was the condemned criminal Pasquier Joris from Iperen. The penalty of death by hanging was carried out on March 29th. In the five days that followed his death, his corpse was used by Ruysch to give his anatomy lessons in the dissecting-room of the Surgeons' Guild. The most remarkable fact is that the body appears to be virtually intact. Injuries resulting from the method of execution, even the welts of the noose, are conspicuously absent. Furthermore, the raised right leg is not compatible with the lifeless state of the body, due to rigor mortis. The idealized representation of the body is more reminiscent of a man who is asleep rather than that of a corpse being subjected to anatomical dissection. Backer has done his utmost to detract attention away from the body's lifeless state. This might have been a deliberate choice, possibly partly because of Ruysch's request, in order to draw the focus to his revolutionary preparation and preservation techniques.

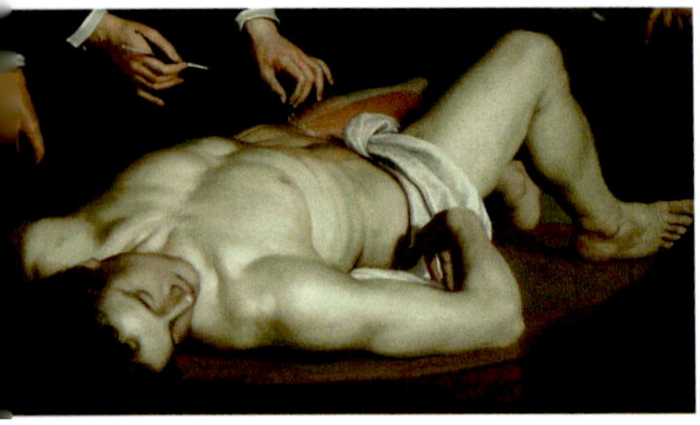

Pasquier Joris, the condemned criminal in *The Anatomy Lesson of Frederik Ruysch.*

As mentioned before, Ruysch had won both national and international fame for his new methods of conservation, which enabled him, so to speak, to breathe new life into his anatomical specimens. By injecting the blood vessels with a rapidly solidifying wax, he was able to preserve his anatomical specimens, while the addition of dyes produced a lifelike effect. Perhaps this is what made it possible to organize anatomy lessons in months other than those of winter. In 1696, a notice was even published in the *Amsterdamsch Courant* (Amsterdam Journal) announcing that Ruysch was planning to give anatomy lessons in the summer months using preserved anatomical specimens. In fact, of the thirty-one documented anatomy lessons given by Ruysch and recorded in the Anatomy Book, six were given during the other seasons. In the case of Pasquier Joris, it is not very likely that Ruysch had preserved the body before the lesson, as just one day would have been too short a time between the execution and the lesson.

▸ **Anatomy** The public anatomy lesson which Ruysch gave in the spring of 1670 presented an opportunity for him to have himself and a group of surgeons immortalized in a painting by Adriaen Backer. The painting shows how Ruysch conducted an anatomical dissection on the lymph nodes of the left groin. However, it can never have been intended to be a trustworthy representation of the lesson, as it is unlikely that Ruysch would have begun with the dissection of the inguinal lymph nodes with the rest of the corpse still intact. Instead, he would have adhered to the usual order, which required that the most perishable organs of the abdominal and thoracic cavities be removed first. That Ruysch is portrayed during a carefully composed demonstration of the lymph nodes is no coincidence: the anatomical procedure shown in the painting is a strong reference to the pioneering research that Ruysch had conducted on the structure of the lymphatic system.

Nowadays, it is known that lymphatic fluid or 'lymph' is carried to the lymph nodes through a fine network of lymphatic vessels, which are to be found virtually everywhere throughout the body. Well-known localizations of lymph nodes are the groin, the arm pits, the neck and the organs of the abdominal and thoracic cavities. Lymph plays an important role in creating immunity against pathogens. In the stomach, the lymph primarily transports fats absorbed

Anatomical dissection of the inguinal lymph nodes in the left groin by Frederik Ruysch. The skin on the inside of the upper thigh has been removed.

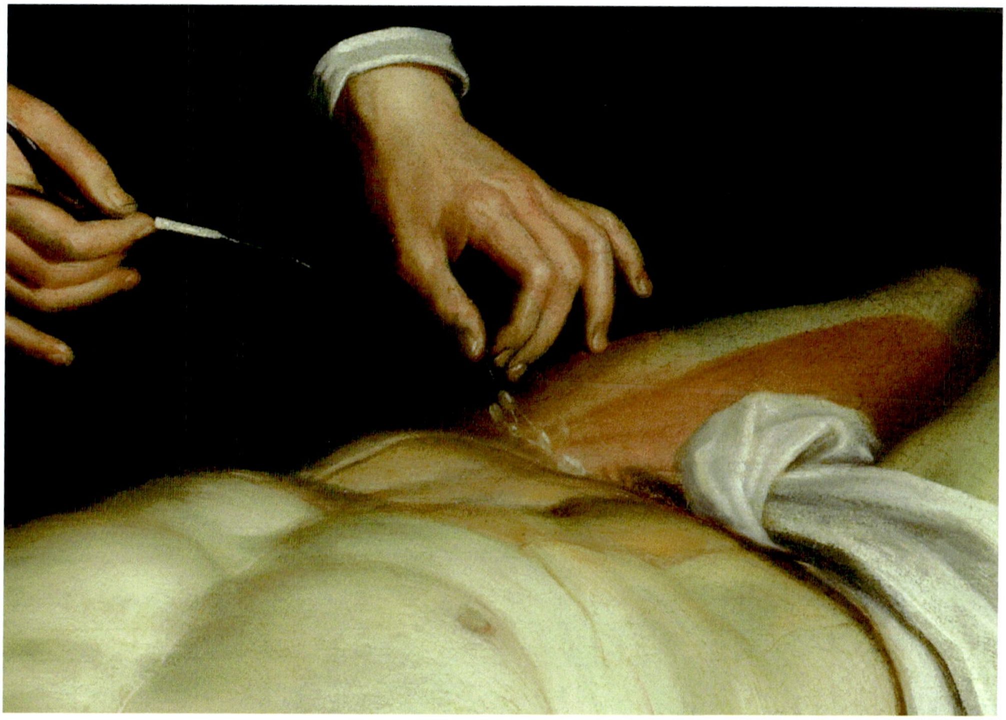

from ingested food. This causes the lymph vessels in the intestines to take on a milky colour (*chyle*). All the lymph accumulates in one large lymph vessel, the *ductus thoracicus*, and eventually ends up in the venous system.

The discovery of the lymphatic system is attributed to various scholars. In the seventeenth century, one was still fairly ignorant about the anatomy and pathophysiology of the lymphatic system. Research into the lymphatic system proved very difficult because of the very fine and transparent texture of these vessels. During an anatomical dissection, most of the fluid from the lymph vessels drains away, making them impossible to locate. In 1622, during the dissection of a live dog straight after it had eaten, the Italian professor of anatomy and surgeon Gasparo Asellius (1581-1626) discovered 'white vessels' in the mesentery (*mesenterium*) of the intestines. When he cut into the vessels, a milky fluid oozed out. This showed that there was yet another vascular system functioning alongside the circulation of the blood: the lymphatic system. Shortly afterwards, the English-born doctor William Harvey (1578-1657) discovered the mechanisms that explained the circulation of blood. In contrast to blood which is pumped by the heart, lymph is not set in motion by a pump. At that time, it was not yet clear how the lymphatic fluid circulated through the body, and which routes it took.

From the beginning of the seventeenth century, knowledge of the lymphatic system was expanded on by the following scholars: the German anatomist Johann Vesling (1598-1649), the French physician Jean Pecquet (1622–1674), the Swedish professor Olaus Rudbeck (1630–1702) and Professor Thomas Bartholinus (1616–1680) from Denmark. Most of their observations were based on anatomical dissections of living animals. During an anatomical dissection in the *Theatrum Anatomicum* in Leiden in 1651, Ruysch's teacher, Professor Johannes van Horne (1621-1670), demonstrated the presence of the thoracic duct (*ductus thoracicus*) in the human body. When he was a medical student in Leiden, Frederik Ruysch attended Van Horne's anatomical dissections. The latter encouraged him to delve deeper into the study of the lymphatic system. It was presumed that the lymph vessels must have valves in order to regulate the flow of the lymphatic fluid. However, very little was known about these valves, because nobody had yet succeeded in making the delicate lymph vessels visible. Ruysch devoted himself to research on the lymphatic system, and he was the first to succeed in preparing, and then demonstrating the valves in the lymph-vessels. He published his results in *Dilucidatio valvularum in vasis lymphaticis et lacteis* (Elucidation of the Valves in the Lymphatic and Lactic Vessels), a short manual which appeared in 1665. A Dutch translation was included in Ruysch's collected work of 1744.

In his preparation of the lymphatic vessels, Ruysch used extremely fine syringes. After tying off each end with a ligature, he filled them with air. He then prepared the air-filled vessels by excising them from the surrounding tissue and drying them in the sun. Then came the exciting moment at which, for the very first time, he observed the crescent-shaped valves in the lymphatic vessels. Ruysch began to comprehend in which direction the lymphatic fluid flowed. During an anatomical dissection of the liver of a horse, he took the opportunity to investigate the animal's lymphatic vessels and lymph nodes. His next step was to prepare the lymphatic vessels in the horse's mesentery. Three hours after the animal had eaten, he opened the stomach and tied off the 'white vessels' of the mesentery. He used the fine syringes to fill the lymphatic vessels with air. Ruysch also found lymphatic vessels in the prepared spleen of a calf. Two hours after the calf had eaten, he took out the spleen and prepared the lymphatic-vessels using the same method. He observed that the lymphatic vessels continued right into the centre of the organ. As said, Ruysch assembled an impressive anatomical collection. In the collection's catalogue, he describes various anatomical specimens demonstrating prepared lymphatic vessels, for instance, a small skeleton of a four-month-old fetus clutching a bunch of prepared lymphatic vessels in its hands. Ruysch mentions that twenty-five years after he had prepared the lymphatic vessels, the valves still remained visible. Unfortunately, his specimens of the fragile lymphatic vessels did not survive for long at the *Kuntkamera* in St Petersburg.

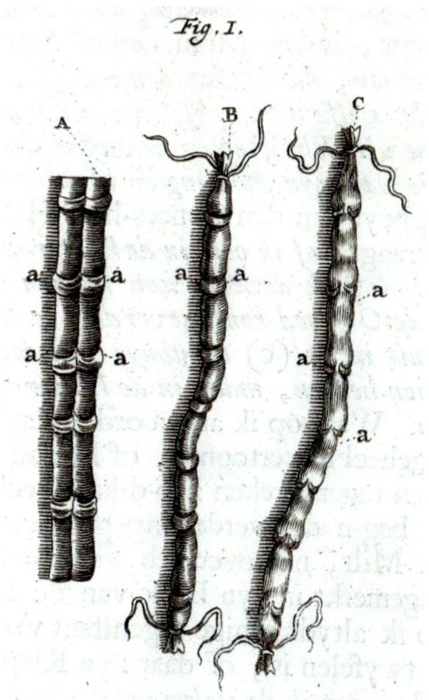

Anatomical dissection of the ligated lymph-vessels filled with air by Frederik Ruysch. Longitudinal section of a lymphatic-vessel [A]; side-view [B]; front view [C]. The valves are marked with an **a**. From: *Alle de ontleed-, genees-, en heelkundige werken van Frederik Ruysch* (1744).

Frederik Ruysch was among the pioneers who made it possible to display the lymphatic system more explicitly. His discoveries were based on meticulous anatomical observations. Using his innovative preservation techniques, for the first time in history he succeeded

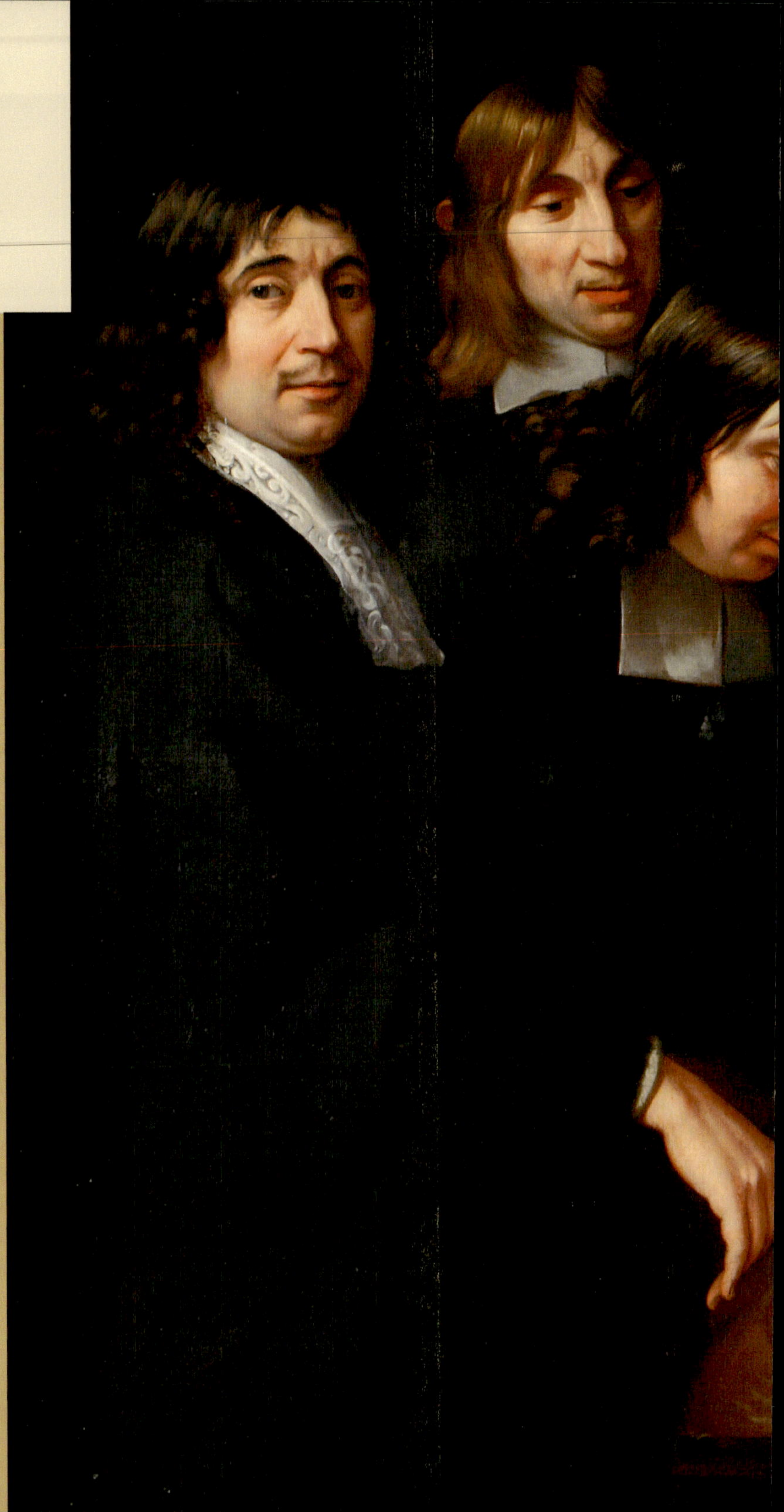

Jan van Neck, *The Anatomy Lesson of Frederik Ruysch*, 1683. Detail, Collection Amsterdam Museum.

7

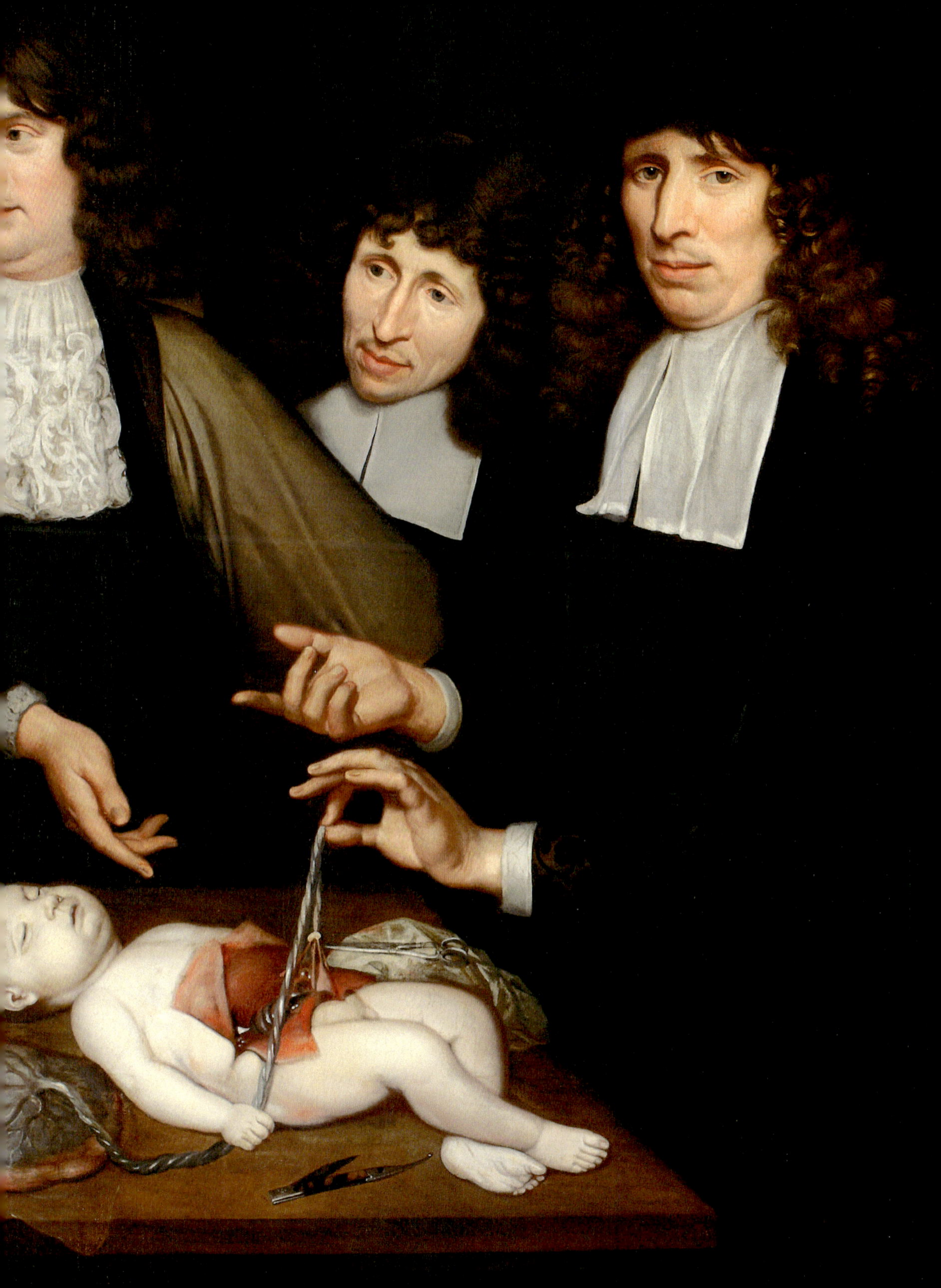

Frederik Ruysch [2]

The Anatomy Lesson of Frederik Ruysch,
painted by Jan van Neck in 1683.

▸ **The Painting** In 1683, thirteen years after Adriaen Backer had immortalized the Guild's members of the Board, Jan van Neck painted a second group portrait of the same gathering of men. Once again, the main character was the *praelector*, Frederik Ruysch. In the painting *The Anatomy Lesson of Frederik Ruysch*, he is depicted performing an anatomical dissection on the body of a newborn baby. He looks directly at the observer, recognizable from the hat he is wearing. There are five members of the Guild's Board standing on his right side, grouped around the dissecting-table, while on his left stands a boy holding the skeleton of an infant. This is his son, Hendrik.

The anatomical dissection of a newborn baby in the presence of a child would seem to be rather unconventional. It is remarkable that the *subjectum anatomicum* in this portrait is a baby, while those in all the preceding 'anatomical lessons' were the bodies of adults; the majority of which were executed criminals. In the surgeons' Anatomy Book, in which the Guild documented all its anatomy lessons, there is no record of an anatomy lesson in 1683, the year in which the painting was completed. An anatomy lesson is recorded in the previous year of 1682, but it does not mention any anatomical demonstration conducted on a newborn baby. This suggests that it was probably not intended to be an exact representation of a documented anatomy lesson, but is instead a studiously composed group portrait, painted to depict the *praelector* and the newly appointed members of the Board.

Whatever the case, the choice of a newborn as the *subjectum anatomicum* was not a random one. By choosing to perform an anatomical dissection on a child, Ruysch publicized his interest in human development, one of the central themes of his private collection of preserved specimens. He was particularly interested in the different stages of pregnancy and the blood circulation in the foetus. There is no doubt that Ruysch played an instrumental role in the education and examination of Amsterdam's midwives. Bearing this in mind, the painting can be considered an affirmation of his involvement in obstetrical education in Amsterdam.

▸ **The Painter** The commission for the painting of this second anatomy lesson by Frederik Ruysch was awarded to the artist Johan, or Jan van Neck (c. 1635–1714). Van Neck, the son of a physician, was born in Naarden. While he was young, he was apprenticed to Jacob Backer, who had also taught Adriaen Backer, the artist who painted the first anatomy lesson of Frederik Ruysch. According to the artist's biographer, Arnold Houbraken, Van Neck adopted his master's 'bold brush-strokes' and 'powerful style of painting'. He was a courteous, kindly man, and a regular church-goer. His 'entertaining stories' ensured that his company was always appreciated. Van Neck's daughter, Siebregje, would later marry Frederik Ruysch's son, Hendrik. In the 1683 painting, Hendrick is shown as a young boy holding an infant's skeleton.

Jan van Neck is known for his splendid portraits, his paintings of historical scenes and for his allegorical murals and ceiling

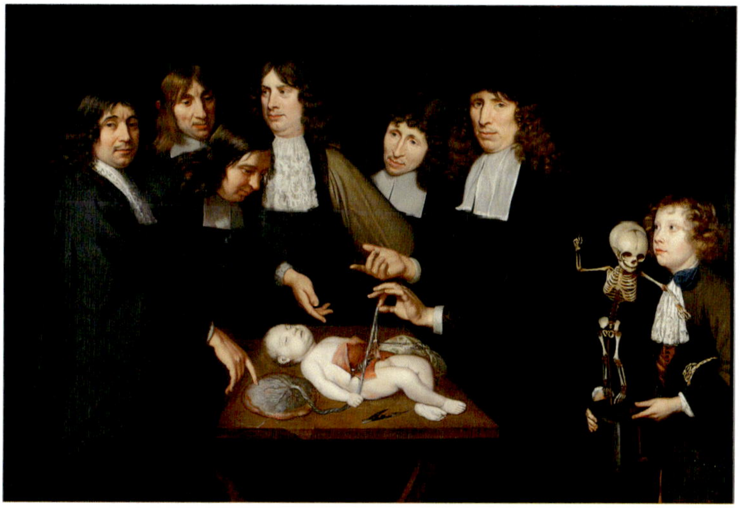

Jan van Neck, *The Anatomy Lesson of Frederik Ruysch*, 1683. Collection Amsterdam Museum.

paintings. His work can be found across the world in both public and private collections. The artist died in Amsterdam at the age of seventy-nine.

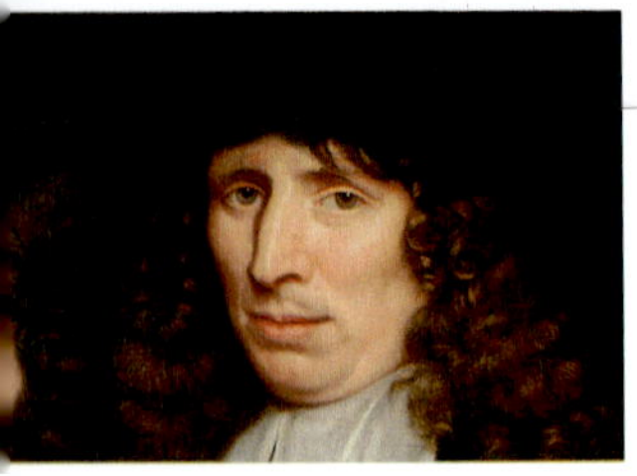

Frederik Ruysch (1638–1731)

▸ **The Dissector** It was no coincidence that the anatomical dissection of a newborn child was chosen as the central theme of the painting, especially as one considers that Ruysch had been appointed chief obstetrician of the city of Amsterdam in 1672. Traditionally, this position was held by a surgeon. Ruysch was the first physician and *praelector* to hold this function. The chief obstetrician was consulted in the event of a difficult delivery. His position also meant that Ruysch was responsible for the education and examination of Amsterdam's midwives. The anatomical dissection of a newborn baby is a clear reference to Ruysch's ambition to improve the quality of obstetrical education.

In 1668, they made it compulsory for midwives in Amsterdam to take an examination. A total of 134 midwives were registered that year, this number grew by another fifty-four in the next decade. One of the midwives who successfully passed her exam, — conducted

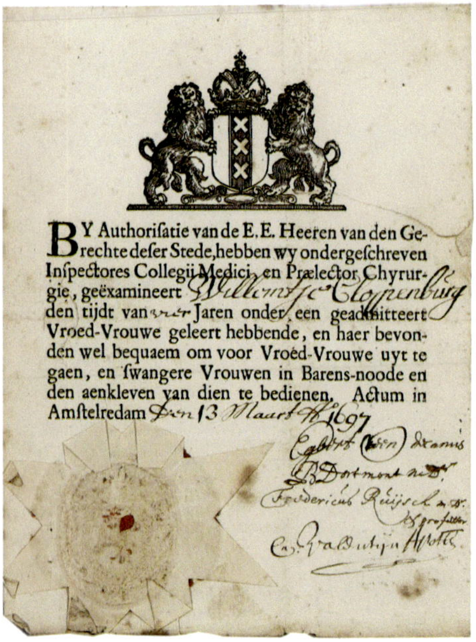

BY Authorisatie van de E.E. Heeren van den Gerechte deser Stede, hebben wy ondergeschreven Inspectores Collegii Medici, en Prælector Chyrurgie, geëxamineert Willemtje Cloppenburg den tijdt van vier Jaren onder een geadmitteert Vroed-Vrouwe geleert hebbende, en haer bevonden wel bequaem om voor Vroed-Vrouwe uyt te gaen, en swangere Vrouwen in Barens-noode en den aenkleven van dien te bedienen. Actum in Amstelredam den 13 Maart A° 1697

Midwifery certificate awarded to Willemtje Cloppenburg, signed by Frederik Ruysch as well as other examiners. Municipal Archive Amsterdam.

by Frederik Ruysch — was Willemtje Cloppenburg. Her certificate was co-signed by Frederik Ruysch in 1697.

The standard of the midwives' anatomical knowledge had always been lamentably poor. In 1674, the mayor of Amsterdam gave Ruysch permission to give the midwives four anatomical lessons per year. In order for him to do this, the Sint-Pietersgasthuis (St Peter's Hospital) provided him with the body of a deceased woman several times a year. The bodies were specifically to be used for instruction in anatomy. Apart from these anatomical sessions, the midwives and their apprentices were obliged to follow regular lessons in obstetrics given by the chief obstetrician. Under the terms of a regulation laid down in 1682, their absence was penalized with a fine of 12 *stuivers*. A list of exam questions dating from 1700 gives an insight into the subjects and provides an idea of what subjects were on offer: 'molar pregnancies, also known in Dutch as "bunch of grapes" pregnancies (*druiventroszwangerschappen*), miscarriages, breech births, or "what to do when the child does not present itself properly, what signs to look for to see if the foetus is alive or dead, what to do if the waters rupture prematurely, and how to expel the placenta".

In his advice on that last topic, Ruysch recommended waiting patiently after the child was born for the spontaneous expulsion of the placenta, which he also referred to as the *moederkoek* or 'mother cake'. He even claimed that he had discovered a special muscle in the uterine wall (which he called the *musculus Ruyschianus*) whose specific task was to expel the placenta. Ruysch did not propagate the forcible removal of the placenta. And yet, impatient midwives regularly proceeded to remove the retained placenta manually. In such cases, the midwives would use her finger to trace the direction of the umbilical cord till she reached the uterus. She would then pierce the placenta with her finger in order to detach it from the uterus wall. In his collected works, Ruysch shows a placenta with a 'tear made by the index finger of the midwife, so that she could detach the placenta'.

As chief obstetrician and forensic examiner, Ruysch had access to a large number of dead embryos, foetuses and newborns. He prepared these to form a unique, extensive collection of anatomical specimens which illustrated the stages of human development. He was the first person in history who had documented the successive stages of foetal development so thoroughly. He kept his specimens in the anatomical museum which he set up in his own home on

Placenta with a tear caused by its manual removal by a midwife. Ruysch notes the rotation of the blood vessels in the umbilical cord. It was thought that the number of twists in the umbilical cord was an indication of the number of children the woman would eventually bear. From: *Alle de ontleed-, genees-, en heelkundige werken van Frederik Ruysch* (The complete anatomical, medical and surgical works of Frederik Ruysch), 1744.

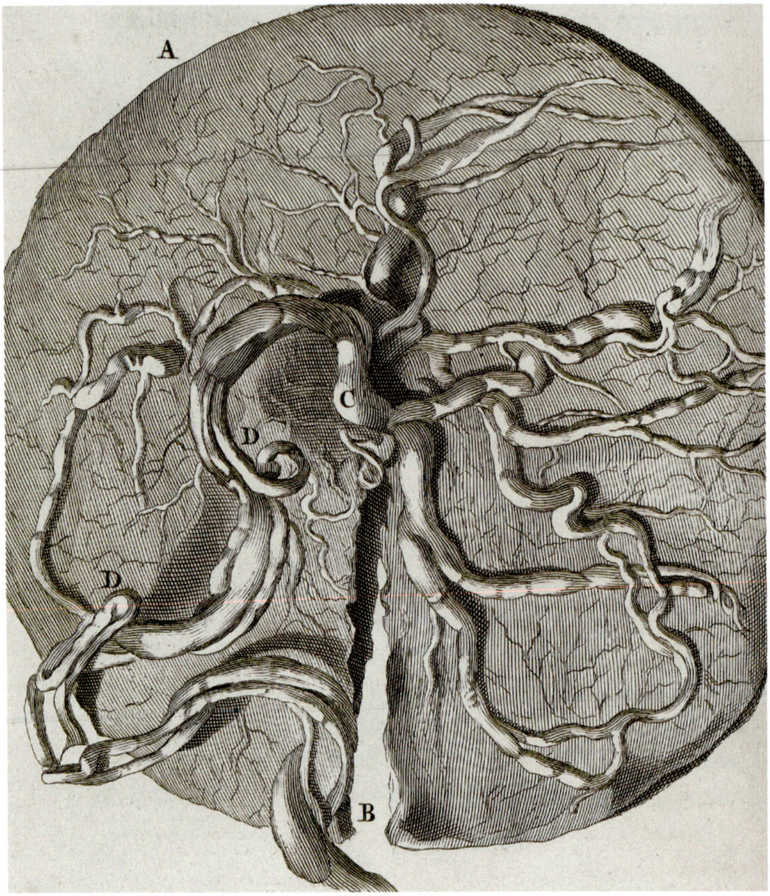

the Bloemgracht. Among them were the preserved/embalmed embryos, foetuses and limbs of children at various stages of development. His revolutionary technique of injecting the blood vessels with coloured wax was one of the keys to his success, and it was Ruysch who laid the foundations for scientifically preparing and preserving 'anatomical specimens'. His method of preservation allowed him to keep his anatomical specimens in order to study them in depth and to use them for teaching purposes, without the concern that the rapid onset of decomposition might destroy his work. The anatomical knowledge he acquired he put to good use in the lessons he gave to the surgeons and the midwives.

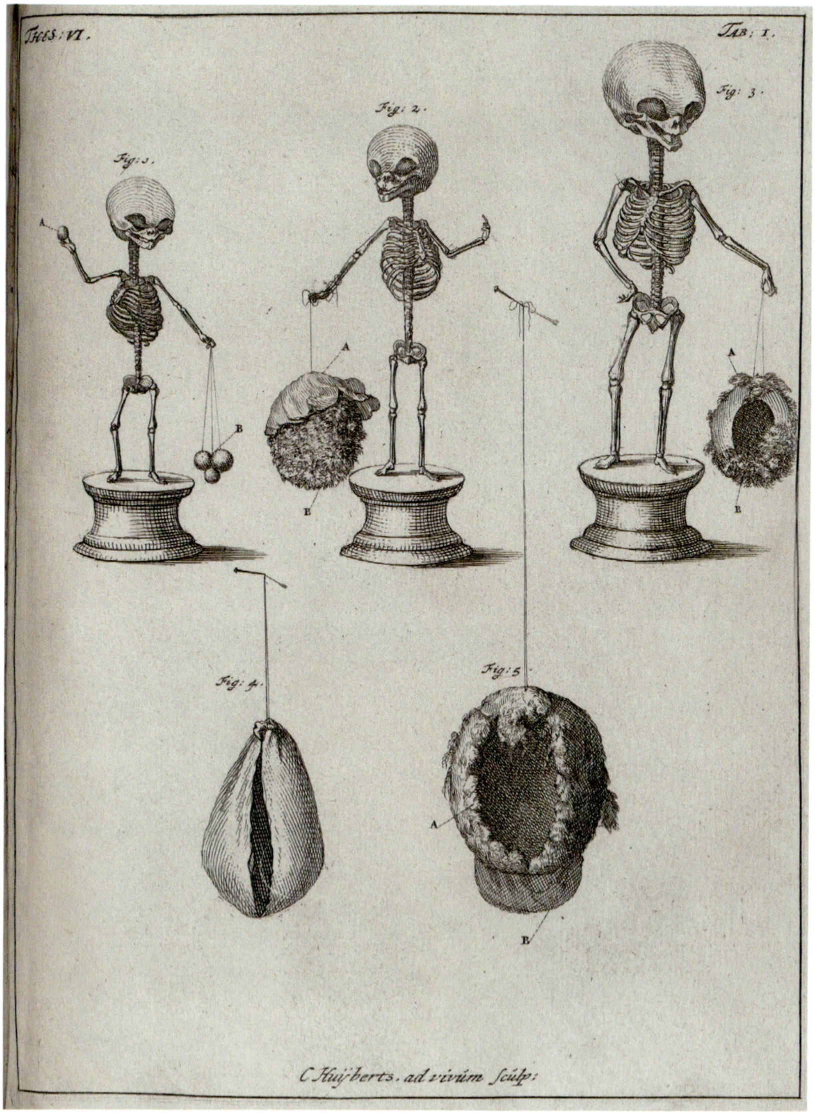

Exhibition of the development of a human being from the sixth cabinet of Frederik Ruysch. On the left-hand side is a skeleton the size of the little finger holding unfertilized ova in its hands. The tiny skeleton next to it holds a fertilized ovum and a placenta at an early stage of its development. The last skeleton grasps a similar structure, this time cut open by Ruysch. Below left is an example of a miscarriage. Below right is an illustration of the placenta at an early stage. From: C. Huijberts, *Alle de ontleed, genees-, en heelkundige werken van Frederik Ruysch* (The complete anatomical, medical and surgical works of Frederik Ruysch), 1744.

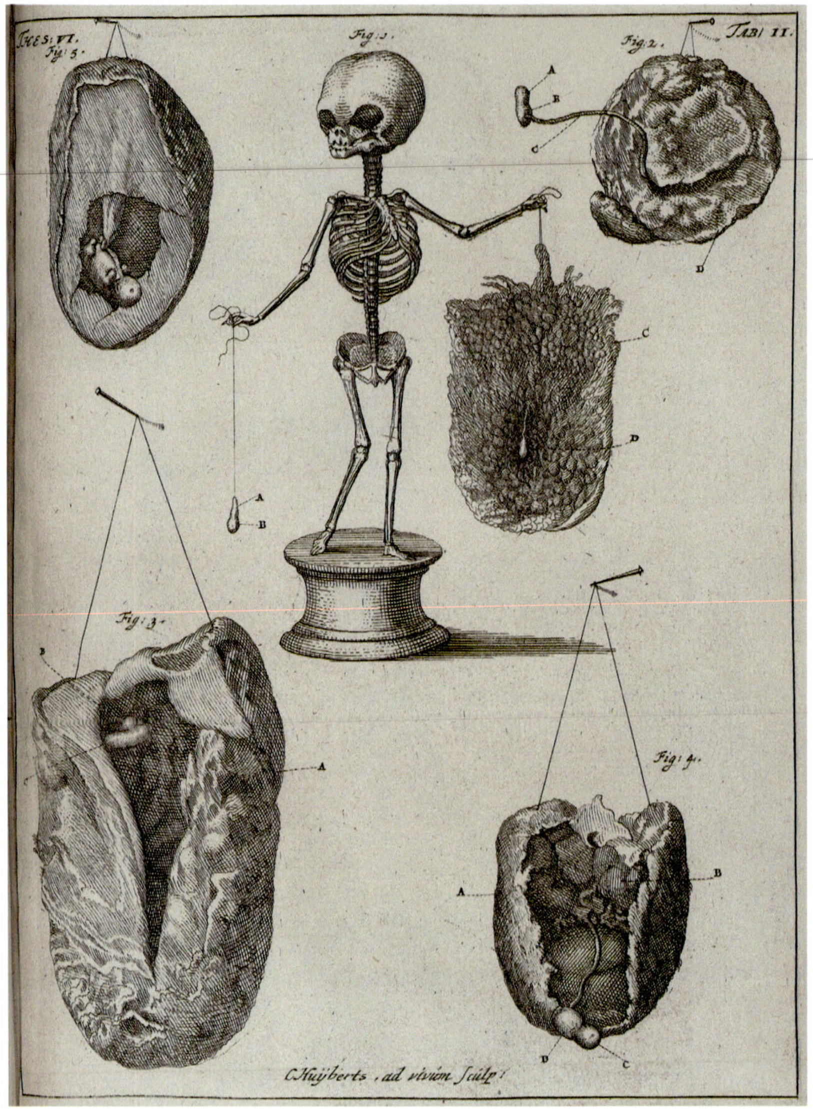

The small skeleton of a three-month-old holding an embryo the size of an aniseed in its right hand. In its left hand, it holds an embryo the size of a louse, attached to the placenta by the umbilical cord. Above right, Ruysch illustrates an embryo the size of a grain of barley. The images seen below left to below right and then to above left, illustrate the successive stages of embryonic development. The 'tiny human creature' was said by Ruysch to be about an 'inch big'. C. Huijberts, from: *Alle de ontleed-, genees-, en heelkundige werken van Frederik Ruysch* (The complete anatomical, medical and surgical works of Frederik Ruysch), 1744.

7 *Frederik Ruysch* [2] *1683*

▸ **Surgeons and others represented in the painting** The surgeons whose likenesses are portrayed in the painting are Anthonie van Paamburg, Abel van der Horst, Pieter Adriaanszn, Andries Boekelman and Jean de Milly. All were members of the Surgeons' Guild's board. Although we know their names, we do not know which name belongs to whom, with the exception of two people: Frederik Ruysch (the *praelector* wearing the hat) and his son, Hendrik Ruysch (the boy on the far right). As described in his collected works, Ruysch regularly collaborated with all the directors portrayed.

Anthonie van Paamburg Van Paamburg was the dean, or Head of the Surgeons' Guild. Apparently, he had his hands full with administrative affairs, because Ruysch doesn't mention his surgical activities anywhere.

Abel van der Horst Abel van der Horst was the Chief Tutor. In this position, he spent his time preparing and conducting the examinations for the trainee surgeons. Ruysch wrote one description of a surgical operation which he performed together with Van der Horst. One day, they were summoned to see a woman who was in torment due to a painfully distended abdomen. As time progressed, she was afflicted by 'fire' or an infection around the navel. This then led to a 'violent eruption' of fluid from the abdomen. Van der Horst, whom Ruysch judged to be an experienced surgeon, succeeded in stopping 'any further leakage with bandages and adhesive plaster'. The fluid that flowed from the abdomen exuded a foul stench. Four or five days after the rupture of the abdomen had occurred, 'the poor creature' died.

Her family gave permission for a post-mortem to be held on the dead woman's body. In the abdomen, Ruysch and Van der Horst discovered 'a tumour the size of a fist from which, after being cut open longitudinally, a rather whitish porridge-like substance initially flowed'. After all this substance had been removed, 'they found nothing less than a hard ball, consisting of old, matted hair.' They examined the 'hairball' under a magnifying glass and came to the conclusion that these were from the head. The hairball (*bezoar*), which had caused obstruction and possibly an intestinal perforation into the abdomen, must have been caused by the frequent and compulsive ingestion of hair.

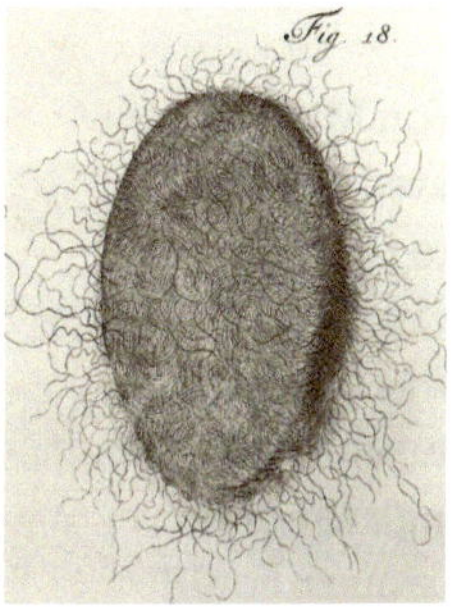

The hairball which Ruysch and Abel van der Horst discovered in the abdomen of a patient during an autopsy. From: *Alle de ontleed-, genees-, en heelkundige werken van Frederik Ruysch* (The complete the anatomical, medical and surgical works of Frederik Ruysch), 1744.

The affected palate had to be cauterized and the accompanying tumour excised. In order to obtain a good view of the area to be operated, Adriaanszn and his colleague Cyprianus first extracted some of the lawyer's teeth and molars. Using a small curved sharp scalpel, they excised the tumour and then inserted glowing hot cauterisers into the mouth to treat the damaged palate. On another occasion, Adriaanszn was taken to a woman who had a large swelling around her jaw. It had 'grown to such a size that it covered her entire jaw, and extended from the ear to near the eye down to the mouth, and thence downwards to the neck and throat.' He tied off the swelling and treated it with a caustic substance. A few days later, he cut it away. It took several months for the wound to heal.
Pieter Adriaanszn enjoyed an excellent reputation as a surgeon, not least because he introduced Amsterdam to a new technique for the amputation of the lower leg. His inspiration for this had come from an English surgeon. Till then, the usual method was to cut straight through the skin, muscles and bones. In the new method, the calf muscles were used to form the stump. Adriaanszn described his discoveries in *Een nieuwe manier van 't afzetting in 't been* (New Way of Amputating the Leg). A very similar operative technique is still used for an amputation of the lower leg even today.
As his reputation as a surgeon grew, Adriaanszn was invited to perform operations throughout the country.

Andries Boekelman The professional skill of Andries Boekelman is quoted many times in Ruysch's collected work. Boekelman was also appointed associate municipal obstetrician, working alongside Ruysch. This appointment aroused the envy of various Amsterdam medical men, who also had an eye on this position. They seized every opportunity to discredit Ruysch and Boekelman.
In 1677, Ruysch and Boekelman were summoned to see the twenty-eight-year-old Lysbeth Jans after she had gone into labour. She emanated a terrible stench, caused by her seriously infected vagina and the dead infant in her womb, which had reached an advanced state of decomposition. Boekelman set to work professionally and delivered her of the dead child. The protracted obstruction caused by the dead child had torn the perineum (the section between the vagina and anus). This had gradually devel-

oped into an unnatural, incurable connection between the rectum and the vagina, known as an *anovaginal fistula*. One of the physicians at the hospital, a certain Dr Van Dortmondt, alleged that this tear was the fault of the combination of ignorance and incorrect use of obstetrical instruments by Ruysch and Boekelman. These two gentlemen dismissed the accusations as unfounded, and countered that the fistula had developed due to the patient's lack of knowledge and neglect. The whole affair led to a hefty row between the two parties, producing a flood of accusatory pamphlets back and forth. All the more reason for Ruysch and Boekelman to be more careful in their handling of any subsequent obstetrical cases.

On another occasion, Ruysch asked Boekelman to come and give his opinion on the case of a farmer who lived just outside Amsterdam. The man had a malignant growth on his penis. They both concluded that the amputation of the penis was the only possible treatment. The operation was carried out as follows: 'Once the catheter had been introduced into the cavity of the bladder via the urethra, we bound off the penis just behind the aforementioned tumour, tying it off with a thin but very strong ligature and pulled this tight.' After five days, they used a scalpel to sever the atrophied penis with the tumour on it. Two days later, the urinary catheter was taken out and the patient recovered quickly after that. In order to urinate, 'without wetting his clothes', the gentlemen presented him with an ivory urinary cannula.

Jean de Milly The Anatomy Book of the Surgeons' Guild reveals that Jean de Milly was one of the student surgeons whom Ruysch had given the chance to demonstrate his practical skills during a public anatomy lesson. In this case, in 1694, the corpse of the hanged criminal Jacob Roelofse was made available 'to be dissected by the Professor of Anatomy Frederik Ruysch, for public benefit and learning'. This lesson was spread over a total of nine days. On the third, fifth and seventh days Ruysch delegated the dissecting work to De Milly. This gesture was an enormous compliment to the aspiring surgeon. Pieter Adriaanszn was responsible for the dissection on the first and second days. In total, the lesson raised 188 guilders. The report in the Anatomy Book was signed by the incumbent members of the Board Van Paamburg,

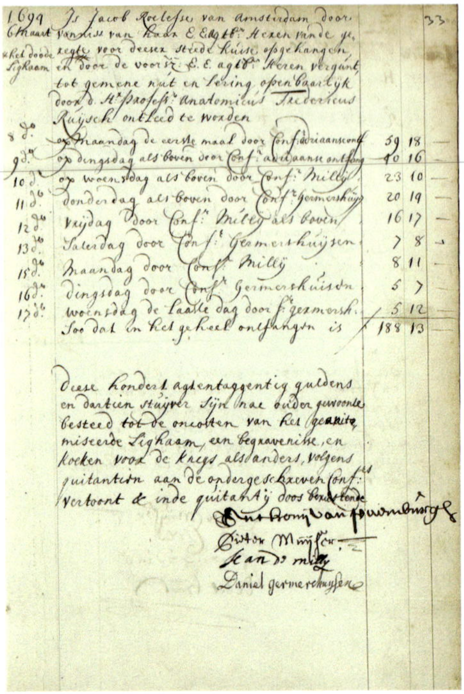

1694 Is Jacob Roelofse van Amsterdam door
6 Maart vonnisse van Heeren E. Edlagtb. Heeren van de ge-
het doode regte voor deeser stede huise opgehangen
Lighaam en door de voorsz. E. E. agtb. Heeren vergunt
tot gemene nut en leering openbaarlyk
door d. Hr Professr Anatomicus Fredericus
Ruysch ontleed te worden

8 do	op maandag de eerste maal door Confr Adriaansz ontf	59	18
9 do	op dingsdag als boven door Confr Adriaansz ontfang	40	16
10 do	op woensdag als boven door Confr Milly	23	10
11 do	donderdag als boven door Confr Germershuysen	20	19
12 do	vrijdag door Confr Milly als boven	16	17
13 do	Saterdag door Confr Germershuysen	7	8
15 do	maandag door Confr Milly	8	11
16 do	dingsdag door Confr Germershuisen	5	7
17 do	woensdag de laatste dag door Confr Germersh.	5	12
	Soo dat in het geheel ontfangen is	188	13

Deese hondert agtentaggentig guldens
en dartien stuyver sijn nae ouder gewoonte
besteed tot de oncosten van het geexecuteerde
Lighaam, een begravenisse, en
koeken voor de knegs als anders, volgens
quitantien aan de ondergeschreven Confrs
vertoont & inde quitantij door [illegible]

[illegible]
Pieter Muijser
Jan de Milly
Daniel Germershuysen

Report of the 1694 anatomy lesson in the Anatomy Book of the Surgeons' Guild. On a number of days, Ruysch delegated the dissection, or a part thereof, to the surgeons Jean de Milly or Pieter Adriaanszn. Municipal Archive Amsterdam.

Muijser, De Milly and Germershuysen. The fact that Ruysch was willing to delegate dissections only goes to show how much confidence he had in his student surgeons.

Hendrik Ruysch The boy standing next to Frederik Ruysch holding a foetal skeleton, is his son Hendrik (1673–1727). From an early age, Hendrik showed an interest in anatomy and botany. Before establishing himself as a physician in Amsterdam, he studied medicine in Amsterdam and Franeker. He regularly assisted his father with his lessons in anatomy, botany and obstetrics and he helped his father perfect his methods for preserving anatomical specimens. One of his father's students described Hendrik as 'your beloved and only son, a courageous successor and champion of his father's virtues, and a faithful companion of your work'. Following in Frederik Ruysch's footsteps, Hendrik was appointed chief obstetrician in Amsterdam, which gave him the authority to instruct midwives and to conduct their exams.

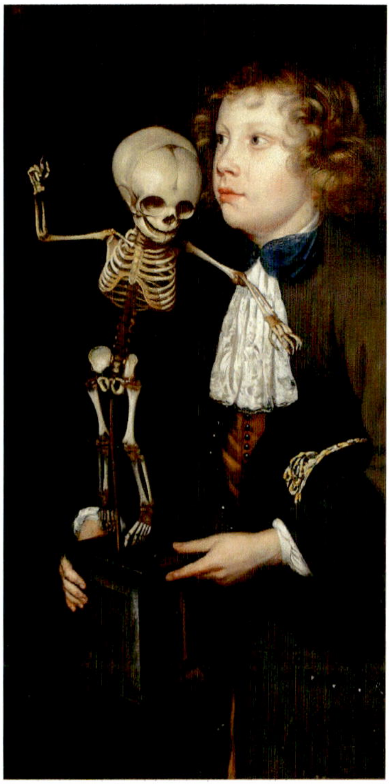

Despite his own skills and qualities, Hendrik always remained in the shadow of his famous father, and his life was not an easy one. Nearly twenty years after the painting was completed, he married the artist's daughter, Siebregje van Neck. Hendrik and his bride went to live on the Prinsengracht, opposite his old family home on the Bloemgracht in Amsterdam. Siebregje died five years later. Hendrik suffered regular bouts of depression and died at the age of fifty-four.

When the painting was completed in 1683, Hendrik was still a child. His presence on the canvas could indicate a more profound significance of the scene. Hendrik is holding a plinth on which a foetal skeleton is mounted, while he holds a hat under his left arm. With its left arm, the baby skeleton seems to be making a grabbing motion towards the hat, while with its right hand it points to the hat of the *praelector*: the one his father is wearing. In those days, wearing a hat was a privilege reserved for physicians. By its gesture, the skeleton is linking father and son and thereby suggesting that Hendrik was destined to follow in his illustrious father's footsteps. Undoubtedly, one of the specimens from Frederik Ruysch's collection will have served as the model for the tiny skeleton shown in the painting. A similar skeleton is still kept at the Peter the Great Museum for Anthropology and Ethnography (*Kunstkamera*) in St Petersburg.

Hendrik Ruysch (1673–1727)

The foetal skeleton in the painting is also a reference to the fabled technique developed by Ruysch in order to preserve the fragile skeletons. It was so refined, that it enabled him to retain even the most vulnerable ligaments and cartilage of the foetus. Last but not least, the small skeleton could also be an allusion to the symbol of vanitas (vanity), or the transitory nature of life in this world. All the foetal skeletons in Ruysch's museum were set in allegorical arrangements, expressing moral proverbs about the transient nature of our existence in accompanying texts written by Ruysch. In contrast to the gloomy *memento mori* – 'remember that you will die' –, the tiny skeleton in the painting is bursting with the joy of life.

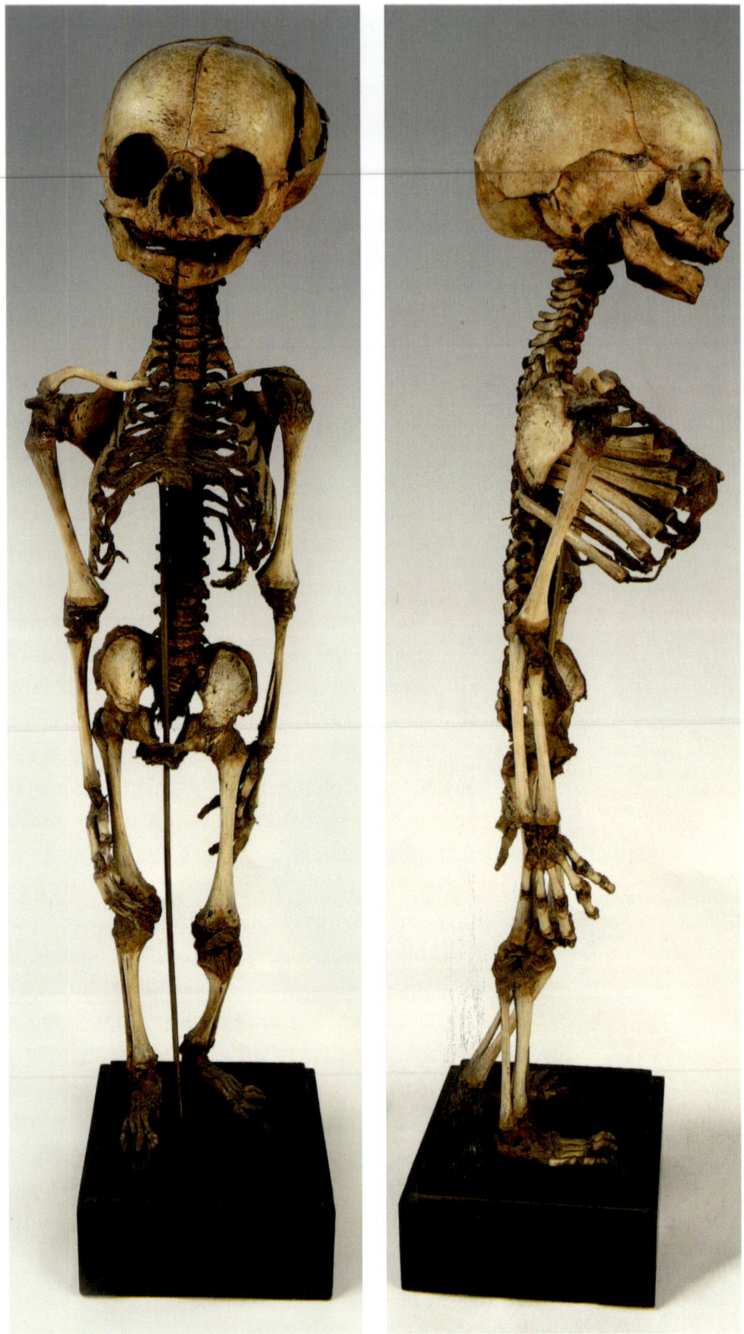

Foetal skeleton with meticulously preserved ligaments from Frederik Ruysch's collection. Peter the Great Museum of Anthropology and Ethnography (*Kunst-kamera*), Russian Academy of Sciences, St Petersburg.

▸ **The Corpse** The identity of the baby whose body features in the painting is unknown. The search for its identity proved to be futile, because the painting cannot be related to any records of the anatomy lessons in the Guild's Anatomy Book. It is a well-preserved body exhibiting no external signs of death; in fact, it looks more like a child peacefully asleep than the corpse of a child. This idealized representation of the body is also a characteristic element in Adriaen Backer's 1670 portrait (see p. 142). The lifelike appearance of the newborn child on the dissection table is perhaps symbolic of Ruysch's expertise in the field of preservation techniques, which he used, as it were, to resurrect his anatomical specimens from the dead.

▸ **Anatomy** In the painting, Ruysch uses the dissected body of the child to draw attention to the foetus' blood circulation. After all, the presence of a properly functioning blood circulation was essential to the healthy development of the baby. In 1628, the British biologist and physician William Harvey (1578–1657) discovered how the circulatory system functioned in an adult. However, knowledge of the blood circulation of a foetus was still very limited. Ruysch devoted himself entirely to making the blood vessels visible. The blood circulation of the foetus was therefore a fitting theme for this anatomical lesson. Nowadays, it is known that oxygenated blood of the placenta, which Ruysch called the *moederkoek* in Dutch, is transported to the

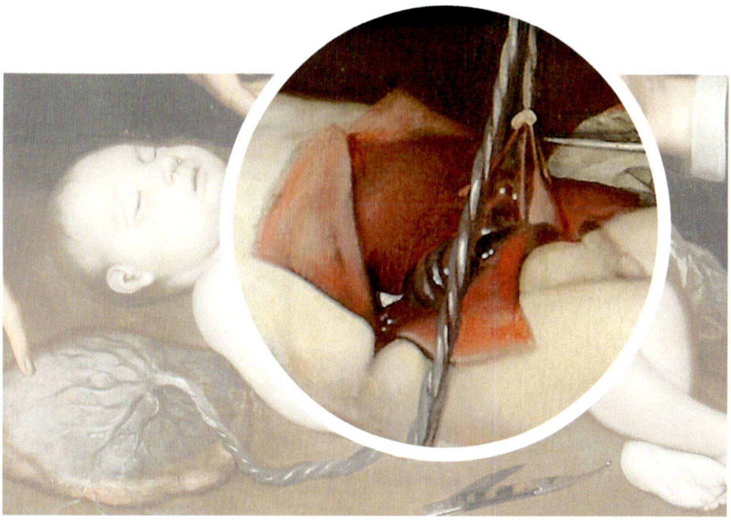

Anatomical structures in the abdomen of the child on the dissection-table.

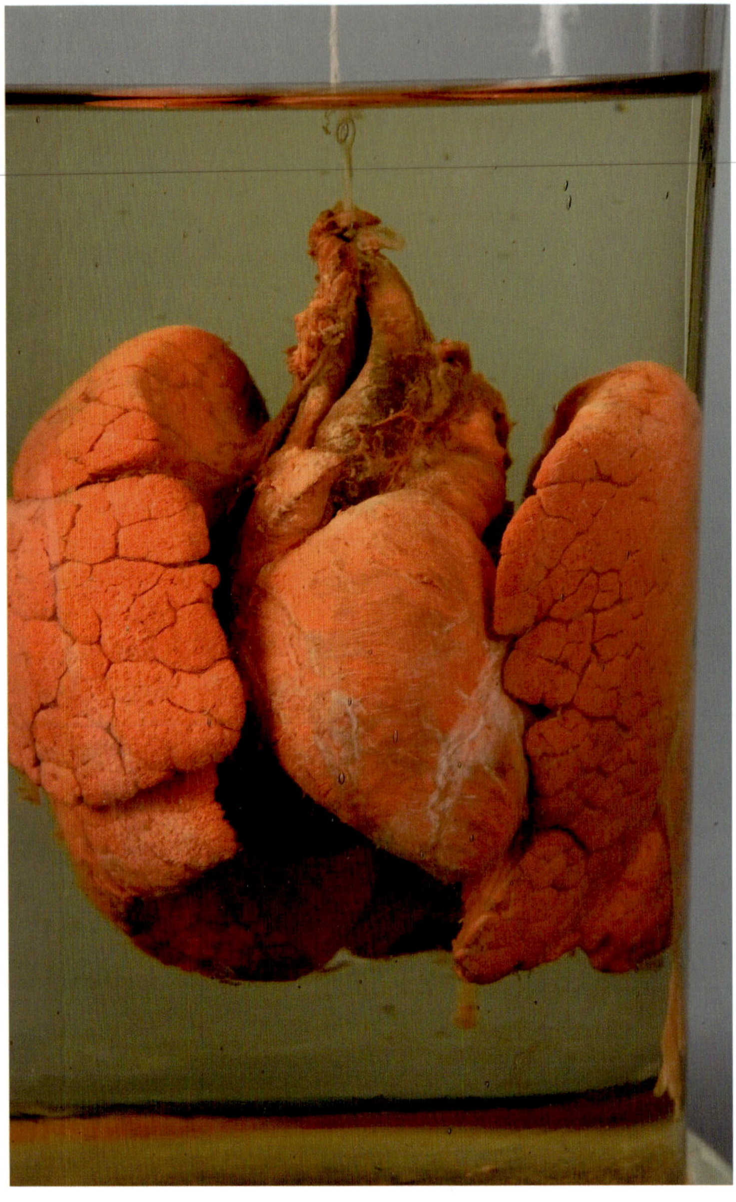

The heart and lungs of a newborn from the anatomical collection of Frederik Ruysch. The lungs have been injected with a waxy substance which gives them a rosy colour and allows them to retain their natural volume. Peter the Great Museum of Anthropology and Ethnography (*Kunstkamera*), Russian Academy of Sciences, St Petersburg.

7

Frederik Ruysch [2] *1683*

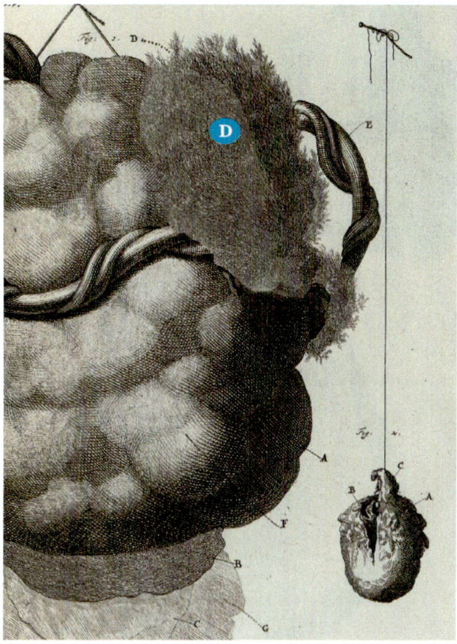

child through the umbilical vein and the deoxygenated blood flows back to the placenta through the paired umbilical arteries. The *urachus* is formed by a canal through which the urinary bladder of the foetus is drained. This structure is part of the umbilical cord and hence forms a connection between placenta and child.

In the first cabinet in his museum, Ruysch exhibited the prepared body of an unborn child that has not yet fully developed, whose umbilical cord and the urachus are clearly visible. The description of the specimen can be found in Ruysch's collected works. In the painting, the umbilical cord clearly consists of four parts, namely: the urachus and three blood vessels. The umbilical vein runs in the direction of the liver, which is shown to be located just above the middle of the abdomen. The spherical structure on a level with the child's pubis is the urinary bladder, which extends into the urachus and is flanked by the paired umbilical arteries. Just above the child's navel, these structures meet. The artist has given an adequate depiction of the various parts of the umbilical cord.

Illustration from the collected works of Frederik Ruysch indicating the various parts of the placenta. The membranes have been peeled back from an upper section of the surface of the placenta [D]. By doing this, Ruysch hoped to demonstrate that the placenta consisted largely of blood vessels. This was completely at odds with the general assumption that the placenta was largely made up of glands. C. Huijberts. From: *Alle de ontleed-, genees-, en heelkundige werken van Frederik Ruysch* (The complete anatomical, medical and surgical works of Frederik Ruysch), 1744.

In his anatomical collection, Ruysch kept a number of impressive specimens demonstrating the blood circulation in newborn babies. He also had mummified children's hearts in his museum. These specimens allowed him to demonstrate the blood vessel (*ductus arteriosus*) which connects the pulmonary artery to the aorta of a foetus. After the birth, its blood begins to flow through the lungs, upon which this blood-vessel should close on its own accord. Inside the heart of the foetus an open connection can be seen between the left and right atria of the heart (*foramen ovale*). This connection should also close shortly after birth. In its right hand, the newborn baby in the painting grasps the umbilical cord, as if it is holding on to his 'life-line' for dear life.

The gaze of the surgeon on the extreme left is fixed on the viewer of the portrait, as he draws our attention to the placenta's blood supply. The remaining amniotic membranes are still attached to the edge of the placenta. Ruysch studied the anatomy of the placenta down to the smallest detail. At the time, it was thought that

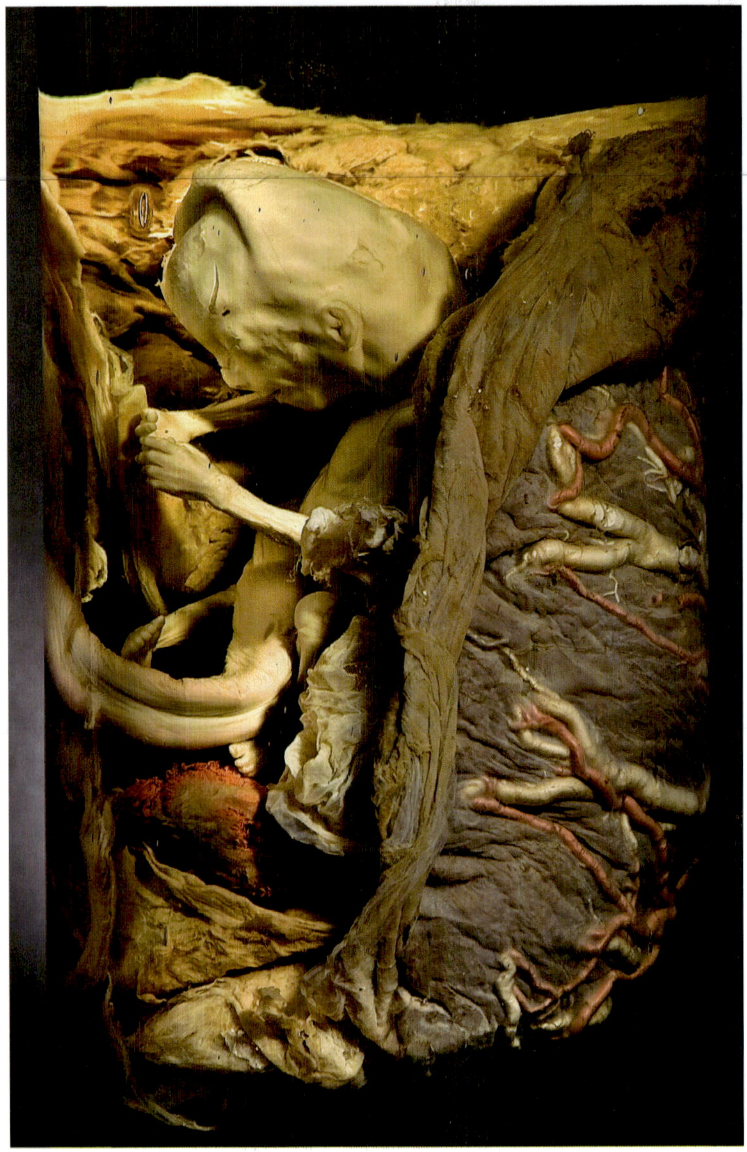

7

Frederik Ruysch [2] *1683*

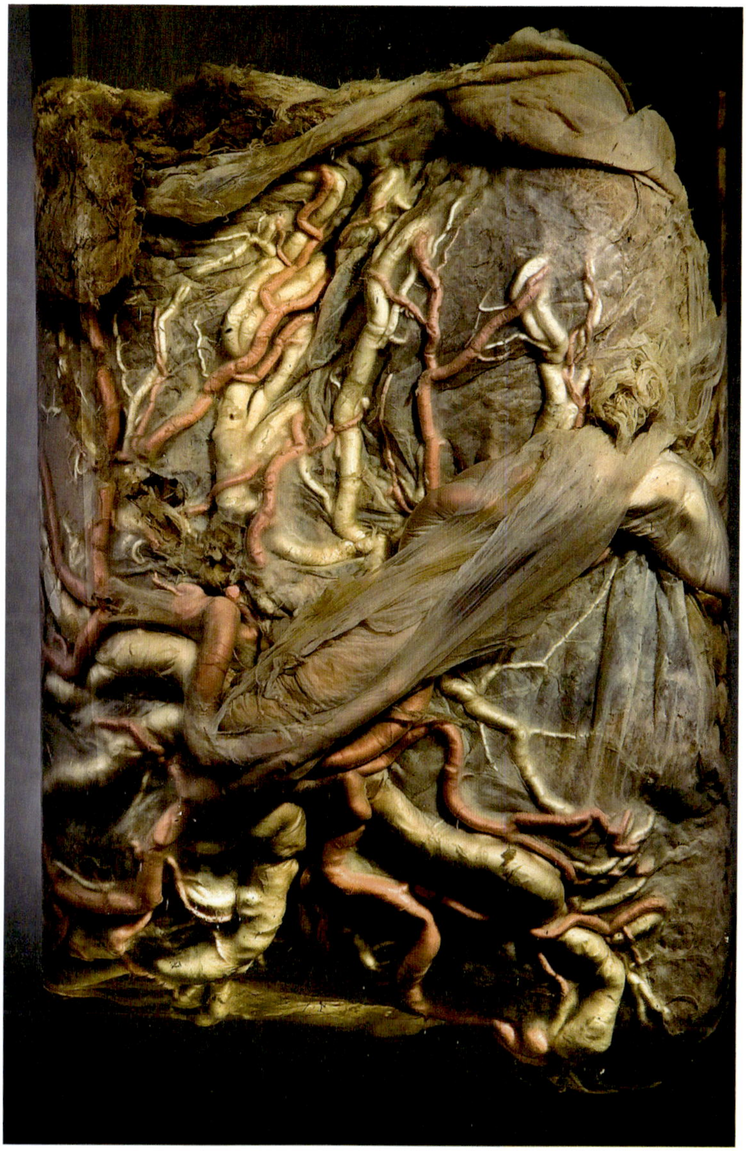

Left and right A three-month-old foetus with a placenta injected with coloured wax from the collection of Frederik Ruysch. Peter the great Museum for Anthropology and Ethnography (*Kunstkamera*), Russian Academy of Sciences in St Petersburg.

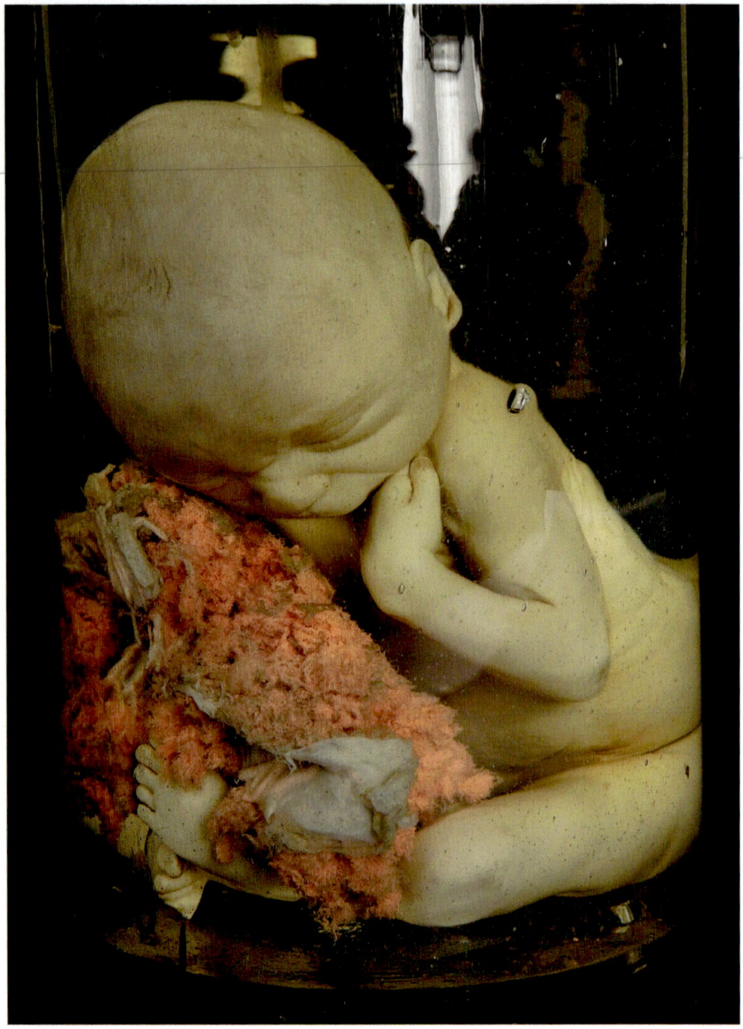

Foetus resting on its red-stained placenta, from the collection of Frederik Ruysch. Peter the great Museum for Anthropology and Ethnography (*Kunstkamera*), Russian Academy of Sciences in St Petersburg.

7

Frederik Ruysch [2] *1683*

the placenta primarily consisted of glands. With the aid of his injection techniques, Ruysch discovered that the placenta was mostly composed of blood vessels.

To this day, a number of the beautiful specimens of placenta that Ruysch preserved around three hundred years ago, are still kept at the *Kunstkamera* in St Petersburg. In this collection we came across a specimen of a three-month-old foetus whose placenta had been injected. Modern research methods have revealed that Ruysch composed a waxy substance consisting of glycerine and mercuric sulphide (cinnabar) to inject into the blood vessels. Ruysch made the distinction between the umbilical artery and the umbilical veins by using both red and white substances to inject into the placenta's blood vessels. The specimen clearly shows that the red (cinnabar) dye penetrated the smallest of capillaries on the maternal side of the placenta, which is situated against the uterine wall during pregnancy. This is distinctly revealed in the fine network of red-stained blood vessels close to the left foot of the foetus. Various placentas with similar colour combinations formed a part of his collection.

Ruysch's collection also contains the specimen of a small child resting on its own red-stained placenta. A fitting description which Ruysch attached to one of his specimens runs as follows: 'A small glass vessel containing liquid, and in it an immature foetus at around the fourth month of gestation, lying gently on the placenta instead of a pillow. It is of the male sex, and has retained its natural colour; its motto being: "Oh, how fortunate am I, now that my bones can lie at rest so peacefully!" Such sentiments were quite typical of Ruysch.

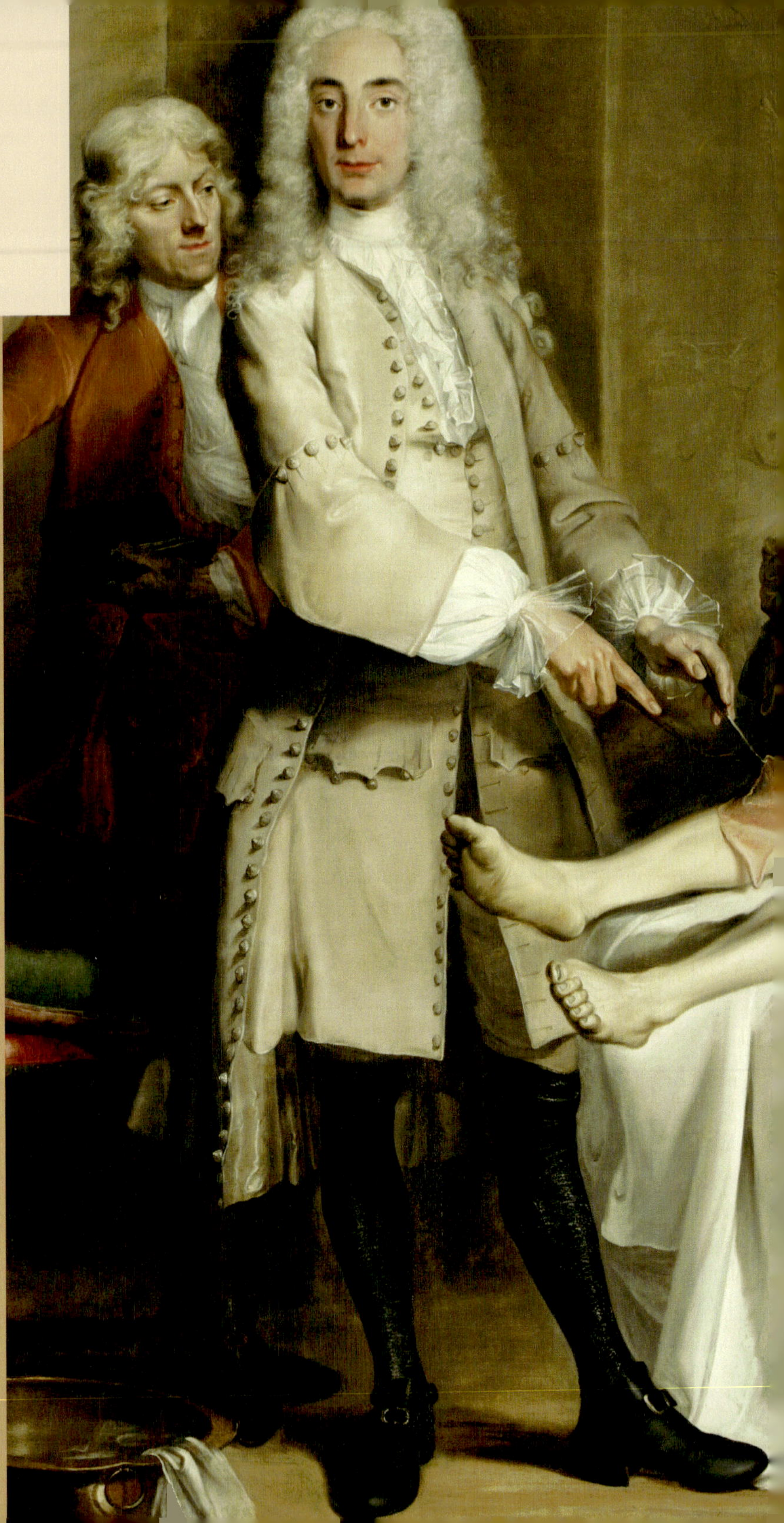

Cornelis Troost,
The Anatomy lesson of Willem Röell, 1728.
Collection Amsterdam Museum.

8

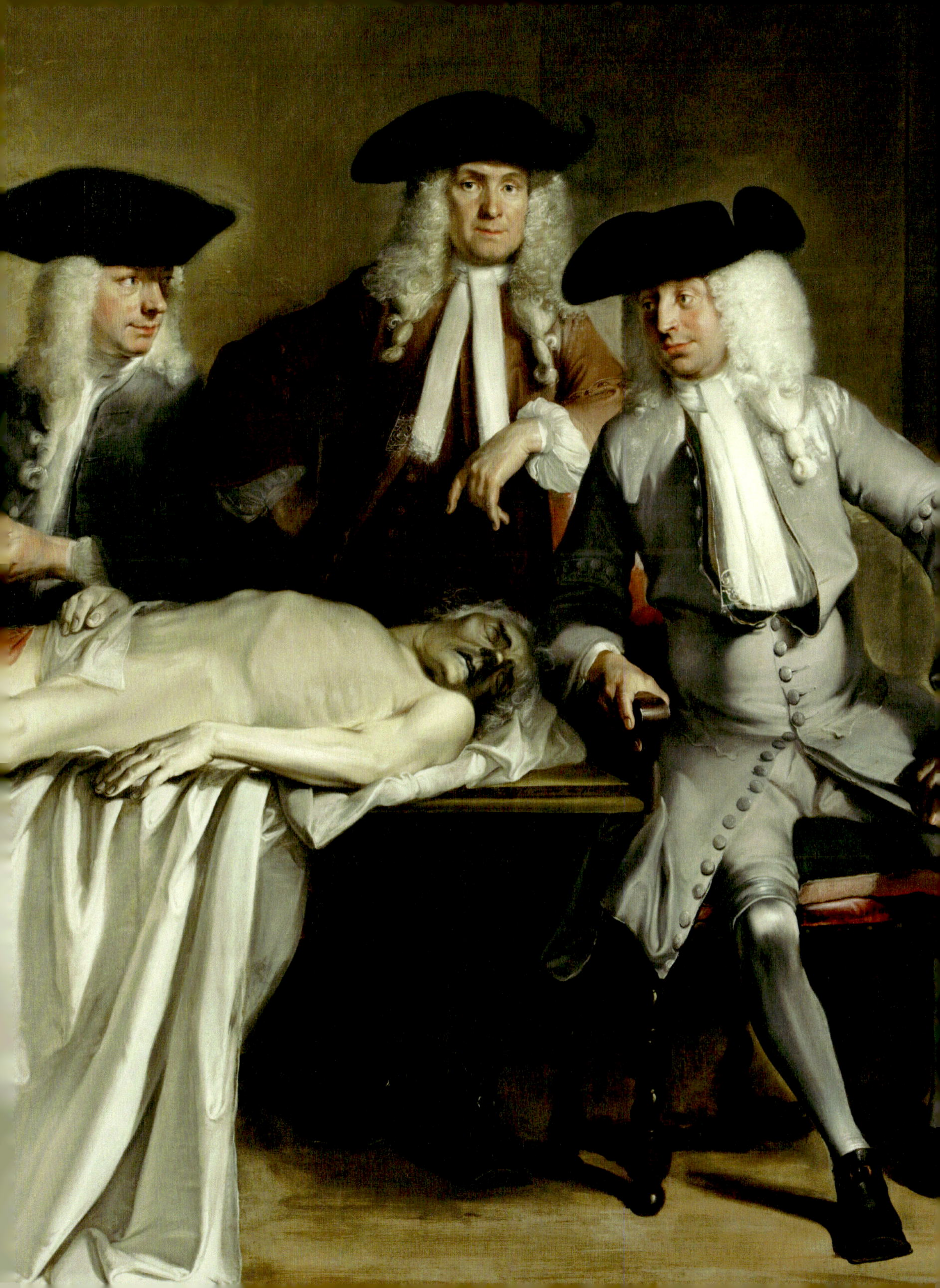

Willem Röell

The Anatomy lesson of Willem Röell, painted by Cornelis Troost in 1728

▸ **The Painting** In 1728, Cornelis Troost painted the eighth 'anatomy lesson' for the Amsterdam Surgeons' Guild: *The Anatomy lesson of Willem Röell*. The artist chose to place his signature along the edge of the dissection-table. In this fine group portrait, we see the *praelector* of the Guild, Willem Röell, dissecting the knee-joint of a dead man in the presence of three members of the Board and a Assistant Tutor (the *praelector*'s assistant).

Before Troost started on the group portrait, he made a sketch of the composition. This preliminary drawing reveals that he had grand ambitions for the painting. In the sketch, the anatomy lesson is being conducted in a framed niche on a raised platform. Behind the *praelector* is a staircase that leads to a tribune where three spectators are sitting. Troost was possibly toying with the idea of introducing a *Theatrum Anatomicum* into the composition. In the past, it has been suggested that, in his composition in the initial sketch, Troost was inspired by Rembrandt's *Anatomy Lesson of Jan Deijman* (see p. 109). The draft sketches of both paintings show some remarkable similarities, such as the niche in which the demonstrations take place, and the features of an anatomy theatre. Perhaps this painting by Troost was intended to replace that of Rembrandt which had hung in the Guildhall and had been seriously damaged by fire a few years earlier. Although Troost clearly had the ambition to create the composition of a grand masterpiece, in the end he decided against it. One possible reason for this, could be that the three potential spectators seated in the tribune had decided not to be included in the portrait because of the artist's fee that they would then no longer have to pay.

→
Cornelis Troost, sketch for *The Anatomy Lesson of Willem Röell*, 1728. Koninklijk Oudheidkundig Genootschap (Royal Antiquarian Society), Amsterdam.

In the end, the painting's final set-up was more modest than was conceived in the sketch. Nevertheless, the central section of the sketch does correspond well with the present painting. When the canvas

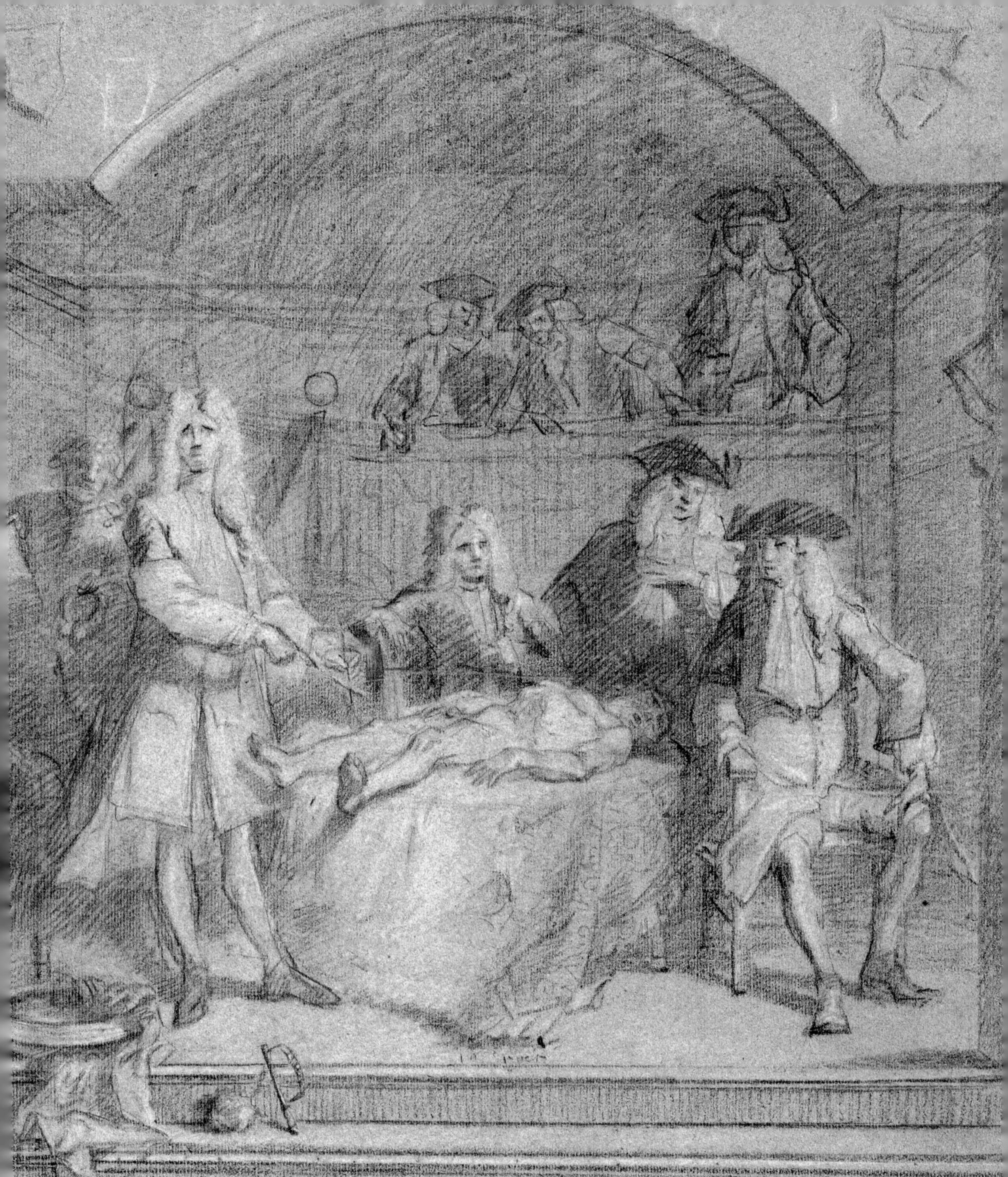

was reframed between 1965–1966, there were no indications that it had ever included the niche, the tribune, and the spectators. Whatever the case, the composition and the execution of this fine masterpiece were done beautifully. The painting is currently on exhibit at the Amsterdam Museum.

▸ **Artist** Cornelis Troost (1696-1750) was born in Amsterdam, the son of the goldsmith Johannes Troost and Barbara Mebeecq. In 1720 he married Susanna Maria van (der) Duyn with whom he had eight children. For a while, the couple lived in Zwolle, but by 1742 they resided on the Binnen-Amstel in Amsterdam and moved to the Prinsengracht in 1747. Susanna had an artistic background, in particular in the theatrical world, and Troost, too, was interested in theatrical arts: he worked in the Amsterdam Theatre, first as a stage designer and later as an actor. When he began, he was paid a fee of one guilder and five *stuivers,* but as time passed, he and his wife earned 6 guilders and 5 *stuivers* for each performance. In the decade of 1710–1720, Troost was taking painting lessons from the portrait painter Arnold Boonen (1669-1729). After 1724, when he began to build a reputation as an artist himself, he bid the stage farewell.

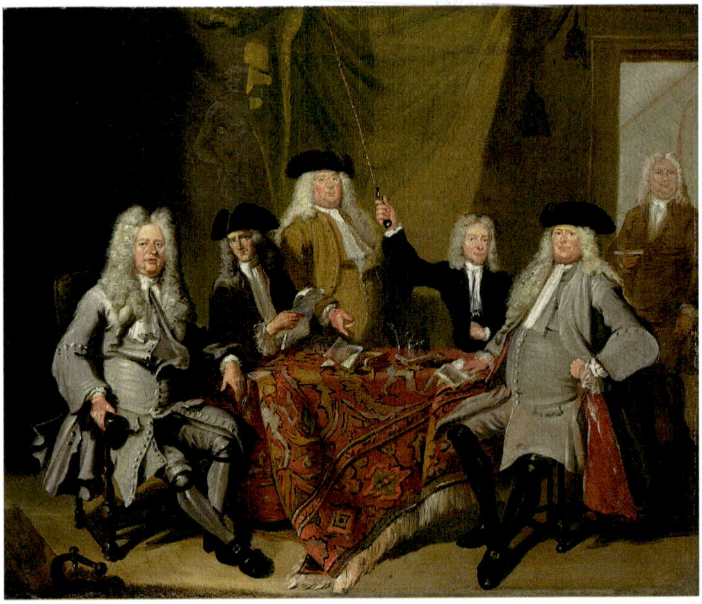

Cornelis Troost, *The Inspectors of the Collegium Medicum in Amsterdam,* 1724. Collection Rijksmuseum Amsterdam.

8 *Willem Röell* 1728

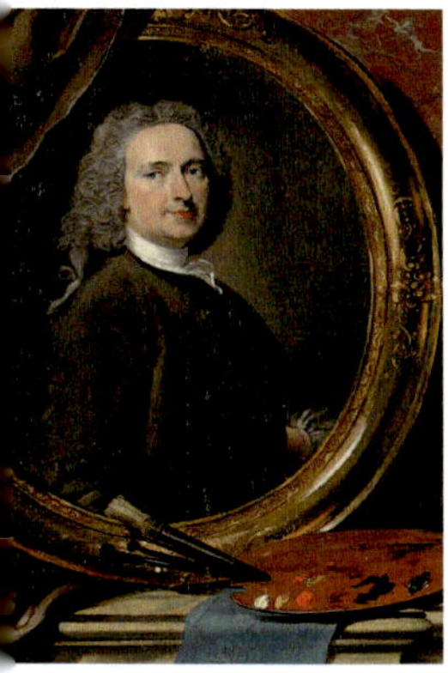

Cornelis Troost, *Self Portrait*, 1739, Collection Rijksmuseum Amsterdam.

Before being commissioned to paint *The Anatomy Lesson of Willem Röell*, Troost had already established his reputation as a portrait painter with the group portrait he made of the five inspectors of the *Collegium Medicum* (Medical Supervisory Board), the influential professional association of *doctores medicinae* and apothecaries living and working in Amsterdam. Four years later, the Amsterdam Surgeons' Guild asked him to paint *The Anatomy Lesson of Willem Röell*. This painting must have been greatly admired by the surgeons because, in 1731, the Guild gave him another commission, this time to paint the portraits of three members of the Board (see p. 224). Besides these three commissions, the Leiden physician and professor – Röell's teacher – Herman Boerhaave (1668–1738) had himself painted by Troost on several occasions. In 1729, Troost once again delivered another prestigious group portrait, this time of the Directors of the Aalmoezeniersweeshuis (Almoners' Orphanage) in Amsterdam. This enormous canvas, measuring more than four by four metres, shows the Directors of this charitable foundation and one orphan boy, arranged around a table set in a deep niche.

Troost's surviving oeuvre consists of around a thousand paintings, executed over a period of thirty years (c. 1720–1750). In a self-portrait

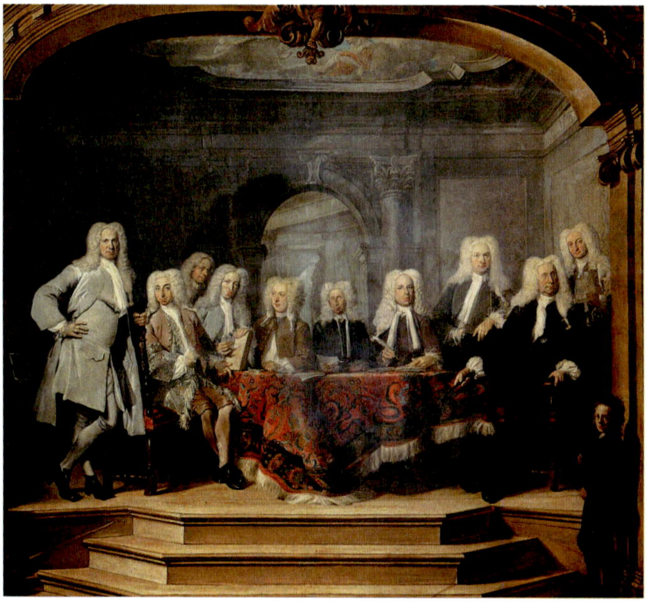

Cornelis Troost, *The Governors of the Benevolent Orphanage and Foundling Hospital in Amsterdam*, 1729. Collection Rijksmuseum Amsterdam.

painted in 1739, he presents himself as an artist; the artist's palette with brushes and the sketch in the foreground a sign of his profession. Troost's work includes a large number of individual portraits of men, women and children, as well as family portraits. His clientele had a wide range and included patrons such as Floris Drabbe (captain in the civic militia), Pietro Locatelli (musician), Johan Jacob Mauricius (Governor-General of Surinam), Isaac Sweers (town councilor and alderman, member of the Council of State (*Raad van State)* and member of the board of the Dutch East India Company [VOC]), Hubertus Vrijhoff (law professor) and Jan Six (burgomaster of Amsterdam). In the period 1733 to 1748, Troost also painted a large number of paintings based on theatrical scenes, including those of comedies and farces, revealing that his passion for the theatre had never truly died. The versatile, multi-talented Troost also produced biblical scenes, domestic interiors, views of cities and towns, military scenes and landscapes. After a prestigious career, he died at the age of fifty-four and was buried in the Nieuwe Kerk (New Church).

▸ **The Dissector** Willem Röell (1700–1775) was born in Franeker in Friesland, the son of the theologian Herman Alexander Röell and Cornelia Bailly. He studied medicine at the University of Leiden, where he earned his his degree of *doctor medicinae* in 1725. He then settled in Amsterdam. In 1733 he married Elisabeth de Farmars (1715–1780) with whom he had one son, Nicolaas.

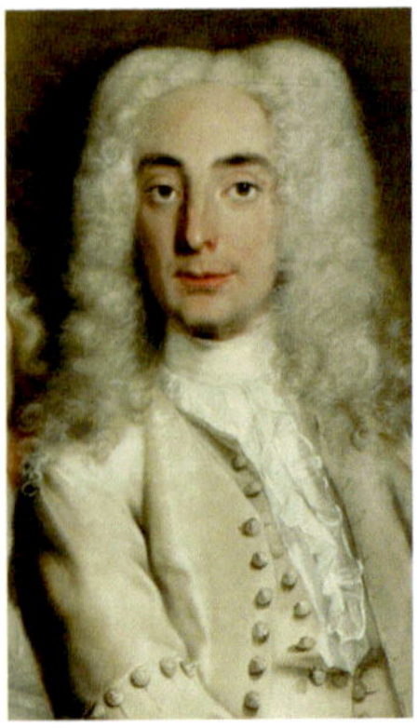

Willem Röell (1700–1775)

In 1727 Röell was appointed assistant to the very elderly Dr Frederik Ruysch. He had probably received very good references from Herman Boerhaave in Leiden, for in that same year, Röell took over the responsibility of the eighty-nine-year-old Ruysch for the surgeons' education, in fact, acting as interim *praelector anatomiae*. While in this position, he had his portrait painted by Cornelis Troost in *The Anatomy Lesson of Willem Röell*. In 1731, after Ruysch's death, Röell assumed most of Ruysch's duties and was officially installed as *praelector anatomiae* of the Amsterdam Surgeon's Guild, municipal obstetrician and forensic examiner. His colleague Johannes Burman (1706–1779), the physician and botanist, took over the Botany lessons given in the Amsterdam Botanical Garden (Hortus Botanicus).

According to the Anatomy Book of the Surgeons' Guild, Röell gave his first anatomy lesson on January 23rd, 1729. Interestingly enough, no anatomy lesson was recorded during the previous year, when

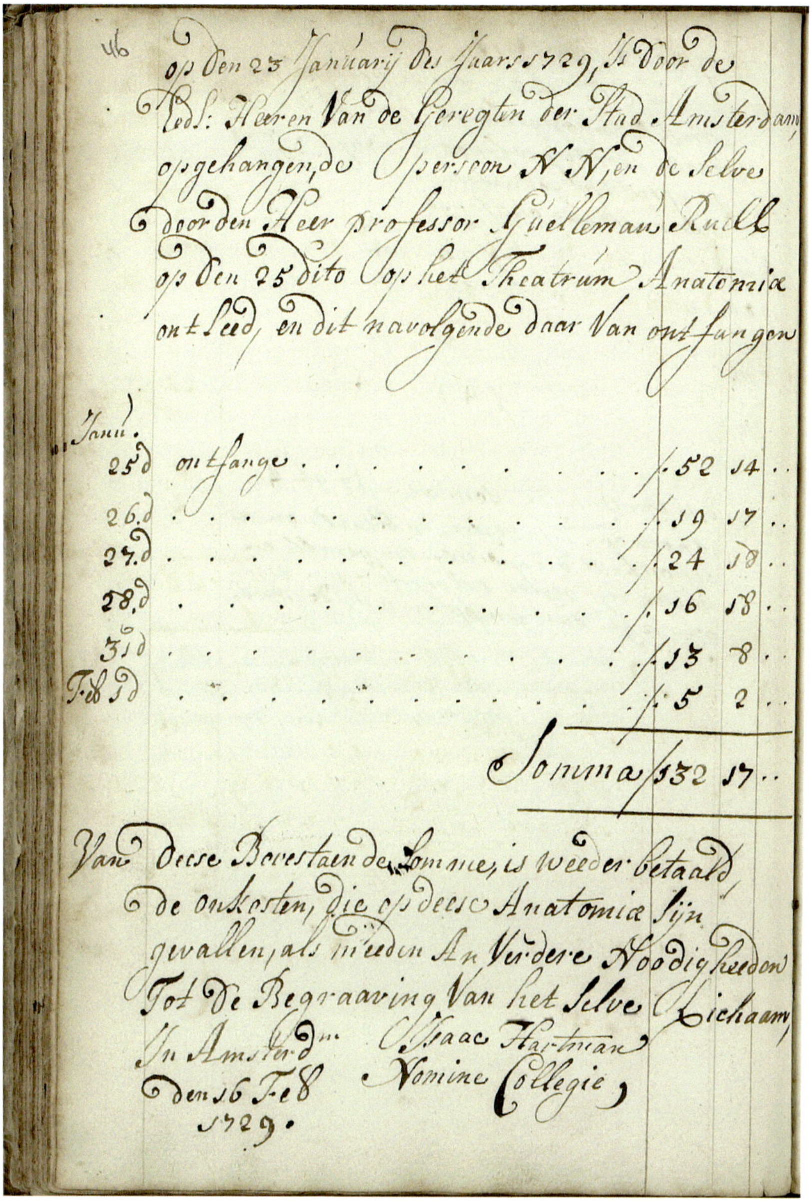

46

op den 23 January des Jaars 1729, is door de
Edl: Heeren van de Geregten der Stad Amsterdam,
opgehangen, de persoon N. N., en de selve
door den Heer professor Guelleman Ruell
op den 25 dito op het Theatrum Anatomiæ
ontleed, en dit navolgende daar van ontfangen

Janu. 25 d	ontfange	f. 52	14 ..
26 d		f. 19	17 ..
27 d		f. 24	18 ..
28 d		f. 16	18 ..
31 d		f. 13	8 ..
Feb 1 d		f. 5	2 ..
	Somma	f. 132	17 ..

Van deese Bovenstaende somme, is weeder betaald
de onkosten, die op deese Anatomiæ zijn
gevallen, als meeden an verdere Noodigheeden
Tot de Begraaving van het selve Lichaam,

In Amsterdm den 16 Feb 1729.

Isaac Hartman
Nomine Collegie,

Record in the Anatomy Book of the Surgeons' Guild of an anatomy lesson conducted by Willem Röell in 1729. Municipal Archive Amsterdam.

The Anatomy lesson of Willem Röell was painted. As early as 1705, his predecessor Ruysch had complained to the municipal council that not enough bodies were being made available for the anatomy lessons. Thereupon it was agreed that, from then on, in addition to the corpses of executed criminals, they would receive four bodies a year from the hospital for dissection purposes. From the time Ruysch had his last anatomy lesson and Röell his first, some six years passed in which the guild organized no anatomy lessons.

Brimming with confidence, Röell recommenced the anatomy lessons in 1729. In the spring of 1729, he dissected the corpse of the hanged criminal 'NN' in the Anatomy Theatre in the Weighing House. The lesson lasted six days and raised a total of 137 guilders. These funds were used to cover the costs incurred by the lesson, as well as those for the burial of the body. In March 1729, Röell gave an anatomy lesson using the body of a person who had died in the infirmary. The lesson lasted only three days and brought in a mere 28 guilders. He carried out a third anatomy lesson in December that same year on 'a female subject from the infirmary of this city'. This lesson was given in the context of training midwives. The sum raised by this lesson was so paltry — only 7 guilders — that the *Collegium Medicum* had to help cover the costs. In 1730 Röell had yet another executed criminal on his dissection-table. The corpse was that of a sheep thief who had been condemned to death by hanging for his offence. In 1731, Röell gave at least three lessons performed on bodies from the infir-

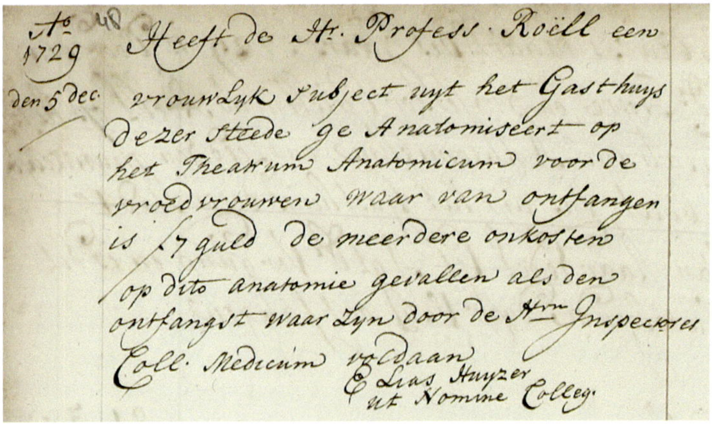
Ao 48
1729 Heeft de Hr. Profess. Röell een
den 5 dec. vrouwlyk subject uyt het Gasthuys
dezer Steede ge Anatomiseert op
het Theatrum Anatomicum voor de
vroedvrouwen waar van ontfangen
is f 7 guld de meerdere onkosten
op dito anatomie gevallen als den
ontfangst waar zyn door de Hrn Inspectores
Coll. Medicum voldaan
Elias Huyzer
ut Nomine Colleg.

Anatomy lesson for midwives given by Willem Röell in 1729. From: The Anatomy Book of the Surgeons' Guild. Municipal Archive Amsterdam

mary. Once again, one of these lessons was intended for the midwives. All that is known of the other lessons given that year is that they raised 89 and 47 guilders respectively, and that the *subjectum anatomicum* was a man. These were the last records in the Surgeons' Anatomy Book of the anatomy lessons given by Röell.

In the time that Röell was *praelector*, the Surgeons' Guild went through a period of great turmoil and unrest. It had come to light that for quite a number of years, the governors had been fraudulent in the issuing of graduation certificates to surgeons who were not properly qualified, and that they had been embezzling money from the treasury. The newly appointed Head of the Guild, Abraham Titsingh, had brought the whole affair out into the open in 1732, resulting in the dismissal of the entire Board, with the exception of Titsingh. The standard of the surgeons' education deteriorated as a result. The Minutes recorded at that time regularly made note of irregularities at the *Theatrum Anatomicum:*

> [...] *the brethren of the guild shall be reprimanded that they, whilst at the location of the Anatomy Theatre, should respect each other and eschew all disorderliness, so that kindness and tranquility will prevail. Refusal to pay fines [and] fisticuffs during the public anatomy lessons were a regular occurrence, while the name-calling and verbal abuse, recorded in the minutes in all its detail, were of such nature, that it would be quite inappropriate for it to be repeated here.*

In the time that Röell was *praelector*, the standard of education left much to be desired and it appears that Röell himself was regularly absent during the final surgeon's qualifying exams. Furthermore, his anatomical lessons were reputed to have been noisy and disorderly. Abraham Titsingh was concerned — probably righty so — about the deterioration of the quality of the education, as well as the surgical care in Amsterdam. In 1730, he even felt compelled to write a book on this problem with the appropriate title *Het verdonkerde heelkonst der Amsterdammers* (The Eclipsed Surgery of the People of Amsterdam).

Röell found himself in a difficult position: on the one hand he was the *praelector* of the Surgeons' Guild, while on the other hand he was — simultaneously — the inspector of the *Collegium Medicum,* the body that represented the *doctores medicinae* (physicians). These two parties were often at odds with one another, while Röell himself often played a part in these conflicts. In 1746, he proposed that 'no one in the city be permitted to hang a signboard announcing his profession as obstetrician on his door, unless, he has been authorized to do so by the Burgomasters upon passing a prior examination conducted by the Professor of Anatomy and the Inspectors of the Medical Supervisory Board'. This did not go down well, as traditionally, obstetrics fell under the responsibility of the Surgeons' Guild, which naturally thought it utter nonsense that 'the examination of Obstetricians' should be handed over to the *Collegium Medicum*. This, plus a fair number of other differences of opinion, probably led to Röell's announcement in 1755 that he wished to resign as *praelector*. However, his resignation was not accepted straightaway, and he therefore continued to preside over the surgical exams for some time. Petrus Camper was appointed new *praelector* to serve alongside Röell. He was made responsible for the theoretical education and the anatomy lessons.

In 1755, Röell was appointed professor of Anatomy at the *Athenaeum Illustre*, what would later become the University of Amsterdam. Seven years later he retired altogether. His coat of arms is painted in the vaulted dome of the former Anatomy Theatre, bearing the inscription: 'W. Röell Anat et Chir Prof, testifying to the prominent positions he filled.

Röell was a wealthy man whose wealth was in part acquired through his wife's inheritance. In 1739, he bought a house on the

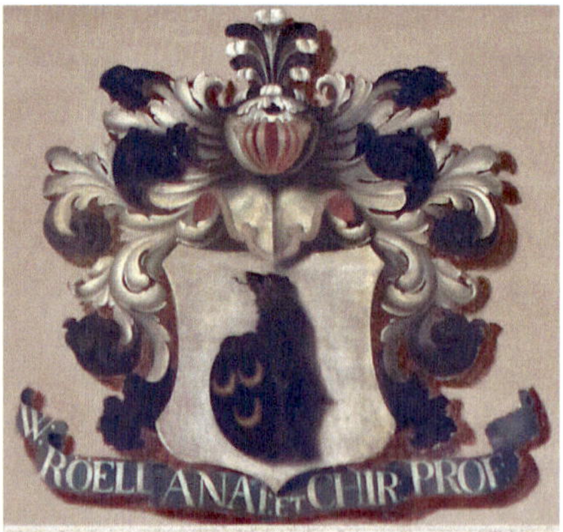

Coat of arms of Willem Röell in the vault of the dome of the Anatomy Theatre at the Weighing House on Nieuwmarkt in Amsterdam.

Keizersgracht for 54,000 guilders (equivalent to 570,000 Euros today). Besides this property, he purchased a country estate on the Keukenhof Estate near Lisse. This estate entailed more than just a villa: it also had stables, a coach house, a gardener's lodge and the farmstead Keukenhof. Nowadays, Keukenhof is famous for its large horticultural park which attracts hundreds of thousands of tourists every year. In 1768, Röell sold the entire estate for 18,000 guilders (175,000 Euros today). Outside of the Netherlands, he also owned two plantations in the colony of Berbice (present British Guyana), where they grew coffee, cacao and cotton. He also filled a number of other posts, such as that of member of the board of the West India Company (WIC), and Director of the Society of Surinam. Röell lived in Utrecht for the rest of his life, where he died in 1755.

▸ **The Surgeons** The three members of the Board who can be seen at the corpse's head in *The Anatomy Lesson of Willem Röell* held office from September 1727 to September 1728. The other three administrators already had their likenesses painted in the group portrait of directors painted by Arnold Boonen (Troost's teacher (see p. 222) in 1715–1716). The three directors on Troost's painting are, from left to right: (probably) Theodorus van Brederode, Anthoni Milaan and Bernardus van Vijve. We know their names from the notes made by the surgeon Monnikhoff, who had copied old pieces of text from the now lost *Groot-Memoriael Gildeboek* (Large Memorandum Book) from 1750. Van Brederode was the first of the three to be appointed Head of the Guild in 1725, while Anthoni Milaan and Bernardus van

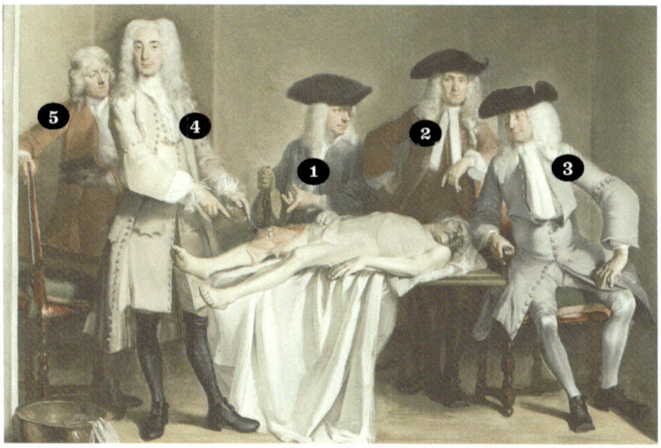

Those portraited in *The Anatomy Lesson of Willem Röell*:

1 Theodorus Van Brederode*
2 Anthoni Milaan*
3 Bernardus van Vijve*
4 Willem Röell
5 Pieter Cleeveringh van Vijve

* The identification of Directors numbered 1 to 3 is based on strong assumptions.

Vijve joined the board two years later. Just above the head of the director portrayed in the middle, the small figure 2 can be seen, while above the head of the director on the far right of the figure 3 is seen. One would therefore expect the number 1 to have appeared above the leftmost governor. There is a very good chance that – on the grounds of seniority – Theodorus van Brederode assumed the number 1 position. After all, he was the longest-sitting member of the Board of Directors. It is therefore highly likely that the other two men follow the sequence in places two and three, in the order in which Monnikhoff mentions them. The man behind Willem Röell is Pieter Cleveringh, Bernard van Vijve's stepson. He held the position of Assistant Tutor, a lesser function that one can ascertain from his subordinate position in the painting, and the small case of surgical instruments he is holding in his hand.

All three directors depicted in the painting are wearing hats, which is somewhat remarkable, as at previous anatomy lessons, the wearing of a hat was the exclusive privilege of the *praelector anatomiae*, a *doctor medicinae* with considerable status. In the *Anatomy Lesson of Nicolaes Tulp*, Rembrandt even had to paint over the hat worn by one of the surgeons for this reason (see p. 96). The elegant dress worn by the gentlemen is also worth mentioning. In earlier paintings, the surgeons either wore sober dark coats, or academic gowns. The stylish clothing is a recurring theme in Troost's work and is always according to the latest fashion of that time. Often, men would also wear the so-called tricorn hat, a hat with three collapsible brims. Later, around 1750, the fashion changed and it became more usual to carry the tricorn in the hand or under the arm, allowing one's wig and face to be seen to their best advantage. The sketch shows that the surgeon who is closest to the dissected knee, was originally painted without a hat. In the final version of the painting, however, Troost gave him a hat, perhaps to conform to the fashionable ideal and the appropriateness of dress at the time.

In the *Anatomy Lesson of Willem Röell*, the three directors proudly pose in their fine apparel, but none of them could have known that the tide would soon turn for them. As respectable are they might appear in the painting, things were quite to the contrary: they were corrupt to the bone in the awarding of surgeon's graduation certificates, and they were embezzling money from the Guild treasury. In 1732, they were all exposed, and all the sitting members of the

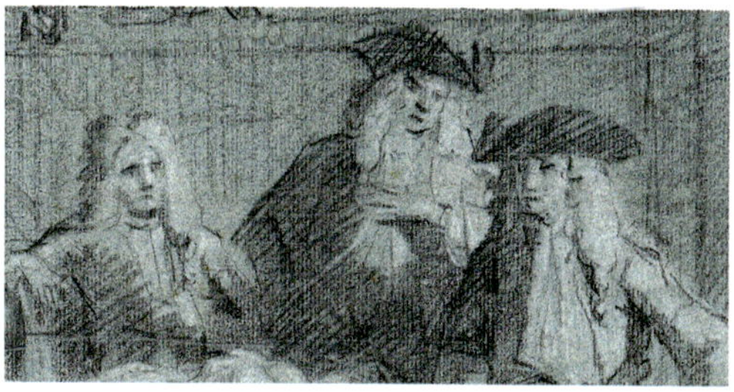

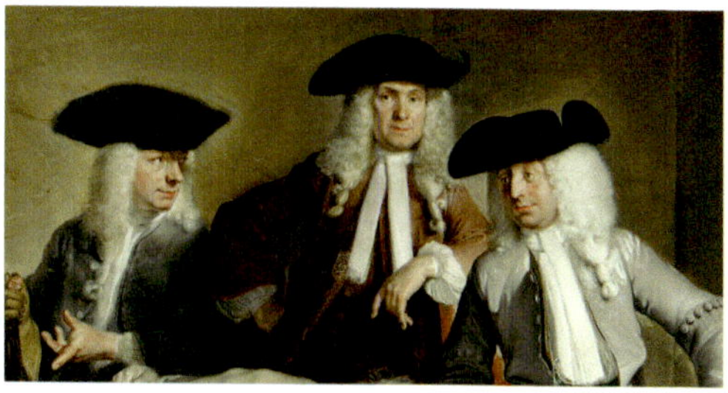

Comparison between the three directors on the sketch (see p. 175) and the completed work of *The Anatomy Lesson of Willem Röell* (see p. 172). In the final version, Troost had given the director on the far left a hat.

Board of that year as well as a number of former directors – among them the three directors depicted in the *Anatomy Lesson of Willem Röell* – were dismissed and no longer eligible for any future nomination. It turned out that they had stolen more than 30,000 guilders (equivalent to 325,000 Euros) from the Guild's coffers. A portion of that money was intended for the pensions of surgeons' widows, who were only receiving one guilder a month, instead of the three guilders a week to which they were entitled. And instead of the statutory three guilders which Guild members were required to contribute every year, they were made to pay five. The corruption affair inspired a stream of satirical poems and pictures. One such example is this poem from the anthology *Lauwerkransen* (Laurel Wreaths):

> *To the painter Troost on account of the work of art,*
> *As painted by him at the Surgeons' Guildhall.*
> *Descendant of Apolles, I see before me a delightful Scene,*
> *Your art defies nature and will endure,*
> *Just as Orpheus is deserving of honour; your artist's paint brush,*
> *Placed on the blue dome of sparkling fires*
> *You only concerned yourself with the son of Asclepius*
> *Your fame would be loftier.*
> *The rest do not deserve to have their image displayed alongside his,*
> *Ignoramuses of the Art* [of surgery], *unworthy of praise:*
> *No, Artist Troost, cover the rest of this scene,*
> *Only His image shall be immortalized by your Brush.*

People were particularly vehement in their criticism of Bernardus van Vijve (1684–1759). His career at the Surgeons' Guild was over, but he had the good fortune that, as a surgeon, he was still permitted

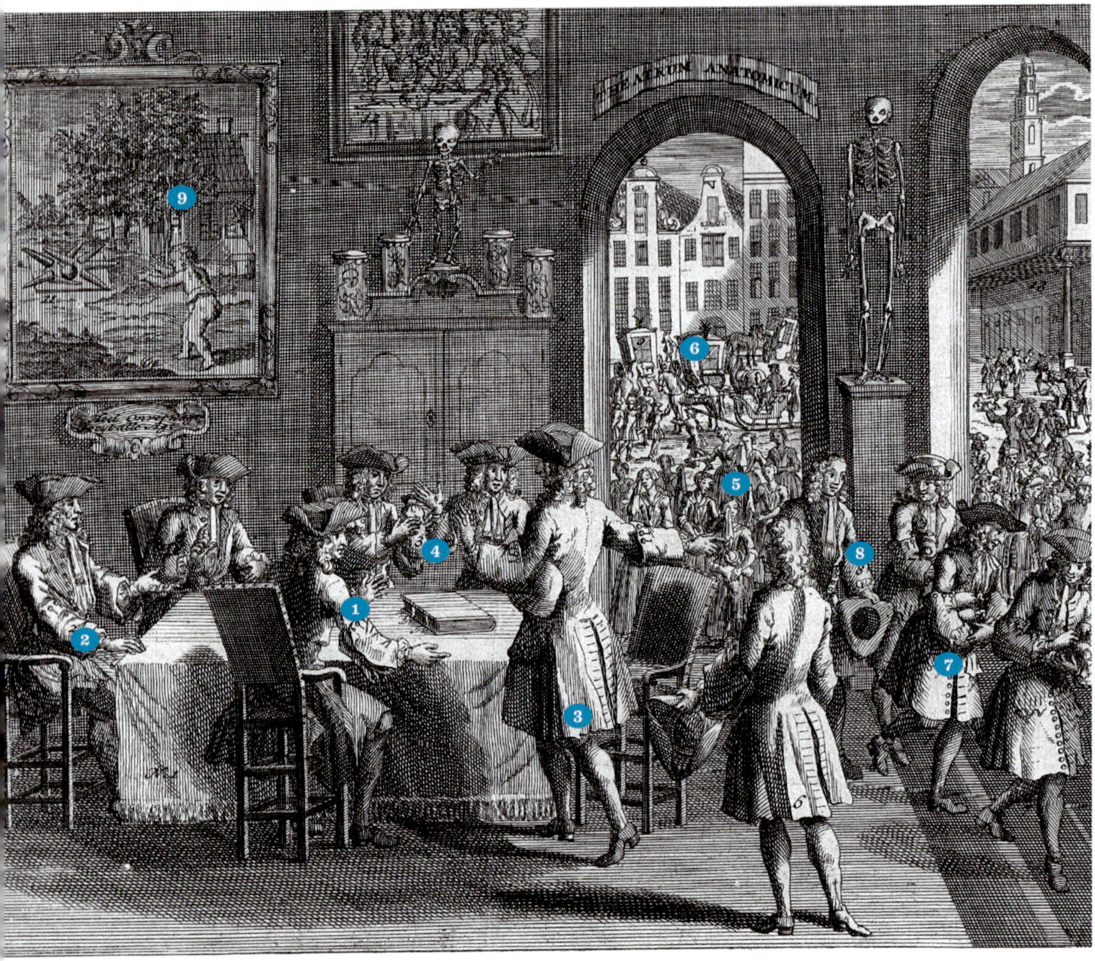

Anonymous artist, satirical print about the sacking of the Board of Directors of the Surgeons' Guild, c. 1732. Rijksmuseum Amsterdam.

Sitting at the table are the corrupt directors [1] and [2]. They are trying to bribe the incorruptible Abraham Titsingh [3] with a bag of money [4]. Just beyond the arch bearing the inscription *Theatrum Anatomicum,* the grieving surgeons' widows gather, having been deprived of their money by the fraudsters [5]. Behind them, we catch a glimpse of the far too expensive carriages belonging to the surgeons [6]. On the right, a few corrupt directors try to leave the Guildhall with bags of money clutched in their hands [7]. They are being ushered out by the Guild servant, who is a part of the conspiracy [8]. On the wall to the left, hangs an allegorical painting of a child who has just knocked over all the skittles in a game [9]. This symbolizes Titsingh overthrowing the corrupt Board of Directors.

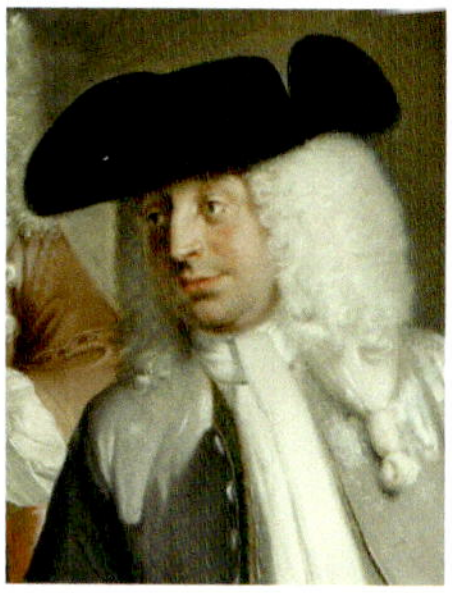

Bernardus van Vijve (1684–1759)

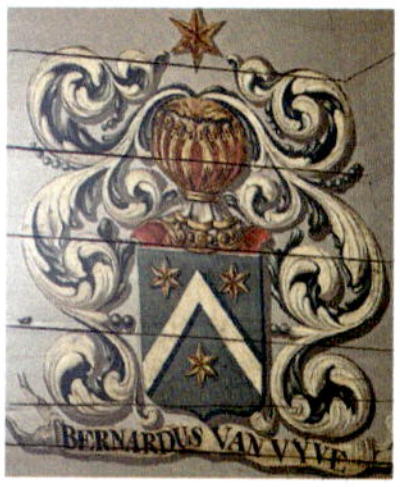

Coat of arms of Bernardus van Vijve, painted on the vault of the dome of the Weighing House.

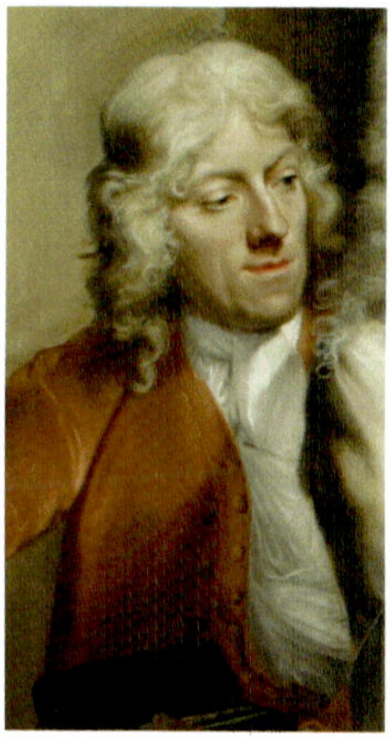

Pieter Cleeveringh van Vijve (1697–1770)

to treat a number of patients in the plague hospital. Despite the fact that his career ended in an infamous way, his coat of arms still adorns the vault dome of the former *Theatrum Anatomicum* at the Weighing House. Shortly after the scandal broke, more satirical poems were written about him. Not only is he depicted in these as a thief, his controversial marriage to Margaretha Schrick (1675–1758) is also ridiculed in detail. Supposedly he used this widow, who was nine years his senior, in order to get his hands on her late husband's surgeon's shop (on the corner of the Binnen Vissersstraat and the Brouwersgracht). Allegedly he had also been unfaithful to his wife. One of the poems about Van Vijve from the *Lauwerkransen* anthology runs as follows:

Cursed Deceiver, are you the reason,
That the Directors are purloining from the Guild coffers,
And share in all the Guild money like thieves?
Are you, oh Renegade, therefore also a Director,
If so, I wish that the Executioner had your healthy bones
Broken on the scaffold a good long time ago.
This is what you deserve, even doubly so,
When you gave your word to a daughter whom you did not intend to maintain,
But bought her off and went and married the "Miss"
Who had first been your whore, why should such a rogue be spared
To be among those directors whose names are as yet untarnished,
And take to the helm as a thief, reigning over the Arts of Healing.

In 1741, after thirty years of marriage to Margaretha Schrick, Bernardus headed for the hills, disappearing for good. On Sunday February 5th of that year, he told his wife that he was going to attend a church service in the Gasthuiskerk but, neither she nor their children ever heard from him again. A month later, Van Vijve turned up in Bruges, where he reported to the local Surgeons' Guild on March 21st. In Bruges he managed to become dean (chairman) of that guild. He died in 1759.

Pieter Cleeveringh van Vijve (1697–1770) — the Assistant Tutor on the far left of the painting — didn't turn out any better than his step-father, Bernardus van Vijve. Pieter tried to earn some extra money by making some shady business deals. By sweet-talking surgeons' widows who were still overwhelmed with grief by the death of their husbands, he tried to talk them into handing over their late spouses' surgeons' shops to him for a pittance. He subsequently tried to sell these shops at a profit to surgeons who were still 'wet behind the ears or bald and stupid'. A couple of his advertisements from the *Amsterdamsch Courant* of 18 March and 10 June read as follows:

> *A thriving Surgeon's Shop for sale, complete with medicine chest, some Surgeon's Instruments, with two Surgeon's signboards: Enquiries to Pieter Cleeveringh van Vijve, Qualified Surgeon and Chief Tutor on the Roosegracht in Amsterdam.*
>
> *For sale, a Surgeon's Shop at a prime location in Amsterdam, equipped with Shop furnishings and a goodly clientele for barbering, with a residence to be rented immediately; enquires to Pieter Cleeveringh van Vijve.*

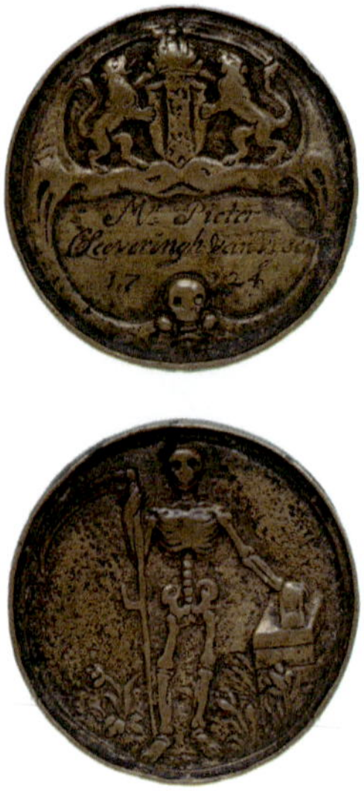

Token with the name Pieter Cleeveringh van Vijve, dating from 1724. Private Collection.

When his activities were exposed, Pieter resigned from the Guild. A very fine guild token which once belonged to him has been preserved as a souvenir of his time with the Guild. He was presented with this token of membership, known as a *presentie-penning*, when he qualified as a surgeon in 1724. Despite his failed career with the Surgeons' Guild, he still prospered after the scandal. In 1742 his annual income was 2,500 guilders. In 1768 he could afford to live on the Prinsengracht, where he died two years later.

▸ **The Corpse** The corpse is portrayed quite realistically. The pallid skin and the blue lips are characteristic of the lifeless condition of the *subjectum anatomicum*. However, the Surgeons' Anatomy Book makes no mention at all of an anatomy lesson in 1728. Hence, it is impossible to trace the man's name.

▸ **Anatomy** Röell has peeled back the skin from the knee and thigh in order to reveal the joint. The tissue which he holds back with a small hook is connected to the shin and the knee-cap. Logically, this would have been done to show part of the tendon between the shin (*tibia*) and the knee-cap (*patella*), the patellar tendon. In order to get a good look at the knee joint, as Röell is doing, it is necessary to sever some of the *ligamentum patellae* and the knee tendon (*retinaculum*

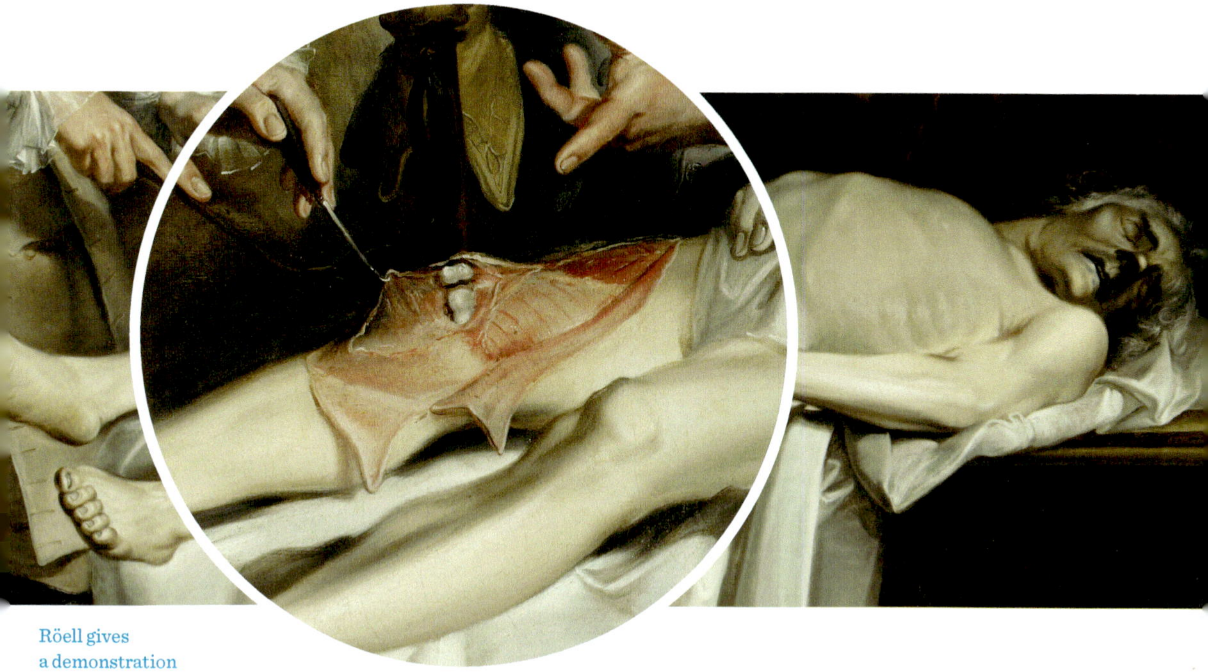

Röell gives a demonstration of the anatomy of the knee.

patellae mediale) longitudinally and push the knee-cap aside. It seems that this is what Röell has done. The picture gives us a glimpse of part of the surface of the joint of the thigh bone (*femur condyls*). At its extremity the thigh bone has two condyles that rest on the surface of the joint of the lower leg (*tibia plateau*). In the joint there are both a lateral and a medial meniscus, plus an anterior cruciate ligament and a posterior cruciate ligament. These are not visible to the onlooker. The anatomical structures in the painting might give a general impression of the anatomy of the area around the knee joint, but they are not an exact representation of reality. Nobody knows why Röell chose this specific dissection of the knee joint, and not some other part of the body.

9

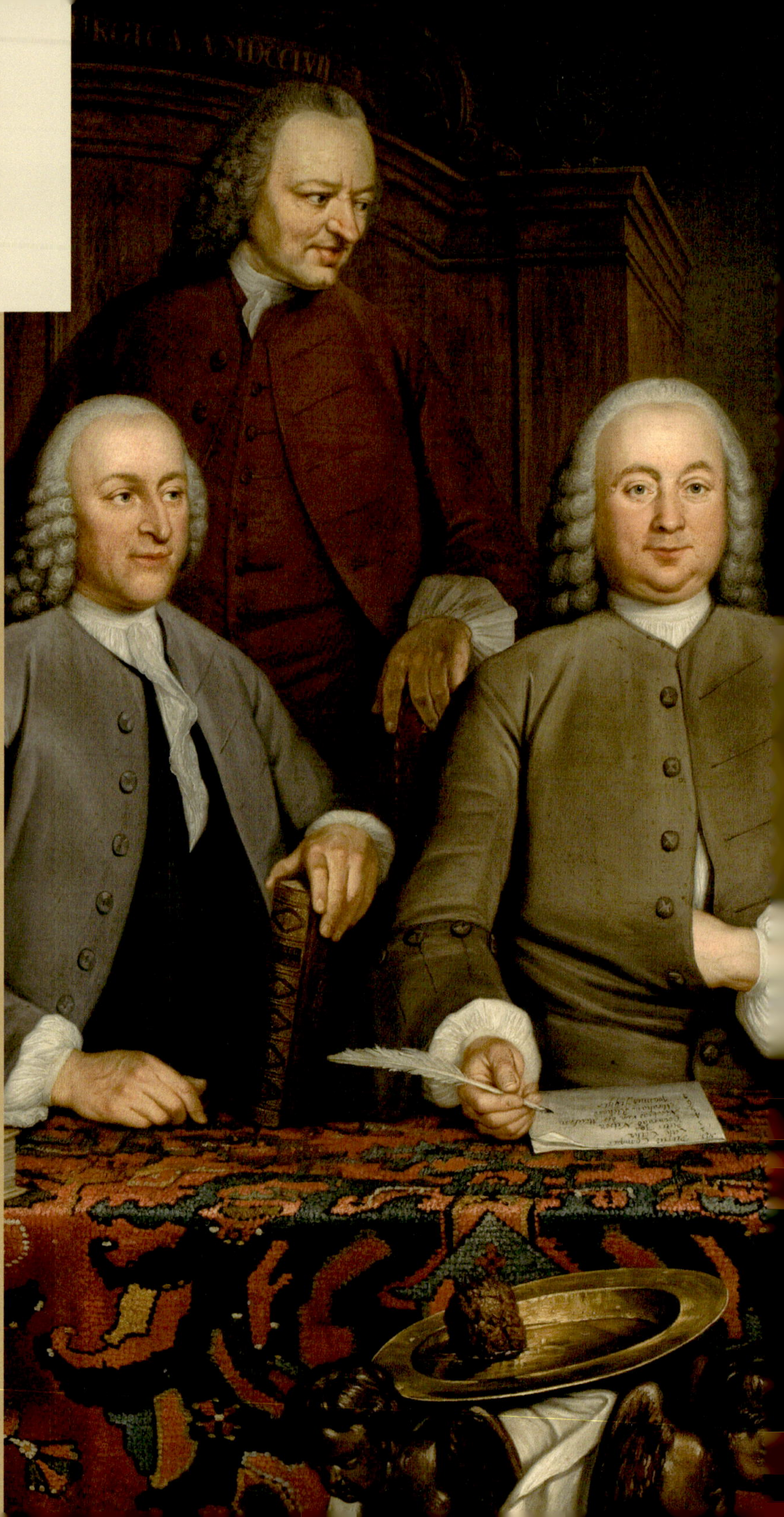

Tibout Regters, *The Anatomy Lesson of Petrus Camper*, 1758. Detail. Collection Amsterdam Museum.

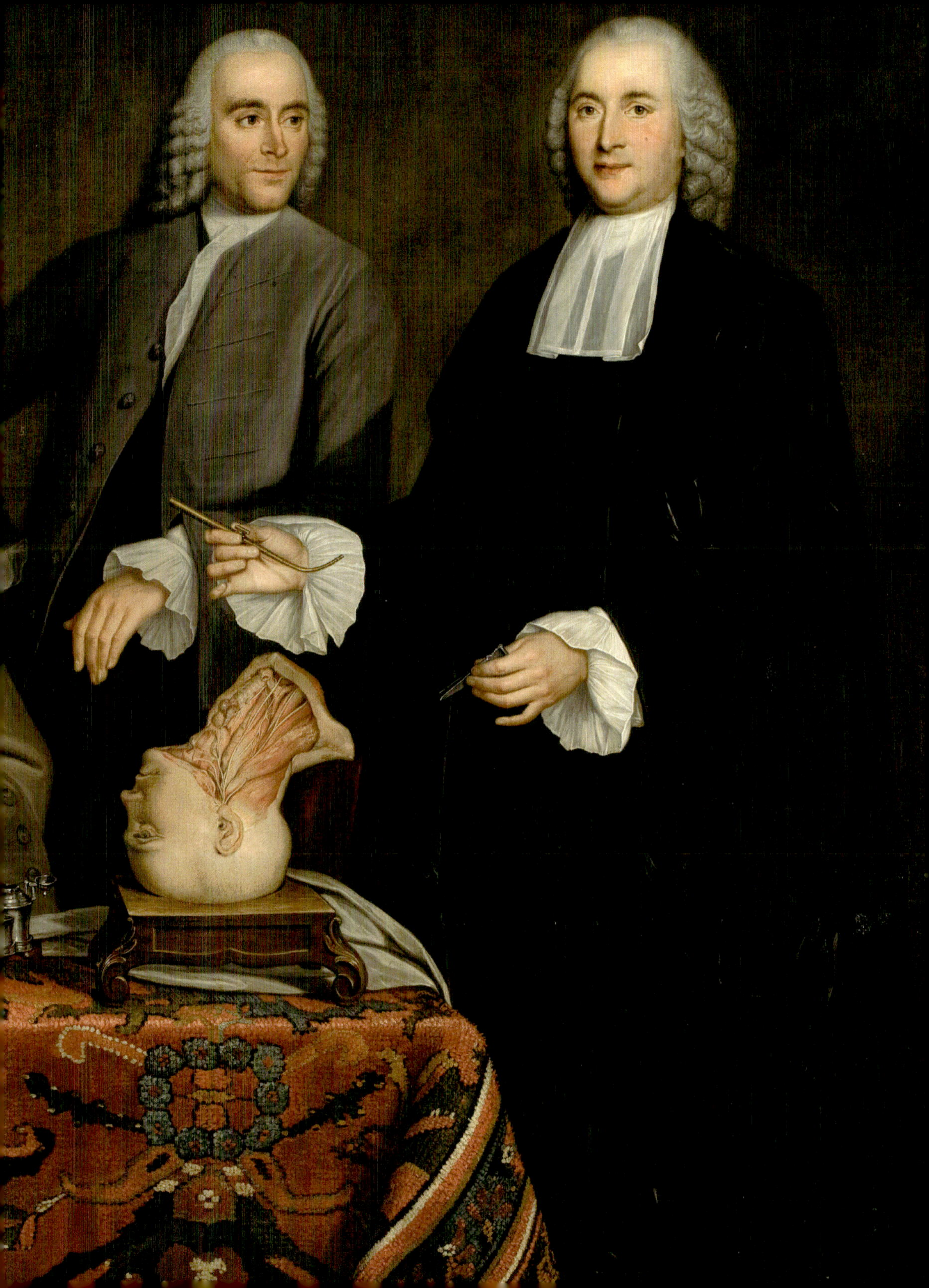

Petrus Camper

The Anatomy Lesson of Petrus Camper, painted by Tibout Regters in 1758

▸ **The Painting** In 1798, the Amsterdam Surgeons' Guild was dissolved. Forty years earlier, in 1758, Tibout Regters had painted the last group painting for the Guild: the so-called *Anatomy Lesson of Petrus Camper*. In the painting, *Praelector* Camper is seen in the company of six other surgeons and a guild servant, posing around a table on which a preserved head/neck is being displayed. Whereas in all the previous anatomy lessons the *subjectum anatomicum* had been a whole body, Camper is displaying only one anatomical specimen: a body part. It is a severed head which has been turned upside down and mounted on a wooden plinth. The dissection table has been replaced by a table covered with a Persian carpet. In the foreground, there is a shaving basin containing a sponge.

It seems that the actual anatomical demonstration is no longer relevant in relation to the rest of the painting. It is obvious that the main focus of attention is on the group portrait, the surgeons formally arranged in order of their importance. Most of them show no interest

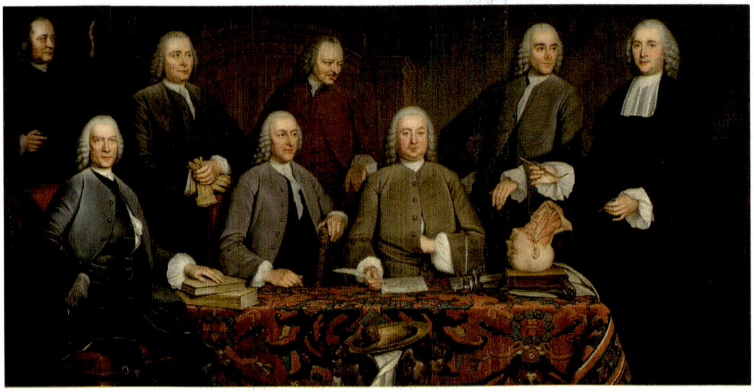

Tibout Regters, *The Anatomy Lesson of Petrus Camper*, 1758. Collection Amsterdam Museum.

whatsoever in the anatomical demonstration, either because they are 'looking at the camera', or their gaze is directed at something beyond our view. The fairly static, formal arrangement of the surgeons is reminiscent of the first *Anatomy Lesson of Sebastiaen Egbertszn* from 1601–1603. (see p. 33).

On the one hand, the presence of the *praelector* and the *subjectum anatomicum* do indicate that an anatomy lesson is being conducted. On the other hand, the composition is more than one might expect to find in a group portrait. The *Anatomy Lesson of Petrus Camper* is a combination of both. The painting is currently part of the collection of the Amsterdam Museum.

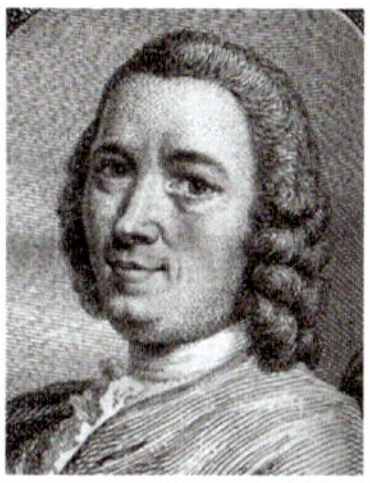

Unknown artist, *Portrait of Tibout Regters* (detail). From: Jan van Gool, *Nieuwe Schouburg der Nederlandsche kunstschilders en schilderessen* (New Gallery of Dutch Painters, Male and Female), 1750–1751.

▸ **The Artist** Tibout Regters (1710–1768) was born in Dordrecht. At the age of two, he moved to Arnhem with his parents. While still very young, he started taking painting lessons from someone called 'ten Haeg'. He must have found these lessons unsatisfactory, because they 'kept him more occupied using a coarse brush rather than using the fine painting brush of an artist'.

At the age of twenty, Regters moved to Rotterdam, where he took painting lessons from an artist called 'Meyer'. Two years later, he left Rotterdam for Amsterdam. Much to his misfortune, he had been 'tricked and deceived', into apprenticing himself to 'the notorious, mediocre bulk painter, Wannenburg'. But it didn't take him long to realize that he had gone from bad to worse, and he quit, upon which he 'finally found a happy arrangement working with the excellent portrait painter J.M. Quinkhard.' Studying under the established portrait painter Jan Maurits Quinkhard (1688–1772) for the next five years, Regters finally had a real chance to develop his talent as an artist. Quinkhard had built up a good reputation with the Amsterdam surgeons, and was commissioned no less than three times to paint the portraits of the Guild's governors (see pp. 226, 229, 232).

Regters became a skilled portrait painter, who produced an impressive number of individual and family portraits. He portrayed a very diverse group of people, including Jan Wagenaar (chronicler of the history of the city), Ludolf Backhuijzen (artist), Evert Jacob van Wachendorff (professor of chemistry and botany), Jan Carel van der Muelen and his family (burgomaster of Utrecht), Gijsbert Antwerpen Verbrugge van Freyhoof and his spouse (merchant-banker) and Jeronimo de Bosch (apothecary and art collector).

Regters also painted — and drew — several official group portraits, among them the directors of the Aalmoezeniersweeshuis (Almoners' Orphanage) in 1751 and the governors of the *Groot-kamersgilde* (textile merchants) in 1766. Two years before the Surgeons' Guild commissioned him to paint the anatomy lesson discussed in this chapter, he made a group portrait of the *Collegium Medicum*, the professional body of the *doctores medicinae* and apothecaries of Amsterdam. His complete oeuvre consists of around 140 paintings, drawings and prints (see also the *Rijksbureau voor Kunsthistorische Documentatie* (Netherlands Institute for Art History). Regters died in Amsterdam on January 26th, 1768, at the age of fifty-eight.

▸ **The Dissector** Petrus Camper (1722–1789) was born in Leiden on May 11th, 1722, the son of the Reverend Florentinus Camper and Sara Geertruida Kettingh. He was born into a well-educated family that valued the upbringing and education of the children. At quite an early age, he was already taking drawing lessons from the even then renowned artist Carel de Moor (1656–1738), one of the founders of the art academy in Leiden. After Petrus Camper had completed the Latin Academy in Leiden in 1734, he enrolled at Leiden University. During his academic education, he attended the anatomy lessons given by Bernard Siegfried Albinus (see p. 66). In 1746, at a solemn ceremony in the great hall of the university, Camper defended two theses about the mechanism of the eye, which earned him the simultaneous titles doctor of philosophy, master in the liberal arts, and doctor of medicine. The awarding of a double doctorate was an exceptionally rare occurrence.

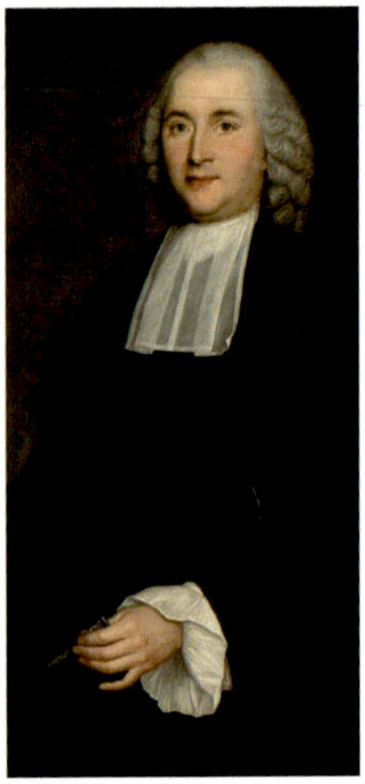

Petrus Camper (1722–1789)

Shortly afterwards, Camper made a study trip to London, where he attended lessons in obstetrics given by the famous obstetrician William Smellie (1697–1763). After this, he moved on to Paris where he honed his surgical skills with Antoine Louis (1723–1792), the renowned master surgeon and secretary of the Académie Royale de Chirurgie. In 1749, after he returned to the Netherlands, he was offered the chair of philosophy at the University of Franeker. Later that year, he was appointed professor of anatomy and surgery by the same university. As far as we know, Camper only gave an anatomy lesson in Franeker once: this was on December 14th, 1750. That same year he returned to London for further training in obstetrics with William Smellie. There he learned how to use the obstetrical forceps which Smellie designed to speed up the birth of a child distressed

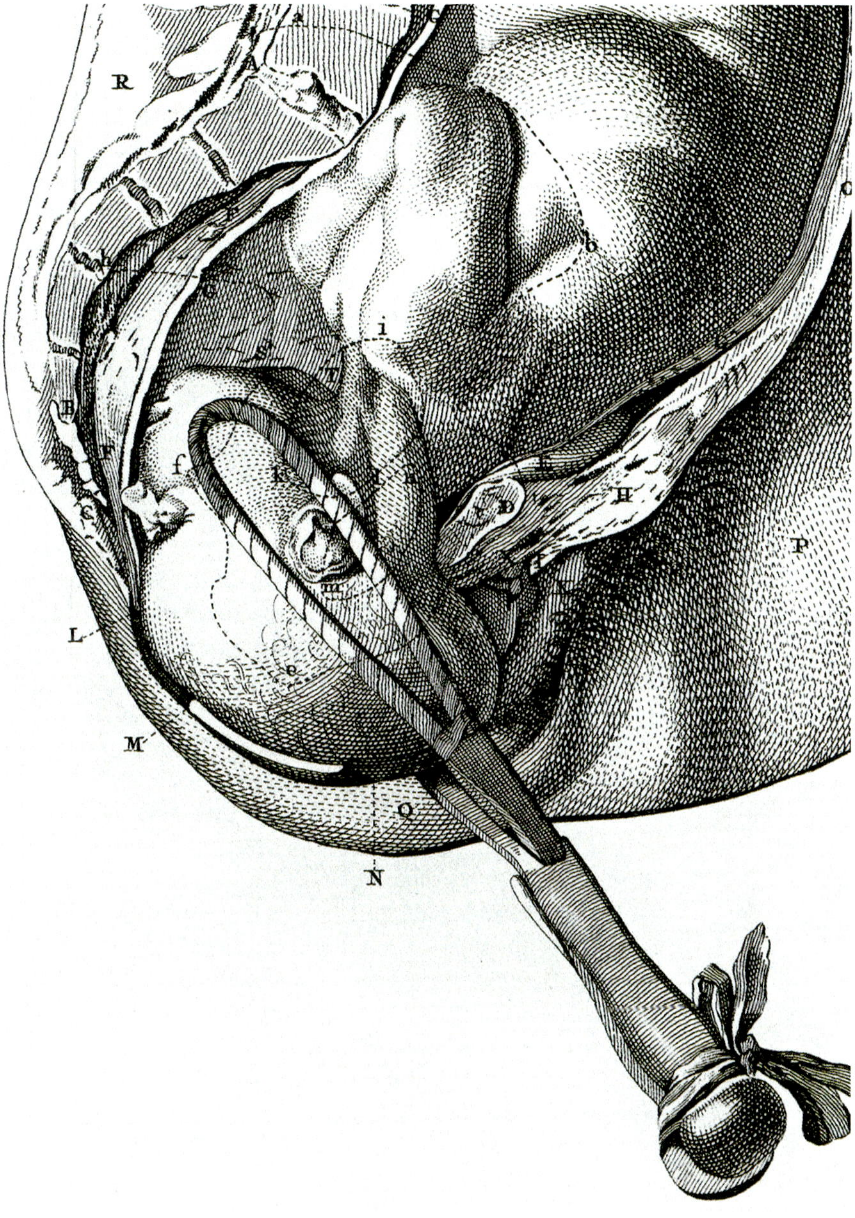

Illustration of the use of a pair of obstetrical forceps drawn by
Petrus Camper for the essay on obstetrics by his teacher William Smellie.
From: *A Treatise on the Theory and Practice of Midwifery*, 1752.
Library Rijksuniversiteit Groningen.

during labour. During this period, his English teacher was just finalizing his *A Treatise on the Theory and Practice of Midwifery* (1752), a weighty obstetrics manual for which Camper had produced a series of anatomical illustrations. One such illustration gives a good insight as to how the two doctors used the obstetrical forceps.

Camper bid Franeker farewell in 1755 and moved to Amsterdam to set up a practice there. Not long after he arrived, he married his sweetheart Johanna Bourboom (1722-1776), the thirty-five-year-old widow of the former burgomaster of Harlingen. The marriage took place in the vicinity of Franeker. They had had five sons, two of which died very young. The family initially settled on the Herengracht and later moved to the Keizersgracht.

At the age of thirty-three, Petrus Camper was appointed *praelector anatomiae* of the Amsterdam Surgeons' Guild, where there was considerable dissatisfaction on the performance of his predecessor, Willem Röell. Even while Röell was still in function, Camper had already been recruited to replace him. Camper's appointment, as well as his salary, caused quite some consternation. Eventually, the town council stepped in and decided that the Surgeons' Guild had to pay him an annual stipend of 1,000 guilders (the equivalent to 10,000 Euros now) and that Röell — whose duties had mostly been taken over by Camper — had to contribute another 306 guilders.

The *praelector* lectured the surgeons on their specialism twice a week. Every year, he was also expected to teach on the structure of the entire human body at the Anatomy Theatre in the Weighing House, 'using as many cadavers as is deemed necessary'. Camper also became actively involved in the education and training of obstetricians and midwives in Amsterdam. He also gave students at the *Athenaeum Illustre* (what would later become the University of Amsterdam), the chance to attend these lessons. In 1758, Camper became professor of medicine at the *Athenaeum Illustre,* and he combined this work with his duties as *praelector* at the Surgeons' Guild. On top of this, he was also consulted regularly in his capacity as municipal forensic examiner.

The ample supply of corpses in the city gave Camper plenty of opportunities to give anatomy lessons at the *Theatrum Anatomicum* on a regular basis. It seems that, within the space of six years (1755–1761), he gave no fewer than forty-six anatomy lessons. According to his own account, in Amsterdam alone, Camper 'had dissected more than fifty bodies in public, while he preferred to remain silent on the

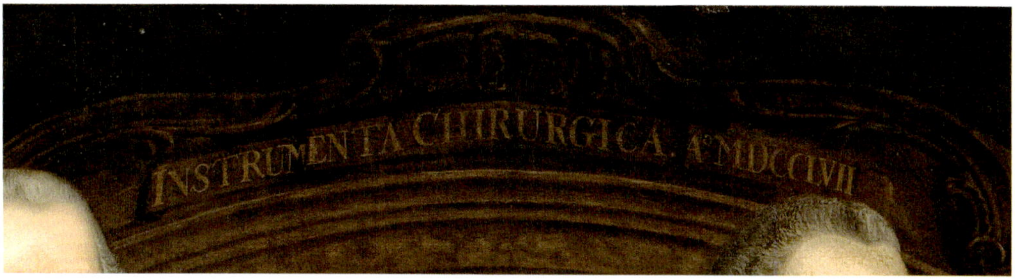

Inscription atop the instrument cabinet of the Amsterdam Surgeons' Guild (detail).

innumerable bodies of children, so as not to seem boastful'. In the winter of 1757–1758, he appears to have given anatomy lessons using ten different corpses. To commemorate this unprecedented number of lessons in one season, on 'Friday June 9th, 1758, the painting, which will serve as a remembrance to posterity, was delivered to the Guildhall, depicting Professor P. Camper [...], painted by the famous, highly esteemed master Thibout Regters.' As mentioned earlier, this was the last group portrait commissioned by the Surgeons' Guild.

A cabinet in the background of the painting carries the inscription *Instrumenta chirurgica, A° MDCCLVII* (Anno 1757). The inclusion of this piece of furniture in the painting is a reference to the cabinet containing surgical instruments which Camper purchased at the request of the Surgeons' Guild. During his anatomical lectures, Camper did not just restrict himself to the anatomy of the human body, he also explained how various operations should be performed.

In his quest to find solutions to certain scientific problems, Camper made good use of the abundant supply of anatomical material that was available in Amsterdam during his time. By dissecting the bodies of deceased persons — both adults and children — he researched, among others, the anatomy of the inguinal canal and the occurrence of inguinal hernias. At that time, people thought that an inguinal hernia occurred because of a 'rupture of the *peritoneum*' (a tear in the peritoneum), but Camper soon determined that this was an incorrect assumption. Treatments of inguinal hernias consisted of non-operative measures such as warm baths, 'hernia ointments', wet bandages and the use of trusses, while there was great reluctance to operate. An operation only took place as a last resort, in the event of a strangulated hernia.

Camper was particularly interested in inguinal hernias in children, as he thought that 'hernias treated with either ignorance or indo-

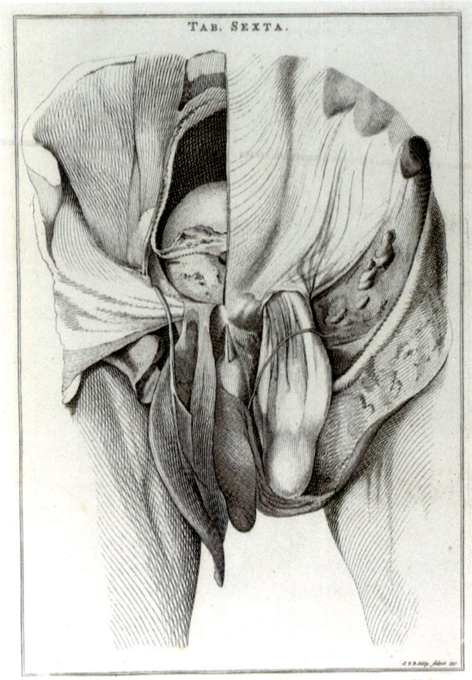

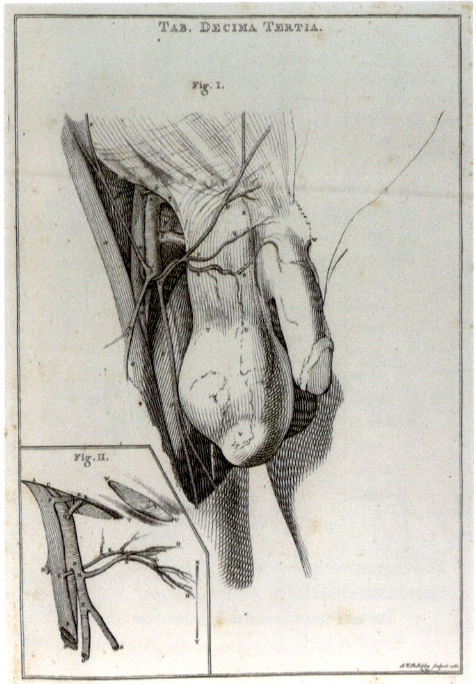

Left Illustration of an inguinal hernia on the left side. The abdominal muscles on the right side have been severed and folded down so that the blood vessels (*epigastric* vessels) which run behind the abdominal muscles are visible.

Right Illustration of an inguinal hernia on the right side which runs deep into the scrotum.

From: Petrus Camper, *Icones Herniarum*, 1801. Special Collections, University of Amsterdam [OTM O 62-2672].

From 1756–1760, Camper carried out a large number of anatomical dissections on corpses of small children in his pursuit of knowledge about the inguinal canal. He noted down the results in two charts. His observations led him to the conclusion that 'this canal (*processus vaginalis*) is natural, [and] should be considered thus in the newly born' and that 'this tube gradually closes around the spermatic cord'. Writing on the etiology of inguinal hernias in children, Camper says: 'Nature does not always appear to synchronize with the timing of birth, and this includes the full maturity of all the parts and, as the result of completely or partially open tubes (*processus vaginalis*) of the peritoneum, provides the opportunity for many hernias [to develop] in small children.' This is in line with the present-day notions on hernias in children. In 1761, Camper gave various anatomy lessons to the general public, in which he demonstrated the inguinal channel and the etiology of inguinal hernias in the bodies of both adults and children, male and female, at the *Theatrum Anatomicum* in Amsterdam.

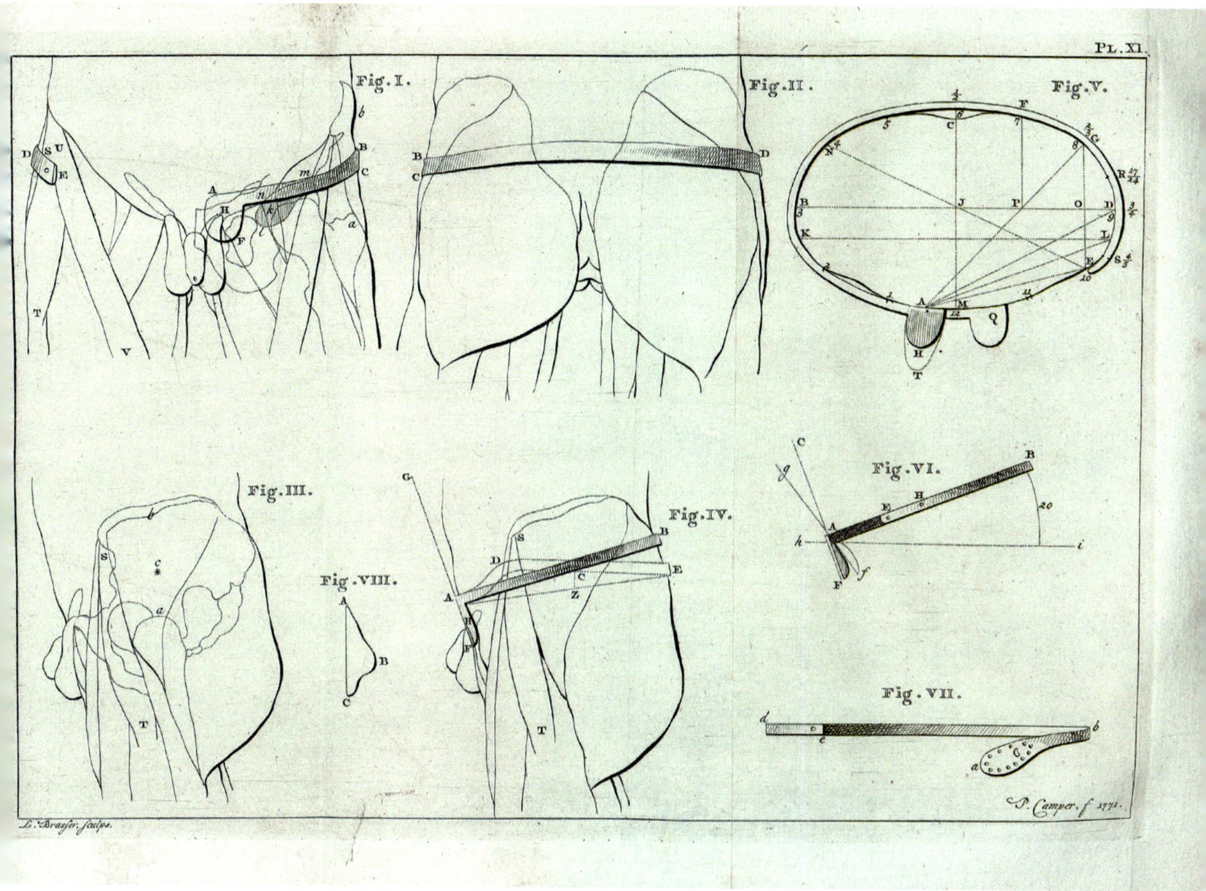

Petrus Camper, designs for Camper's truss. From: Petrus Camper, *Verhandeling over het toestellen van breuk-banden* (Treatise on the Application of Hernia Trusses), 1774. Special Collections University of Amsterdam [UBM DT 839: 1(5)].

Camper's richly illustrated *Icones Herniarum* (Images of Hernias) is probably his best-known publication on inguinal hernias. The anatomical drawings of the inguinal canal and the hernias which can occur in it were collected and published posthumously in 1801 by the German physician, anatomist and anthropologist Samuel Thomas von Soemmerring (1755–1830) – who was an acquaintance of Camper. Camper had made the drawings himself on the basis of anatomical dissections which he had personally carried out.

Camper's artistic aptitude and his talent for drawing proved to be of great advantage to him in this work. His anatomical studies and superb self-drawn illustrations led to a better understanding of the

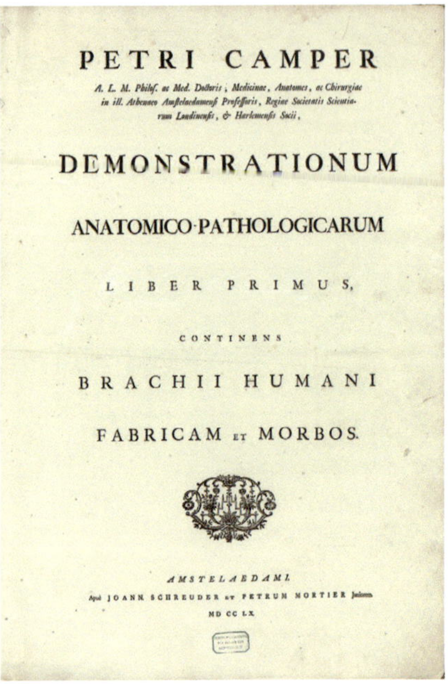

Title page of Camper's anatomical atlas of the arm, entitled *Demonstrationum anatomico-pathologicarum liber primus brachii humani fabricam et morbos* (Anatomical-pathological Identifications of the Structure and Disease of the Human Arm, Volume One (1760). Special Collections University of Amsterdam [OTM OL63-1402].

anatomy of the inguinal region and the etiology of inguinal hernias. Not just in the Netherlands, but also in the rest of Europe.

In order to treat inguinal hernias, he designed the 'Camper's truss', a construction which took into account the geometrical proportions of the pelvis. A truss is a sort of belt or girdle which exerts pressure on the site of the hernia and succeeds in pushing the at times troublesome swelling back in the groin. Hernia trusses are still used by people who prefer not to have their inguinal hernia operated on. Camper even devised a metal truss with a spring and pad (a small cushion which exerts pressure on the hernia) made of cork, wood and ivory. While he worked on the design of this truss, he had examples sent from all over Europe. He used these to test the pros and cons of trusses which had been made by fellow prominent doctors. Poor patients were given these trusses for free, as were sailors. He urged military tailors to make trousers in such a way that they would allow room to accommodate a truss at a later date. In his own day, Camper's hernia trusses were widely used and were greatly appreciated at home and abroad. By sheer coincidence, Camper developed an inguinal hernia himself as he grew older, upon which he ordered a Camper's truss to be made.

During his scientific research into the anatomy of the arm, Camper also made good use of the large number of corpses available in Amsterdam. He used his anatomical dissections in the *Theatrum Anatomicum* in the Weighing House to study the anatomy of the hand and arm. In 1760, on the basis of his discoveries, he published his *Demonstrationum anatomico-pathologicarum liber primus brachii humani fabricam et morbos* (Anatomical-pathological Identifications of the Structure and Disease of the Human Arm, Volume One), an anatomical atlas containing illustrations of dissected arms. He drew the impressive anatomical illustrations for this book himself. The twenty-two-page atlas contains three anatomical illustrations provided with Latin annotations, and was published in folio form (64 × 44 cm). Camper compiled the atlas to serve as a guideline for doctors who treated diseases of the limbs. He shows and describes

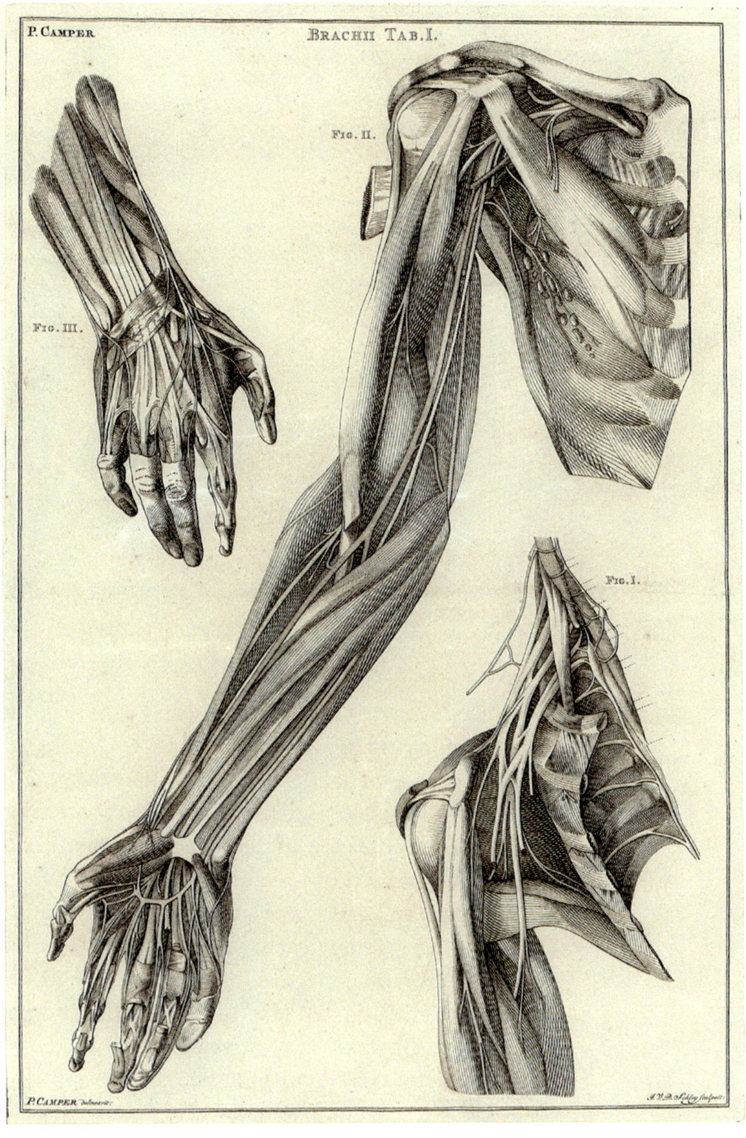

Anatomical representation of the arm, drawn by Petrus Camper. In this illustration, attention is focused on the mutual relationships between the muscles and nerves of the arm. From: *Demonstrationum anatomico-pathologicarum liber primus brachii humani fabricam et morbos* (Anatomical-pathological Identifications of the Structure and Disease of the Human Arm, Volume One (1760). Special Collections University of Amsterdam [OTM OL63-1402].

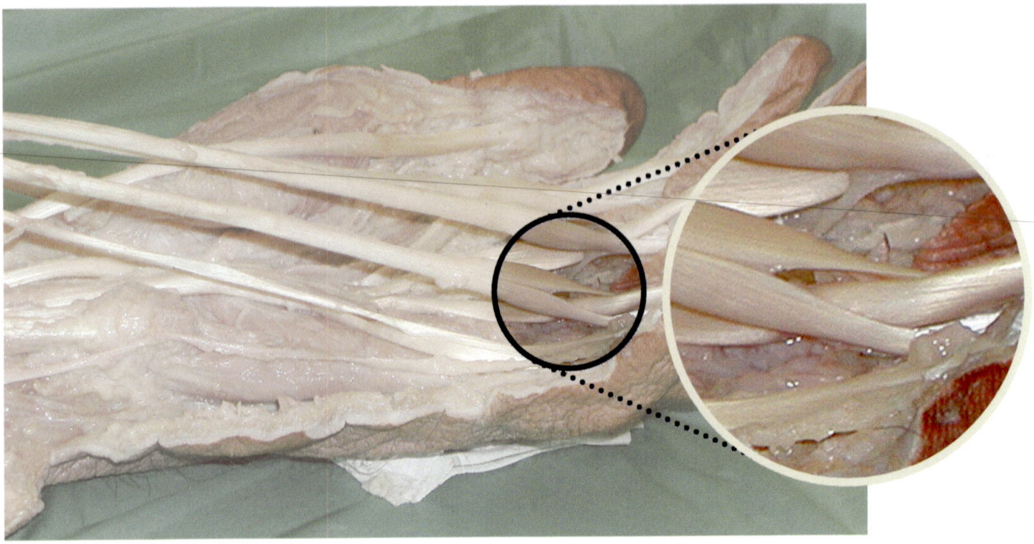

Photograph of Camper's *chiasma tendineum*, the crossing of the anterior and posterior flexor tendons in the hand. (Detail of the illustration on p. 100.)

the muscles, nerves and blood-vessels of the arm and the hand down to the smallest detail.

Camper did not confine himself to the study of the 'healthy arm': he also made the connection between the anatomy and diseases of the arm, for instance, in the case of a *panaritium tendineum* (a serious deep infection which spreads rapidly via the tendon sheaths in the hand). Whenever he came across a case, relying on his anatomical knowledge, he advised making a number of alleviating incisions over the tendon sheaths to allow the pus to drain away. To this day, his name is still associated with an essential anatomical structure of the hand, the Camper's *chiasma tendineum*. This is formed by a crossing of the anterior and posterior flexor tendons in the fingers. The *chiasma* plays an important role in the hand's ability to grip. Camper revealed the anatomy of the *chiasma* in his anatomical atlas and called it one of Nature's works of art.

The Camper family did not reside in Amsterdam for long. In the summer of 1760, he requested the burgomasters of Amsterdam to honourably discharge him from his duties. The reason why Camper wished to leave Amsterdam and return to the Frisian countryside,

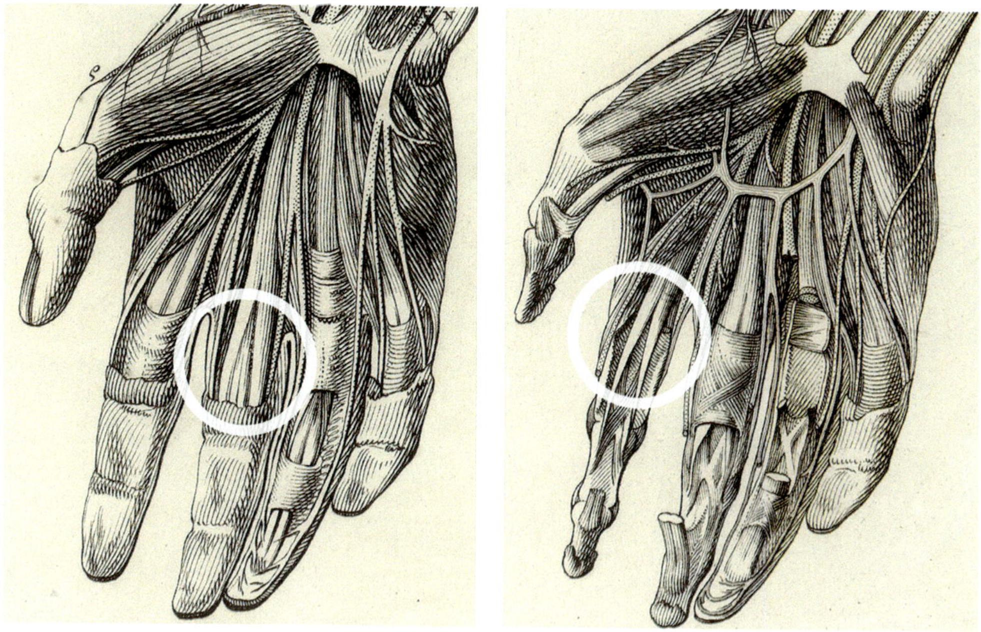

Anatomical illustration of the hand, drawn by Petrus Camper (detail). The circles indicate Camper's *chiasma tendinum*, the so-called crossing of the anterior and posterior flexor tendons in the fingers. From: *Demonstrationum anatomico-pathologicarum liber primus brachii humani fabricam et morbos* (Anatomical-pathological Identifications of the Structure and Disease of the Human Arm, Volume One (1760). Special Collections University of Amsterdam [OTM OL63-1402].

might well have been due to the fact that his wife found it difficult to settle in the big city. The Amsterdam surgeons were fond of him and regretted it when he left the city in April 1761, as Camper's departure would mean a great loss for anatomical education. Camper continued his lessons right up till his departure. The Minutes of the Surgeons' Guild record that Camper gave his final anatomy lesson on Tuesday February 24th, 1761: 'Today, Prof. Camper concluded his anatomy lessons with a recapitulation of all muscles in the human body, with the exception of the larynx (voice-box), pharynx (throat), palate, diaphragm (midriff) and the muscles of the sole of the foot, which the Esteemed Gentleman has shown in the four public demonstrations he has prepared, all within the space of thirty-six hours, by his efforts reaping admiration and delight.' As a token of his appreciation for the 'special regard, courtesies and friendship of the Honourable Gentlemen of the Board of the Surgical College', he presented the Surgeons' Guild with a silver tobacco jar as a farewell gift.

In 1761, the Camper family returned to the small Frisian village of Klein Lankum, 1 kilometre to the west of Franeker. Here, Camper had all the time in the world to immerse himself in the Natural

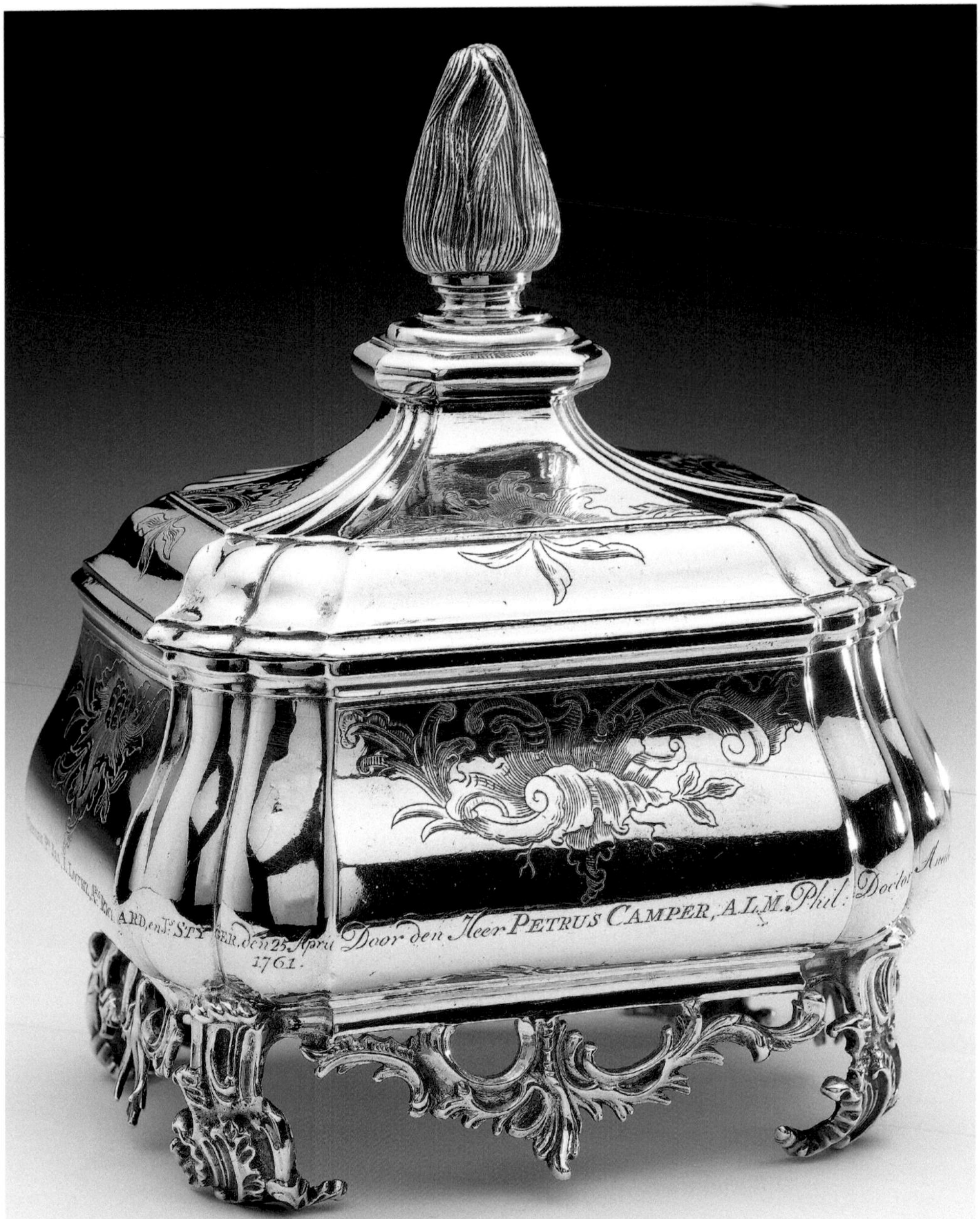

9

Petrus Camper 1758

Sciences. He can justifiably be regarded as one of the most outstanding physicians and scientists of the eighteenth century. He was a member of no fewer than twenty national and international societies, among which the most prestigious: the Académie des Sciences in Paris and the Royal Society in London. Soon after his move to Friesland, he wrote a number of essays on the reproductive system of the Surinam toad, and on the hearing of fish and amphibians.

His quiet life in the small Frisian village didn't last long, however, as in September of 1763, Camper accepted the professorship in medicine, theory (in the art of healing), surgery and botany at the University of Groningen. That same year, Camper and his family moved to the Grote Rozenstraat in Groningen. Shortly afterwards, he was appointed municipal physicist, a job which entailed the function of *praelector* for the surgeons and midwives as well as forensic examiner. In Groningen, Camper introduced the concept of the *collegium causale chirurgicum*, a weekly outpatient clinic which patients could visit without having to pay, and where Camper gave his students training in medical practice. In a period of around ten years, approximately 1,500 consultations were held at this outpatient clinic.

Camper also made an impact on public health. He was very active in propagating the vaccination of people to protect them from smallpox. In 1768, when the provinces of Friesland and Groningen were afflicted by an outbreak of cattle plague, Camper was indispensable in preventing death on a massive scale of the livestock by using vaccinations. The following year, Camper gave a public lecture about the cattle plague in the *Anatomy theatre* in Groningen. By means of the anatomical dissection of a calf, he dealt with the disease very thoroughly. We now know that the cattle plague is caused by the highly contagious *Morbillivirus*.

←
Nicolaes van Diemen (gold-and silversmith), silver tobacco jar of the Amsterdam Surgeons' Guild, 1761. Petrus Camper presented this fine piece of silverwork to the Guild when he resigned in 1761. The name Camper is engraved on the tobacco jar. Also engraved on the jar are the names of the five surgeons who are depicted in the *Anatomy Lesson of Petrus Campers*. Collection Amsterdam Museum.

In 1772, one highly unusual dissection of an animal took place in the *Anatomy theatre* in Groningen: it was a dissection of the head of an African rhinoceros which Camper had been able to acquire through the governor of the Cape of Good Hope, with whom he was on friendly terms. A few years later, the findings made during the dissection led to an original essay on the anatomy of the rhinoceros by Camper.

The subjects he studied during his years in Groningen were very diverse. In a number of lectures, he showed how the shape of the human skull differed between the races, and among different age groups. The concept of 'Camper's facial angle' is derived from this work. This is the angle one obtains when, in the side view of the skull, one connects the root of the nose and the auditory canal on the one hand and, on the other, the front incisors in the upper jaw and the most prominent part of the forehead using imaginary lines. Camper claimed that the facial angle in apes was 40 to 50 degrees, in an 'African Moor' 70 degrees and in a European 80 degrees. In this work, Camper was in fact one of the founders of (physical) anthropology.

In 1773, after having worked at the University of Groningen for ten years, Camper resigned. He returned to Kleine Lankum to devote himself entirely to his family and to science. It was not long before he had published an essay on the 'pneumatic characteristics of avian skeletons' and about 'signs of life and death in newborn children'. Then, in 1774, came the second of his remarkable series of animal dissections. Much to everybody's surprise, the cadaver of an elephant arrived in Kleine Lankum. The dead animal had been put at Camper's disposal for closer investigation by the prince-stadtholder. The anatomical dissection of the elephant — which was conducted in Camper's barn — took three weeks. Camper's discoveries on anatomy of the elephant were published posthumously in 1802 by his son, Adriaan Gilles. A few years after the elephant episode, came the third exotic dissection. Camper was given a dead orang-utan from the prince-stadtholder's zoo in The Hague. The orang-utan underwent the same dissection as the elephant.

The period between 1775–1776 was marred by sickness and sorrow for the Camper family, as, after a long sickbed, Mrs Camper died of breast cancer. In the following years, Camper travelled inside and outside of the country, visiting a number of impressive natural history collections in Germany. He himself had a wonderful private collection of the most exceptional minerals, fossils and skeletons. The last years of his life were dominated by politics. In 1782, Petrus Camper was appointed burgomaster of Workum. In 1787 he was made chairman of the *Raad van State* (Council of State) in The Hague. Camper died in 1789 at the age of sixty-six. He was struck down by severe pleurisy and was buried in the Pieterskerk in Leiden.

▸ **The Surgeons** The Guild's surgeons seen in the painting have been identified using the numbers next to the portraits which correspond to the numbered list of names on the sheet of paper on the table. Petrus Camper (nr 1) is standing on the far right, at the head of the table. The Guild servant, Gerrit van der Weert (nr 8), occupies

Those depicted in *The Anatomy Lesson of Petrus Camper*:

1 Petrus Camper
2 Loth Lothszn
3 Pieter Jas
4 Coenraad Nelson
5 Nicolaes van der Meulen
6 Abraham Richard
7 Joannes Stijger
8 Gerrit van der Weert

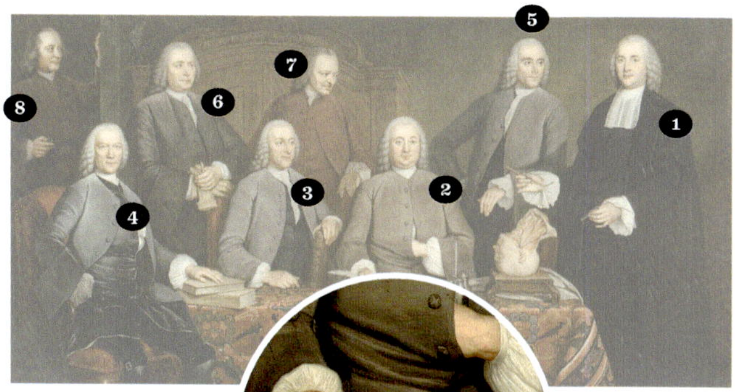

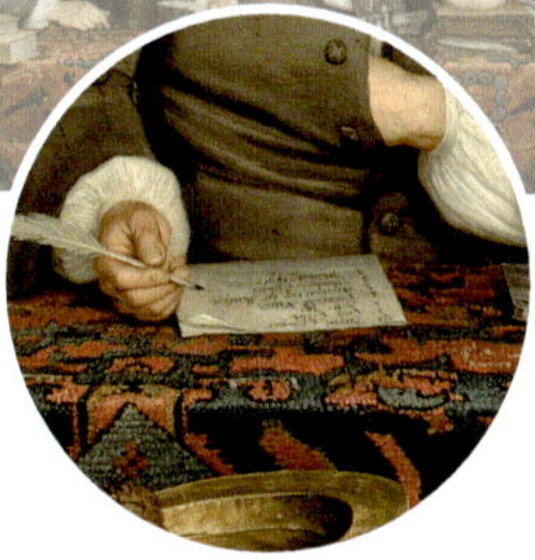

Sheet of paper with the numbered name list of those depicted in *The Anatomy Lesson of Petrus Camper*.

the humblest position within the company, at the back in the left-hand corner. All the gentlemen at the table -with one exception, Joannes Stijger- were members of the Board, and were in function from September 1757 to September 1758.

The fine membership token (or presentation token) of Pieter Jas has survived to this day. He can be seen in the middle of the group of directors, seated at the table while casting a sidelong glance at the anatomical specimen. Jas received his token after passing his final examination to qualify as a surgeon in 1732. Of Loth Lothzn,

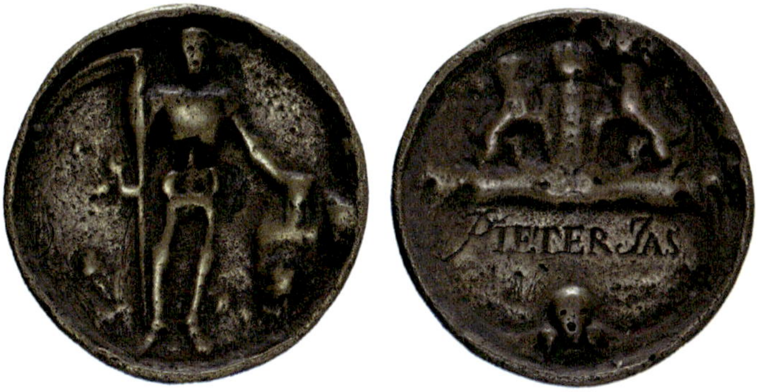

Membership token bearing the name Pieter Jas. Collection Amsterdam Museum.

the director holding the quill and with the list of names in front of him, we know how much he paid the artist for his portrayal: 'I, the undersigned hereby give notice that I have received from Mr Loth Lothzn the sum of eighty-five guilders for the painting of His Excellency's Portrait which was hung in the Surgeons' Guildhall on June 9th. July 10th, 1758. T. Regters.' If all those shown in the painting paid the artist eighty-five guilders, this amounts to a total sum of around 700 guilders (comparable to 6,000 Euros now) for the whole painting.

▸ **Subjectum Anatomicum** The identity of the person whose head – the *subjectum anatomicum* of Camper's anatomy lesson – was used, can no longer be traced. As previously mentioned, Camper had ten corpses at his disposal for his anatomy lessons in the winter of 1757/1758. The dismembered head with the dissected neck in Regter's painting was undoubtedly from one of these bodies.

▸ **Anatomy** While using a head which has been placed upside down on a mount, Camper is demonstrating the complex anatomy of the neck. At the front of the neck, we see the windpipe, where in actual fact a butterfly-shaped organ is located: the thyroid. The thyroid produces hormones which are essential for metabolism. In the painting, two swellings (tumours) are visible on the windpipe. It is possible that these were intended to represent the thyroid, but it is not a realistic representation of the gland. Next to the windpipe, we see a nerve, perhaps the artist meant to depict the *nervus laryngeus recurrens* here. This nerve controls the small muscles around the larynx and is indirectly responsible for managing the vocal cords. One of the complications feared during an operation on the thyroid gland, is damaging this 'vocal cord nerve'. At the base of the windpipe is a severed blood vessel. Normally, the oblique neck muscle (*musculus sternocleidomastoideus*) passes through this region; this begins at the collarbone (*origo*) and runs to the skull base behind the ear (*insertion*). This muscle controls the turning and bowing motions of the head.

→ Petrus Camper demonstrates the anatomical structures of the neck in a head which has been placed upside down.

The oblique neck muscle which is superficially situated is missing in the painting. It is highly likely that Camper had removed this muscle in order to show the structures situated deeper in the neck. Perhaps, with his depiction of the severed blood vessel at the base

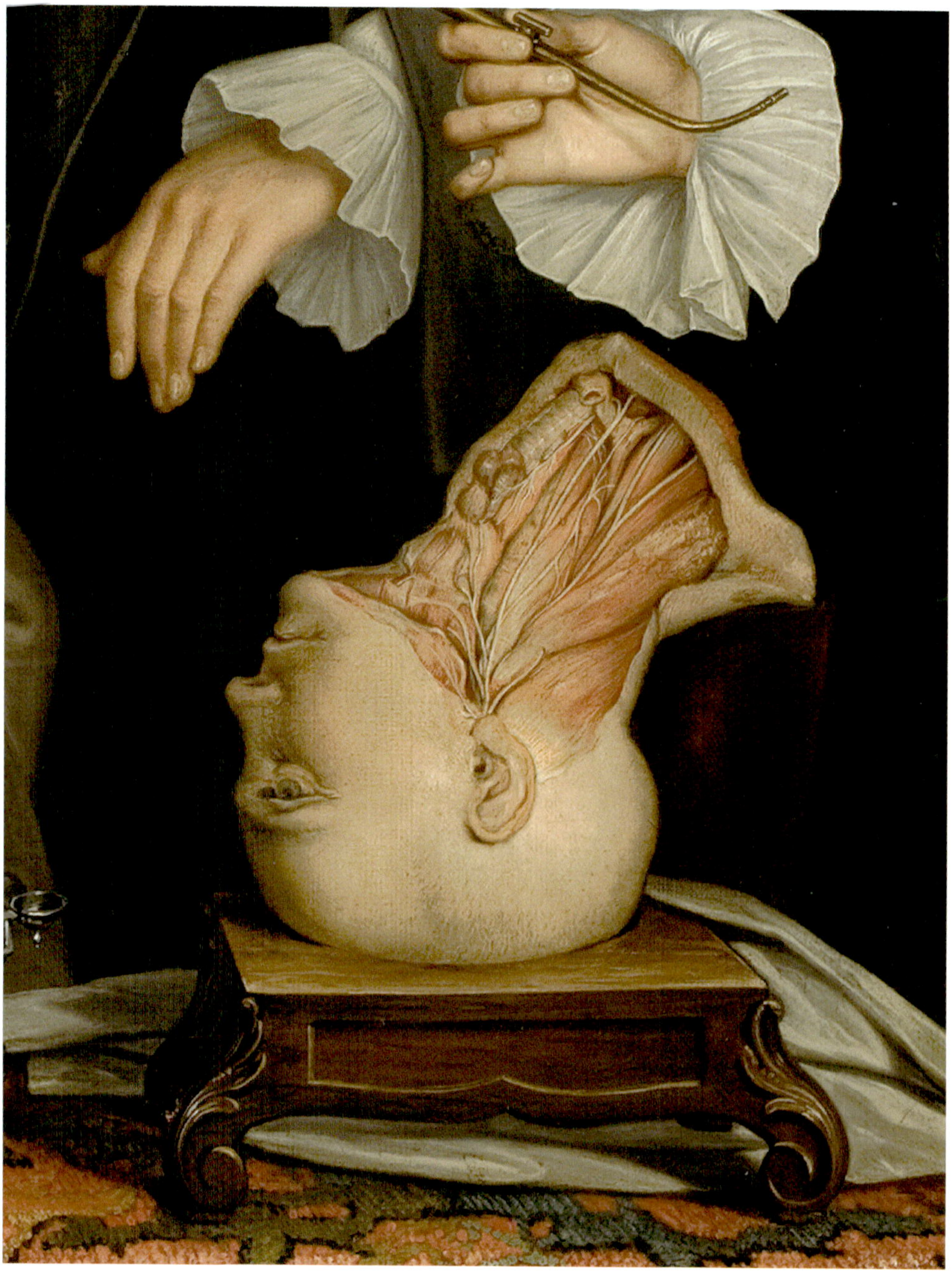

of the windpipe, the painter had actually intended to show the large jugular vein (*vena jugularis interna*). Under the oblique neck muscle – which is missing from the painting – one would expect to find the large blood vessels of the neck (*vena jugularis interna* and *arteria carotis*). However, it is extremely difficult to chart the exact course of these blood vessels in the painting. Behind (dorsal to) the severed vessel, one should see one of the most important clusters of nerves in the neck. This cluster of nerves, the *plexus brachialis*, provides all the nerves in the arm. In the painting, between the anterior and medial scalene muscles (*musculus scalenus anterior* and *medius*), at the place where the plexus should be seen, a structure is visible entering the neck. It is possible that the artist intended this to be the plexus, but, contradicting this argument, the structure shown is connected to the severed blood vessel. A number of other important nerves also pass through the neck, among them the *nervus vagus* (the tenth cranial nerve, controlling various organs), the *nervus phrenicus* (controlling the respiratory muscles) and the *nervus accessorius* (controlling the trapezius muscle, the *musculus trapezius*). In short, the course of the nerves depicted does not fully correspond to reality.

Tibout Regters has made a serious attempt to present an adequate picture of the complex anatomy of the neck. To a certain extent, he has succeeded. Various anatomical structures are certainly recognizable but, as said, the anatomy as shown is not a true representation of the real situation. This is to be expected, because the neck encompasses one of the most complex structures in the human body. Taking into consideration the detailed representation and the fact that some anatomical structures closely approach reality, there is a strong possibility that the artist did see a neck being dissected by Camper with his own eyes.

Even today, the neck is a very challenging part on which to operate. It is may be necessary to surgically remove lymph node metastases in patients suffering from malignant disease in the neck/head region. The most frequent are metastases of tumours of the thyroid, salivary glands (*glandula parotis* or *submandibularis*) and metastases of skin tumours such as melanoma. These operations known as radical neck dissections are invariably complex operations which take several hours and demand an enormous amount of patience and precision work from the surgeon.

Camper is one of the most renowned and famous Dutch scientists of the eighteenth century. Professor P.J. Kuiper (1921–2002), former professor of surgery in Groningen and founder of the Foundation for the Promotion of Medical History – the Petrus Camper Stichting –, described Camper as 'an independent thinker, a solid researcher with an almost boundless curiosity, a highly cultivated man of many interests, who moved in academic circles at a European level.' It would be no exaggeration to say that Camper was extremely fascinated by the complicated anatomy of the neck, and that this was therefore a fitting subject for his anatomy lesson.

Portraits of the Governors

During the seventeenth and eighteenth centuries, a total of eighteen group portraits were painted for the Amsterdam Surgeons' Guild. Nine of these portraits are actual anatomy lessons, all of which have been discussed in detail in the earlier chapters. Almost all of the other group portraits of the governors depict a group of men posing around a table. The theme of the anatomy lesson is absent in these paintings. All attention is focused on the Board of Governors. Objects lie on all the tables to indicate the men's profession, for instance: medical reference books, a page from an anatomical atlas, surgical instruments, bladder stones and bones. The majority of the 'anatomy lesson' painting date from the seventeenth century, whereas most of the group portraits of the governors were painted during the eighteenth century. In a sense, they can be considered the successors to the anatomy lessons. Nevertheless, all portraits share the same purpose — that of a group portrait of surgeons — while the two different portrait types were inextricably linked.

The first group portrait [1], painted by Nicolaes Maes (1634–1693) in the years 1679–1680, depicts six governors gathered around a table. Although it is known who the men in the painting are, it is not known who is who, the one exception being Govard Bidloo. He is the surgeon sitting in front of the table at the left, while looking at the viewer over his right shoulder. Upon being awarded his degree as *doctor medicinae*, Bidloo was appointed professor of anatomy in The Hague (1688) and Leiden (1694). On top of his professorship, he was also personal physician to the stadtholder King William III and 'superintendent-general of all physicians, apothecaries and surgeons in Dutch infirmaries and Dutch military hospitals'. He is known in particular for his book *Ontleding des Menschelijken Lichaams* (Dissection of the Human Body) published in 1690. This was an anatomical atlas containing beautiful illustrations produced by Gerard de Lairesse, the Latin version of which had appeared six years earlier. (see Chapters 2 and 5, pp. 63-65 and pp. 116-118). Because they were quite conscious of their prominent status, the six governors in Maes' painting gave

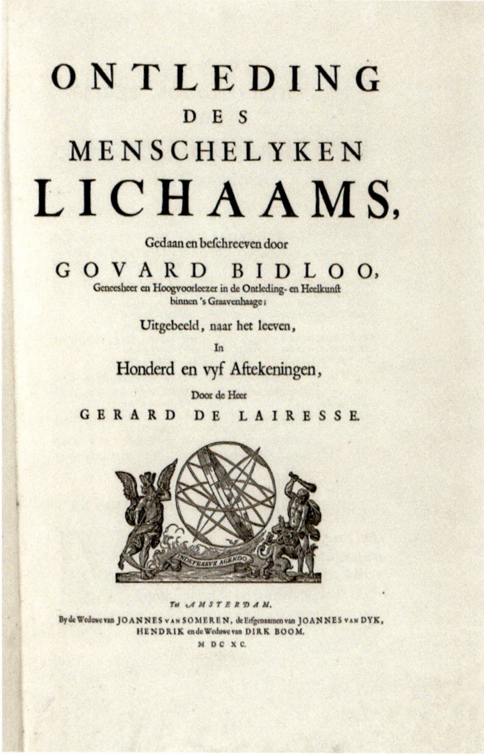
ONTLEDING
DES
MENSCHELYKEN
LICHAAMS,
Gedaan en beschreeven door
GOVARD BIDLOO,
Geneesheer en Hoogvoorleezer in de Ontleding- en Heelkunst
binnen 's Graavenhaage;
Uitgebeeld, naar het leeven,
In
Honderd en vyf Aftekeningen,
Door de Heer
GERARD DE LAIRESSE.

INDEFESSVS AGENDO

Te AMSTERDAM,
By de Weduwe van JOANNES VAN SOMEREN, de Erfgenaamen van JOANNES VAN DYK,
HENDRIK en de Weduwe van DIRK BOOM.
M DC XC.

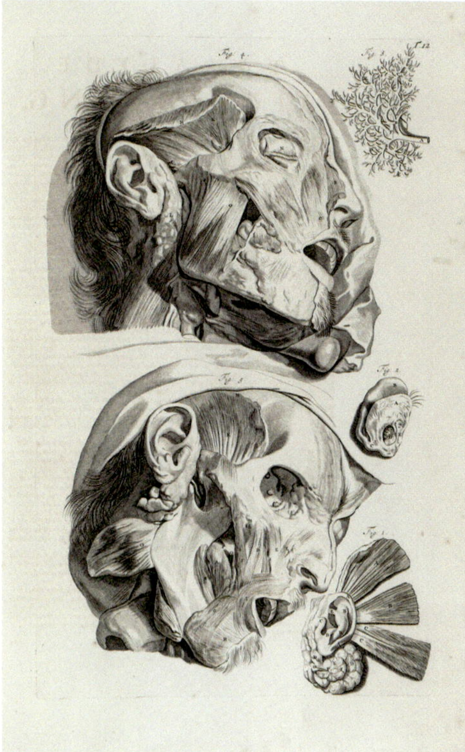

Left Title page of Govard Bidloo *Ontleding des Menschelijken Lichaams. Uitgebeeld naar het leven in honderd en vijf aftekeningen door Heer Gerard De Lairesse* (Dissection of the Human Body shown in one hundred fifty illustrations by Mr Gerard de Lairesse), Amsterdam, 1690.
Right Gerard de Lairesse, illustration of an anatomical dissection of a head. From: Govard Bidloo *Ontleding des Menschelijken Lichaams* (Dissection of the Human Body shown in one hundred fifty illustrations by Mr Gerard de Lairesse), Amsterdam, 1690. Library University of Groningen, Groningen.

their group portrait a prime spot above the mantlepiece in the Guildhall, where the *Osteology Lesson of Sebastiaen Egbertszn* (1619) had once hung. Before long, however, the six men were told by their colleagues that the older masterpiece had to be put back in its place, and that they would have to find another spot in the Guildhall for their own group portrait, to which they complied.

In 1684, three governors commissioned a portrait to be painted of themselves, seated next to a small table with a skull on it [2]. Their names are recorded on the sheet of paper lying next to the skull. Three of their colleagues, who had also sat on the Board from between

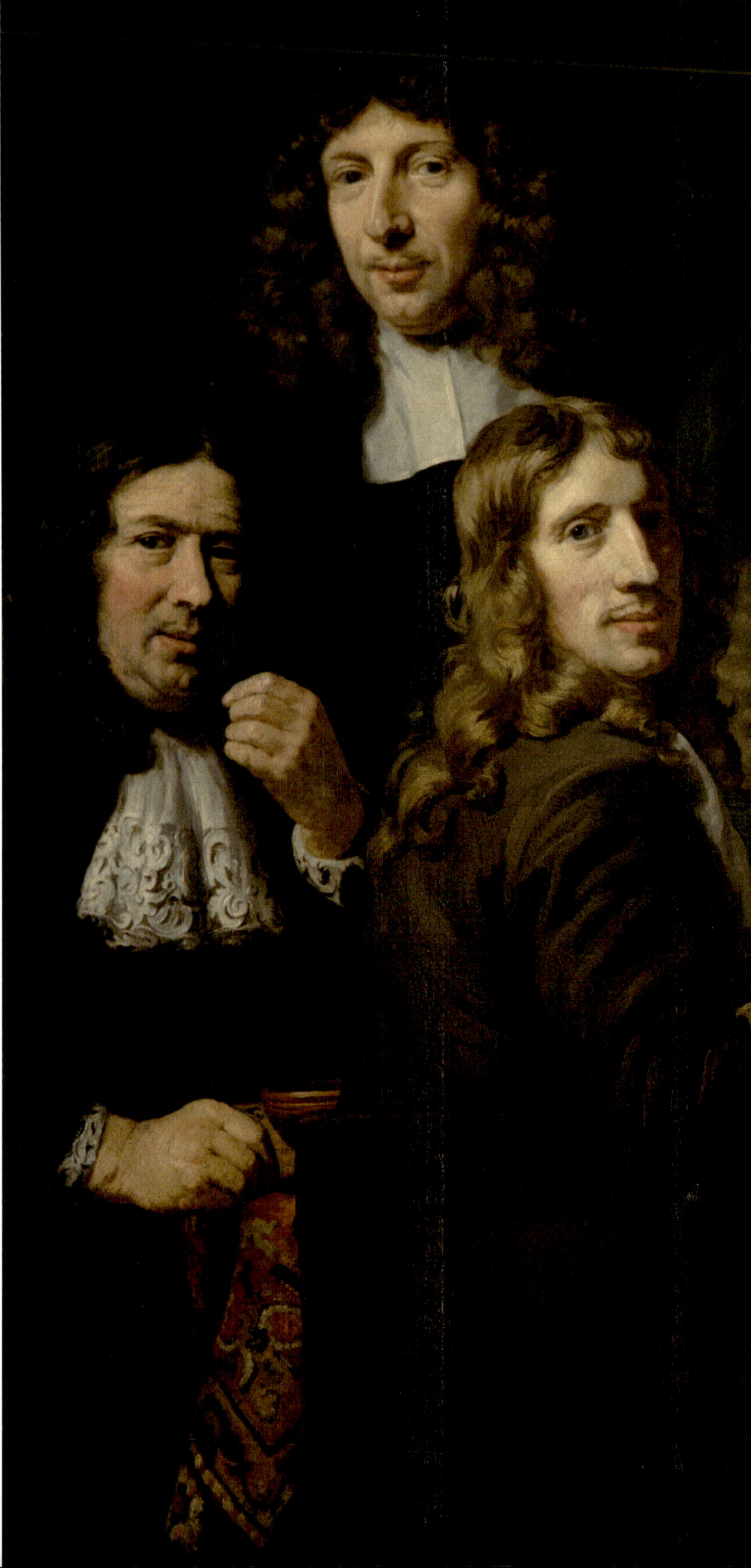

[1]
Nicholaes Maes, *The Governors of the Surgeons' Guild*, 1679–1680. Group portrait of the Governors Govard Bidloo, Jan Koenerding, Gerard Hendrickszn Verhul, Allardus Ciprianus and Isaack Hendrikszn Hartman. With the exception of Govard Bidloo (the person in the foreground), it is not possible to identify who is who. Collection Amsterdam Museum.

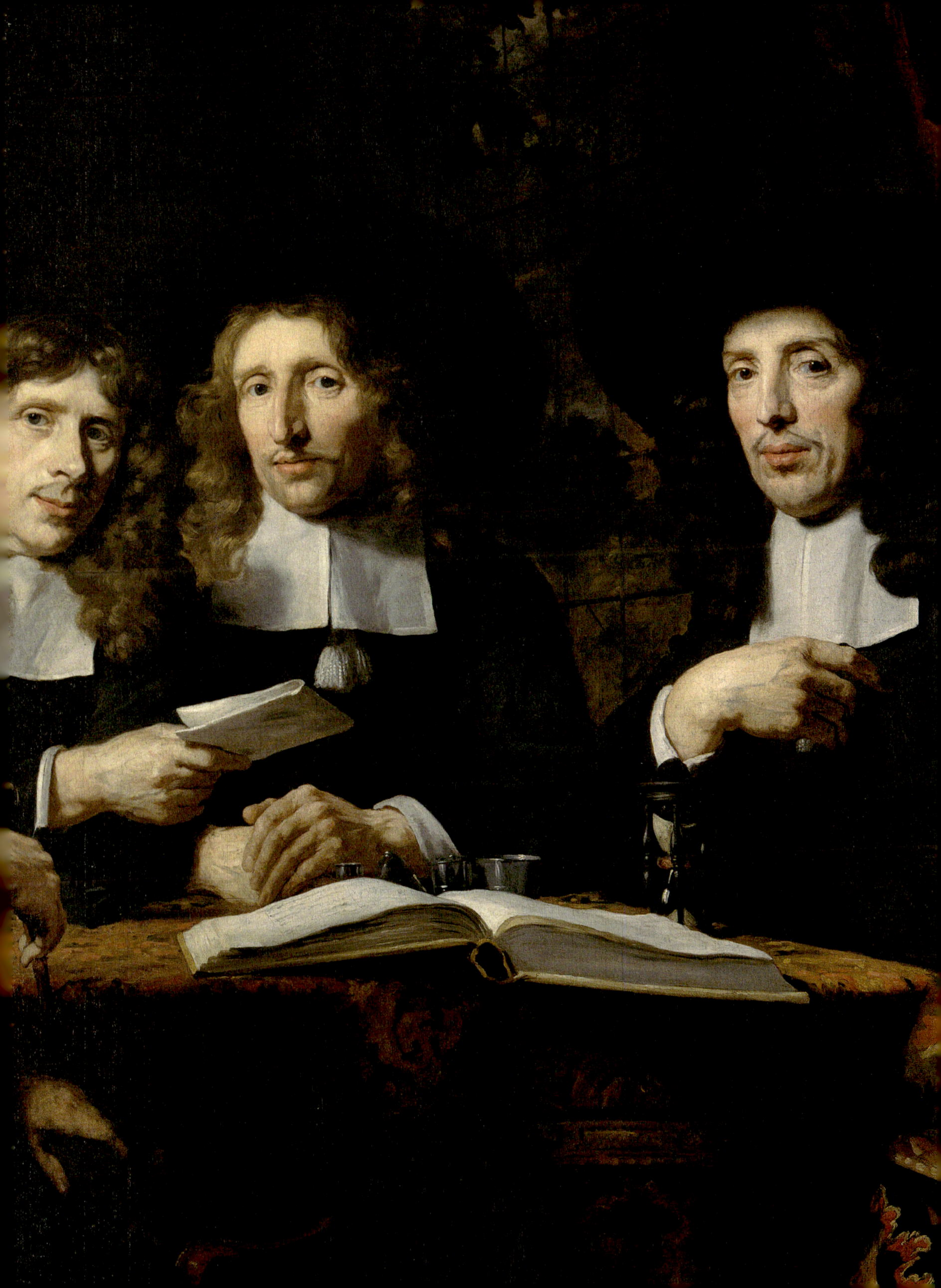

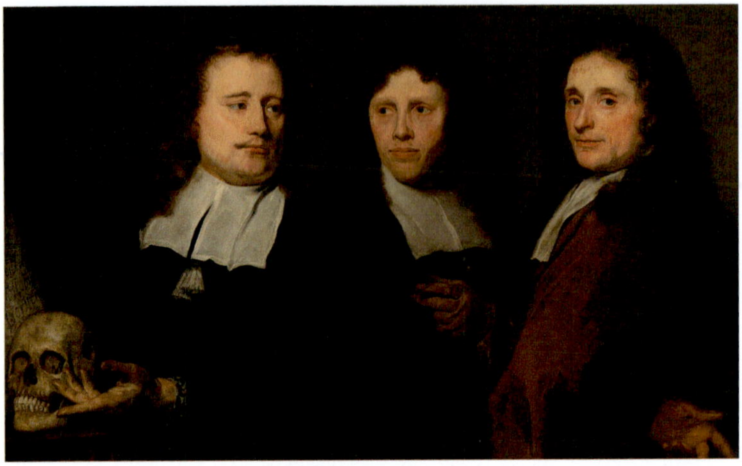

[2]
Unknown artist, *Three Governors of the Surgeons' Guild*, 1684.
Group portrait of the governors (in random order): Jan Willink, Pieter Oosdorp and Gerrit Corver. Collection Amsterdam Museum.

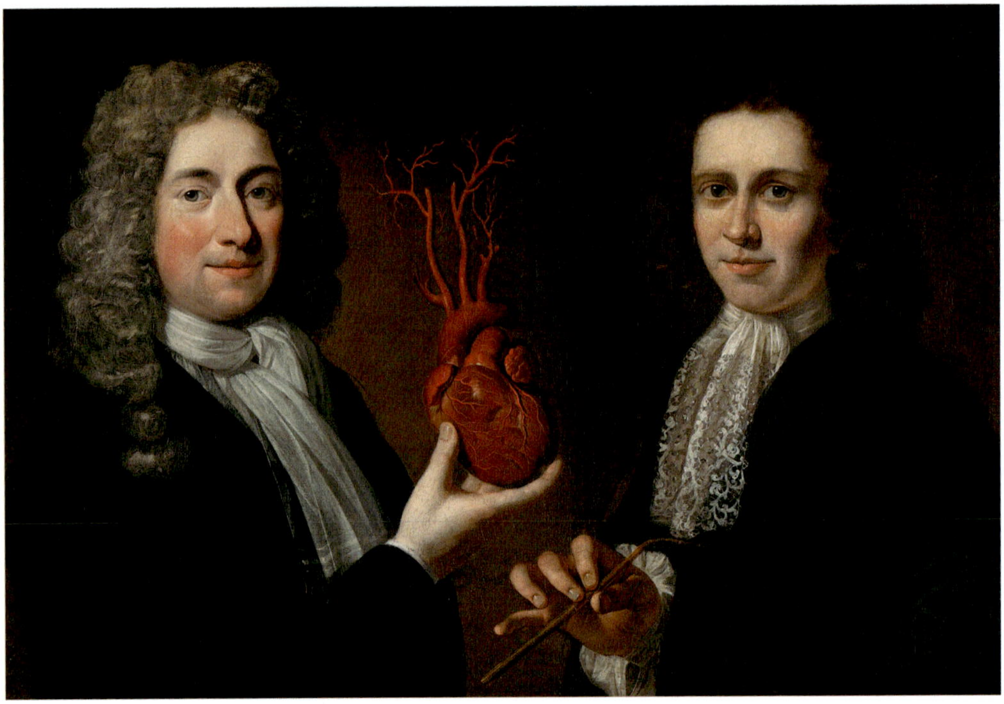

[3]
Jurriaan Pool, *Two surgeons with a preserved heart*, 1699.
Governors portraited: J. Six and C. Boekelman. Collection Amsterdam Museum.

September 1684 to September 1685, had already had their portraits painted in the *Anatomy Lesson of Frederik Ruysch* in 1683 (See Chapter 7).

The next group portrait of Governors, depicting just two men, was painted fifteen years later [3]. The portrait was painted in 1699 by Jurriaan Pool (1666–1745), who was married to the daughter of Frederik Ruysch. The surgeon on the left is holding an anatomical specimen of a heart, most probably a preserved heart from the private collection of Frederik Ruysch. Ruysch had succeeded in giving his prepared anatomical specimens a lifelike appearance by injecting the blood vessels with molten, coloured wax. He succeeded in making even the finest ramifications of the coronary artery visible. He said the following on the subject:(Cabinet IV, specimen N XCVI):

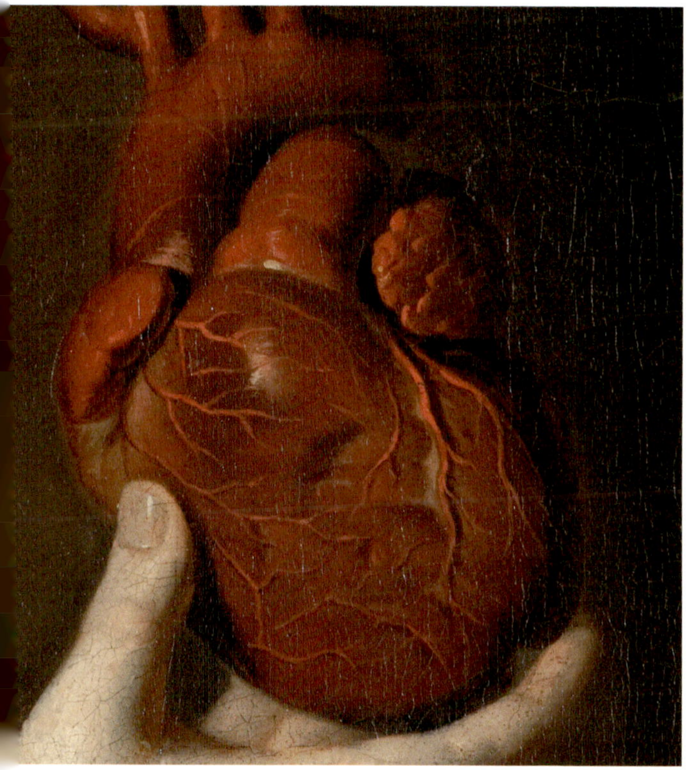

Preserved heart in the portrait of the governors by Jurriaan Pool, 1699.

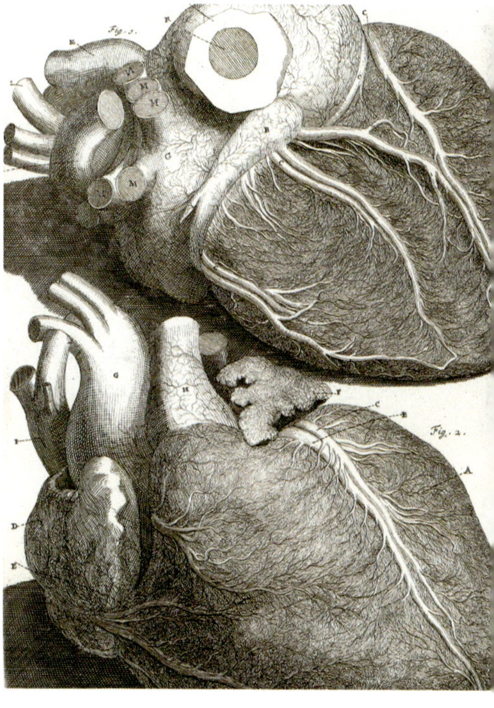

Cornelis Huijberts, Illustration of a preserved heart from the private collection of Frederik Ruysch. From: *Alle de ontleed-, genees-, en heelkundige werken van Frederik Ruysch*, 1744.

> *An embalmed Heart of a human being, which has been dried and kept on a piece of velvet in a small casket of Indian wood. All its blood vessels have been filled with a red waxy substance in such a way that not only the capillary branches (of the very finest hair-like blood vessels), but also their extraordinarily fine extremities are visible to us, as these are also filled with this red substance: and if, when the weather is fine, someone uses a magnifying glass, he will see that this red waxy substance appears to flow out of the heart as it would from a small, downy cloud; in this same way, I assume that whatever flows through the coronary artery serves as nourishment to the Heart,* [...].

A few of the hearts which Ruysch preserved are still kept at the Peter the Great Museum for Anthropology and Ethnography (*Kunstkamera*) in St Petersburg. The coronary arteries of the heart in the painting are a bright red colour which corresponds to the red waxy substance which Ruysch injected into his preserved hearts. When injecting the red preservative, Ruysch used 'small blowpipes', which were made especially for him by the Leiden instrument maker Samuel van Musschenbroek. The surgeon on the right seems to be holding just such a 'blowpipe' – even if it is a bit on the large side.

The next, more modestly sized, fourth group portrait of the governors, in which only three governors are shown, was painted in 1706 [4]. Their names are still faintly legible alongside their images. A '*presentiepenning*' (guild membership token) that once belonged to Hendrik Smeeckes, the surgeon on the left with a skull in his hand, has survived to this day. He was given this token after he had passed his masterpiece and qualified as a surgeon. The token also served as proof of membership of the Amsterdam Surgeons' Guild.

The five Governors on the next group portrait painted in 1715–1716 [5] were members of the Board at that time. One member – Gerret Corver – is absent, perhaps because he had already been included in the portrait of the Board Governors that was painted in 1684. The surgeon sitting in front of the table is holding a trephine drill in his left hand. Among others, this instrument was used to drill holes in the cranial vault of patients suffering from bleeding in the head (*subdural* or *epidural haematoma*). Resting on the table is a medical handbook which has not been identified, open at a page with an anatomical illustration of a skull. Held under the arm of the

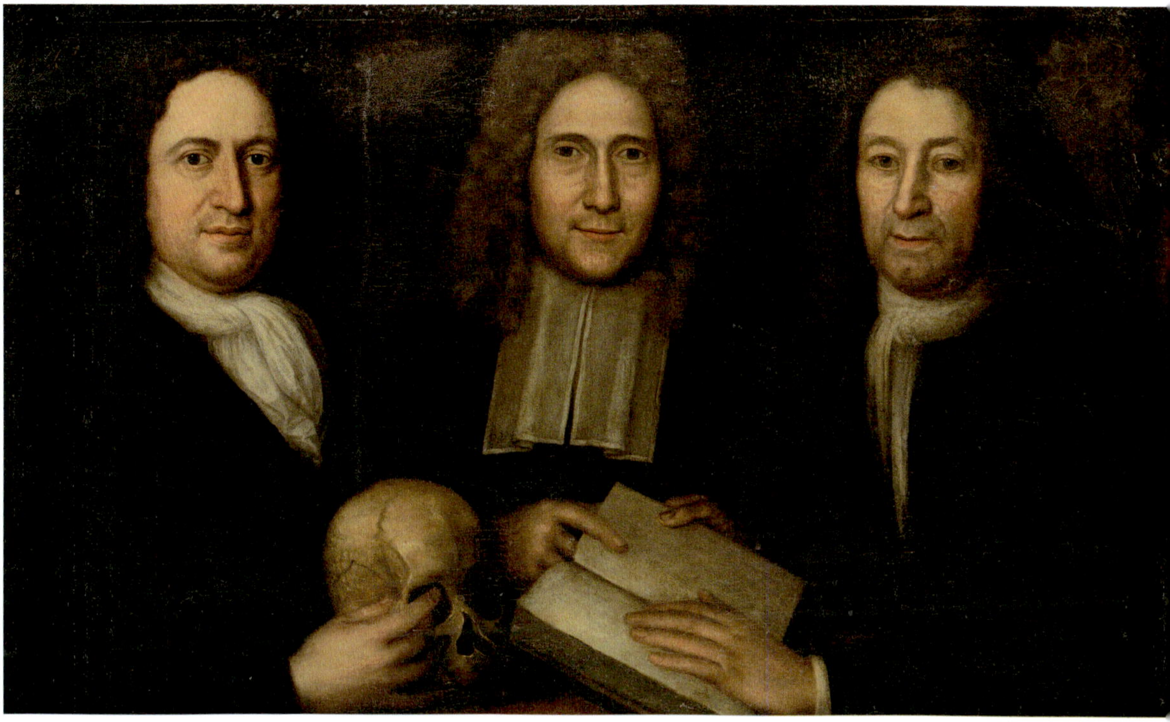

[4]
Unknown artist, *Three Governors of the Surgeons' Guild*, 1706.
From left to right, the surgeons portraited are: Hendrick Smeeckes, Nicolaes Kies and Nicolaes Heems (or Geems). Collection Amsterdam Museum.

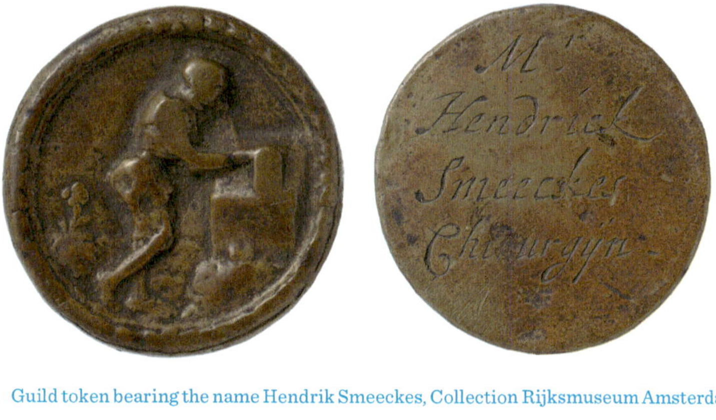

Guild token bearing the name Hendrik Smeeckes, Collection Rijksmuseum Amsterdam.

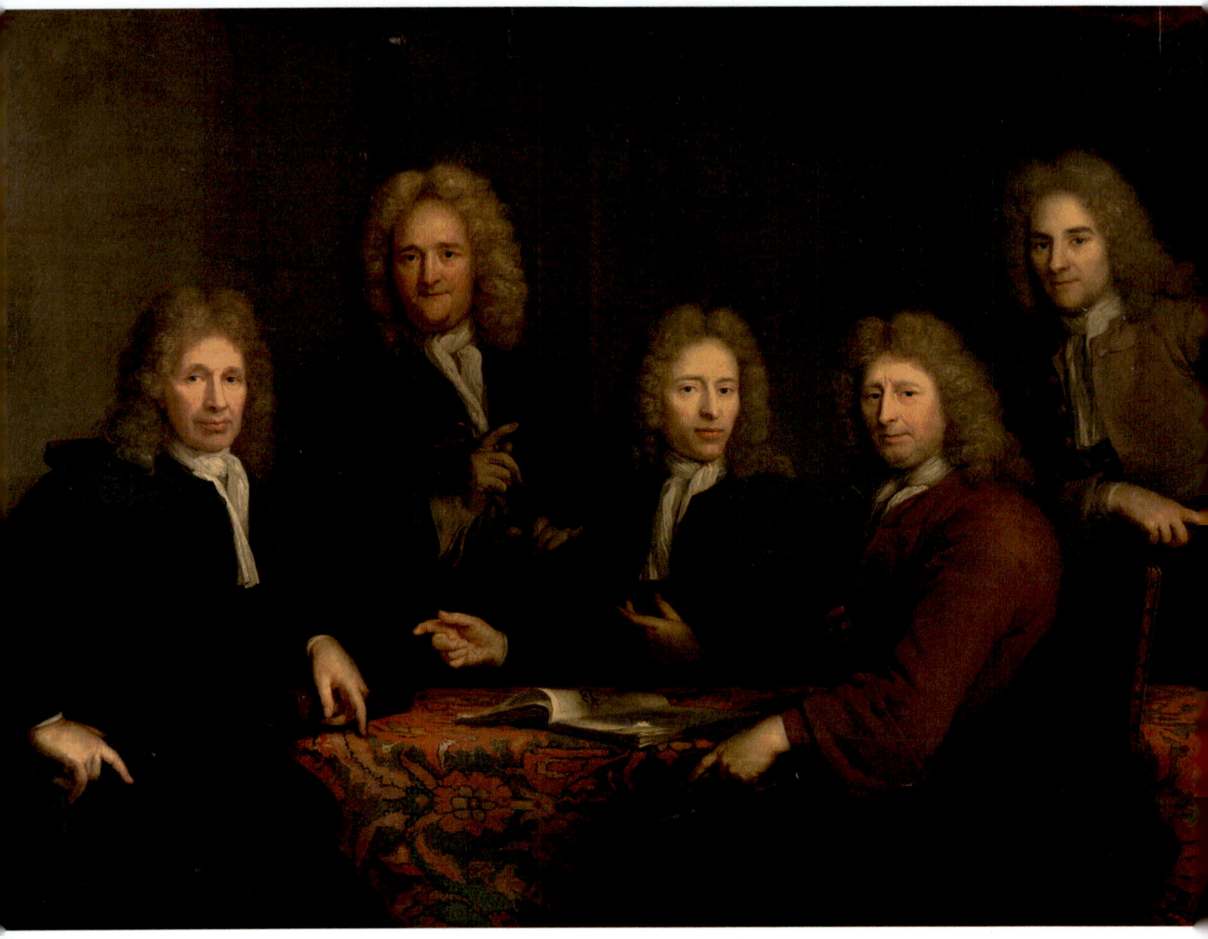

[5]
Arnold Boonen, *Five Governors of the Surgeons' Guild*, 1715-1716.
The Governors depicted are (in random order): Dirck Cloes, Roelof Roelvink, Jan Koenerding, Stilling van Velsen and Benjamin van Tongeren.
Collection Amsterdam Museum.

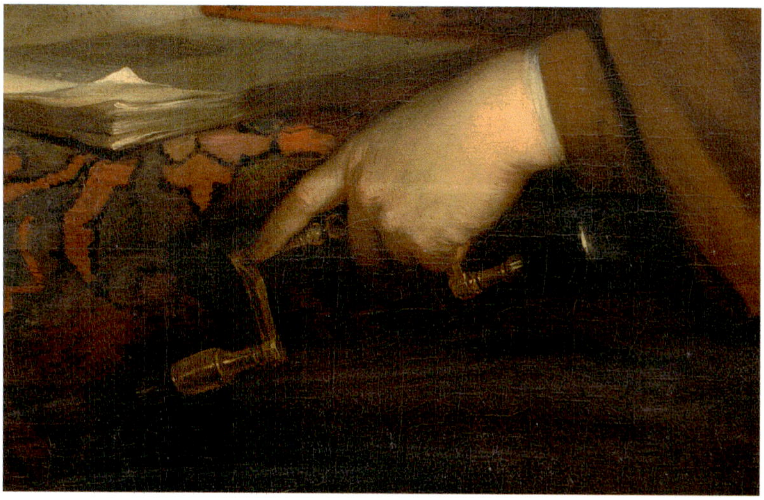

Trephine drill in the portrait of the governors from 1715–1716.

governor seated on the left-hand side of the table is the well-known, influential handbook on surgery by the French surgeon Ambroise Paré (c. 1510–1590).

A new group portrait of the Board of Governors was commissioned in 1731, this time painted by Cornelis Troost (1696–1750) [6]. From left to right, we see the following governors: Isaac Hartman, Elias Huijzer and Adriaan Verduijn. Their coats of arms are displayed on the wall behind them, their names written underneath. These correspond to the coats of arms seen in the third row on the dome vault of the former *Theatrum Anatomicum* at the Weighing House. (See illustration on p. 19 in which the coats of arms of Verduijn and Huijzer can both be seen next to the windows, on opposite sides of each other.) The administrative responsibilities of these Governors are revealed in the painting. Elias Huijzer holds a quill pen in his hand, while Isaac Hartman holds a graduation certificate that was presented to surgeons upon successfully passing their masterpiece (see Introduction, p. 12). No matter how virtuous these surgeons might appear, they were all dismissed one year later by the municipal council for awarding degree certificates in exchange for bribes and for withholding money set aside for the pensions of surgeons' widows. These corrupt practices were exposed by the surgeon Abraham Titsingh in 1731, when he assumed the position of dean and was offered bribes himself.

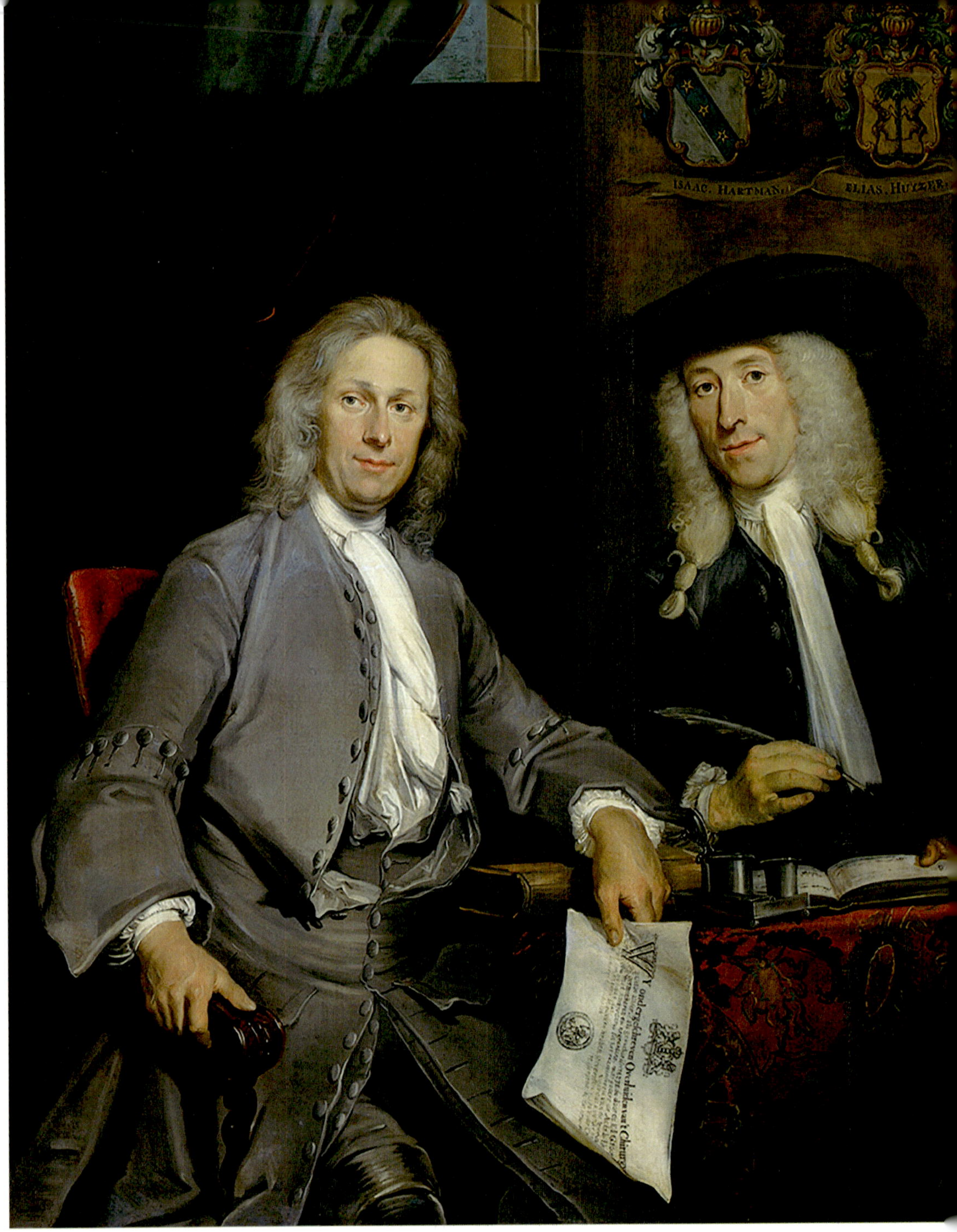

Portraits of the Governors

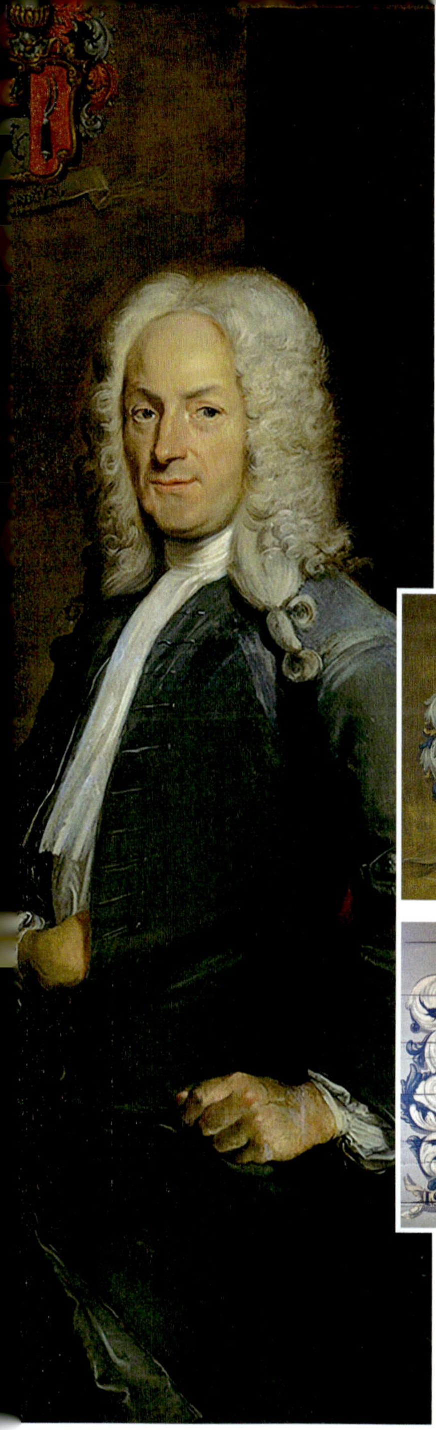

[6]
Cornelis Troost, *Three Governors of the Surgeons' Guild*, 1731. The men portrayed are, from left to right: Isaac Hartman, Elias Huijzer and Adriaan Verduijn. Collection Amsterdam Museum.

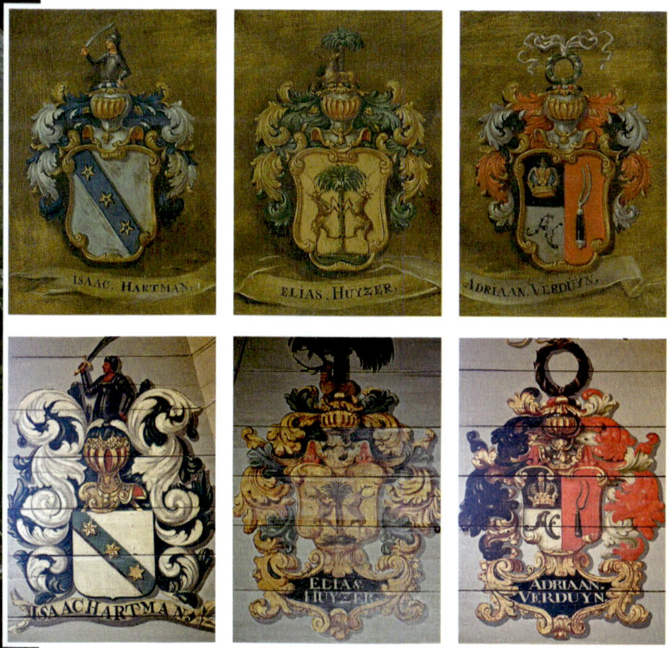

Above The coats of arms of Hartman, Huijzer and Verduijn seen in the background of their group portrait.

Below Corresponding coats of arms of the three governors painted in the dome of the *Theatrum Anatomicum* in the Weighing House.

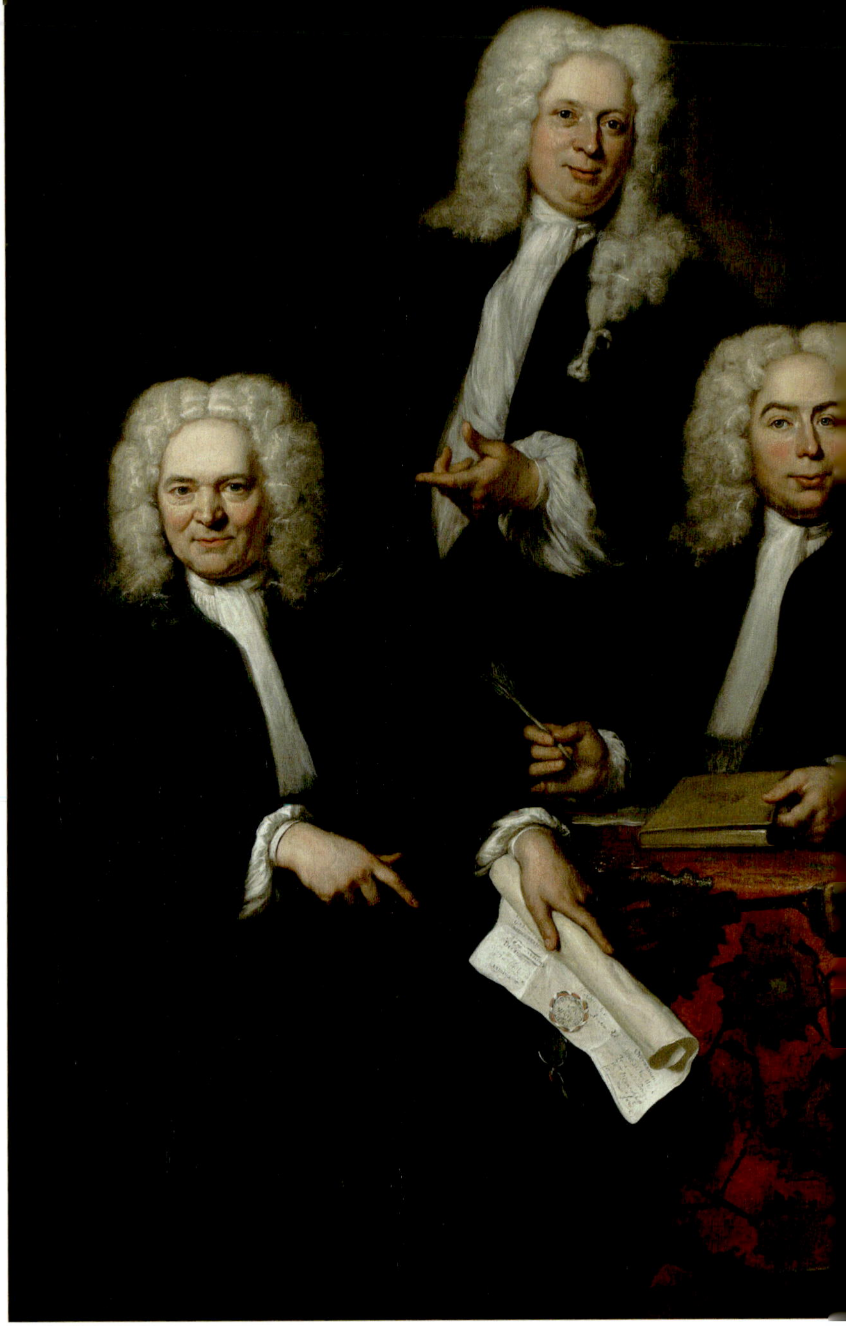

[7]
Jan Maurits Quinkhard, *The Board of Governors of the Surgeons' Guild*, 1732. From left to right: Bartolomeus Vermij, Cornelis van der Swed, Johannes de Bruijn, Willem Monnikhoff, Wichard van Wesik and Abraham Titsingh. Collection Amsterdam Museum.

Inset The degree certificate and coins are a reference to the corruption affair.

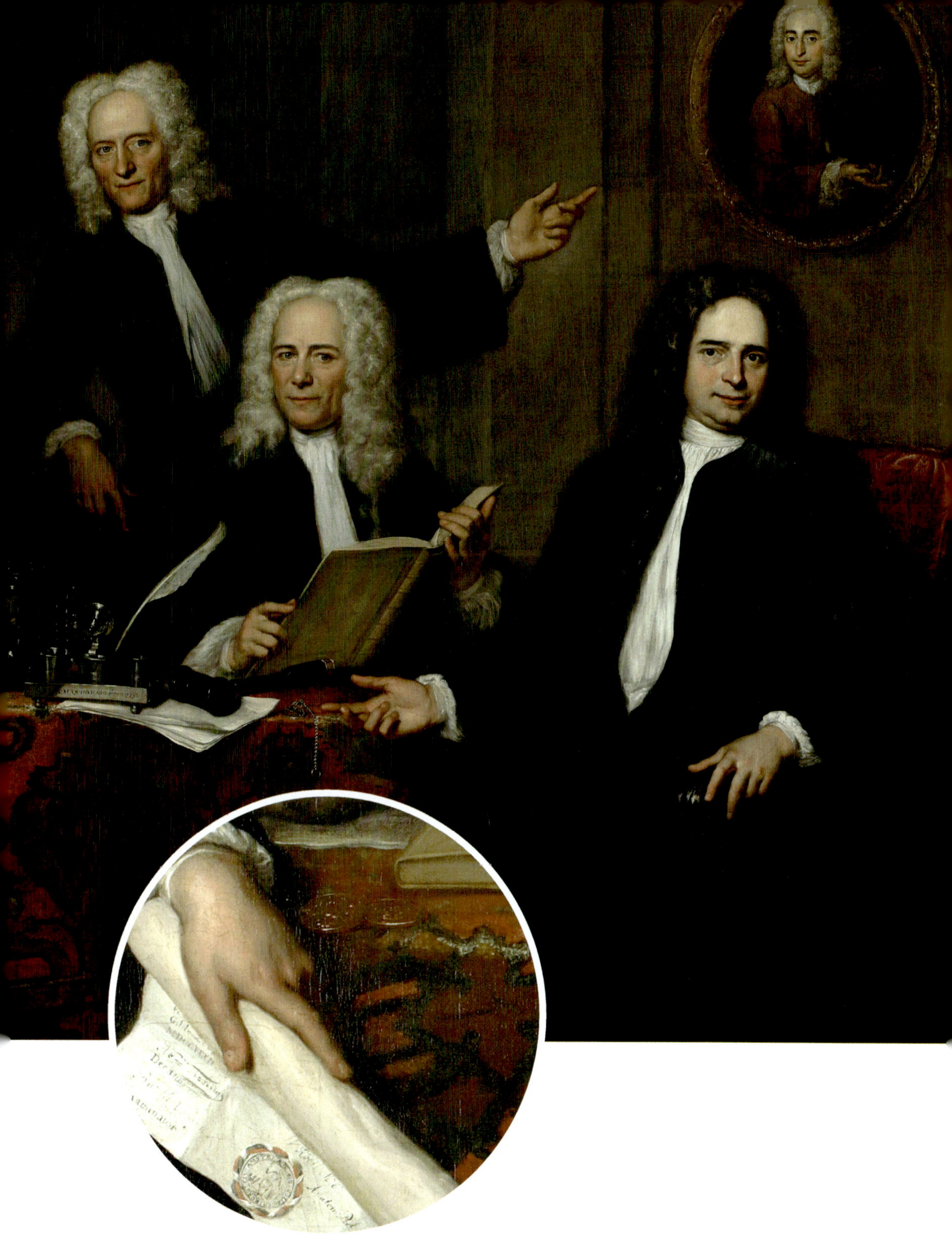

Jan Maurits Quinkhard (1688–1772) painted a group portrait of the Guild's entirely new board in 1732 [7]. Quinkhard signed this group portrait on the silver (or silver-plated) writing set on the middle of the table. The six surgeons portrayed covered the cost of the painting with their own money (they paid the artist a total of 600 guilders), in stark contrast to their predecessors, who had pilfered money from the guild's treasury for this purpose. On the left side of the table sits the oldest governor, Bartholomeus Vermeij, pointing at the document held in his left hand with some emphasis: it is probably a surgeons' diploma. The artist is making a reference here to the preceding board's corrupt practices of awarding degree certificates for money. Once the new board had taken office, such practices became a thing of the past. Just above the degree certificate we can vaguely make out the contours of two coins, perhaps hinting subtly at the bribes accepted by the previous Board. The scene includes more ambiguous elements of significance. On the table, there are three hour-glasses, a chairman's gavel and a small blue notebook, known as a Heerenboekje *(Gentlemen's Notebook)* in which the governors' personal information was noted down. Surgeon Van Wesik holds an open book with the inscription *'grootboek'*; this was the main ledger in which they kept their financial administration. On the right of the table sits Abraham Titsingh, the man who exposed the corruption affair. On the wall behind him, hangs the portrait of the current *praelector* Willem Röell, which carries the inscription *vigilate juste* (be vigilant and just). This suggests that Röell had distanced himself from the fraudulent affair and had sought to associate himself with the new Board of Governors, which was 'as honest as the day is long'. It seems that many of the elements in the painting refer to the financial turmoil in which the Guild's Board of Governors found itself. Fortunately for the Guild, better times were ahead.

The second portrait of the Board, painted by Quinkhard in 1737, shows seven Board members seated behind a table [8]. With the exception of surgeon Leonard Coster (far right), all had been Head of the guild at some point. Coster had been nominated for a Board function, but he was never elected. The coats of arms of the seven men are shown along the border of the carpet covering the table. These correspond to the coats of arms painted in the dome of the *Theatrum Anatomicum* at the Weighing House. Only the unadorned

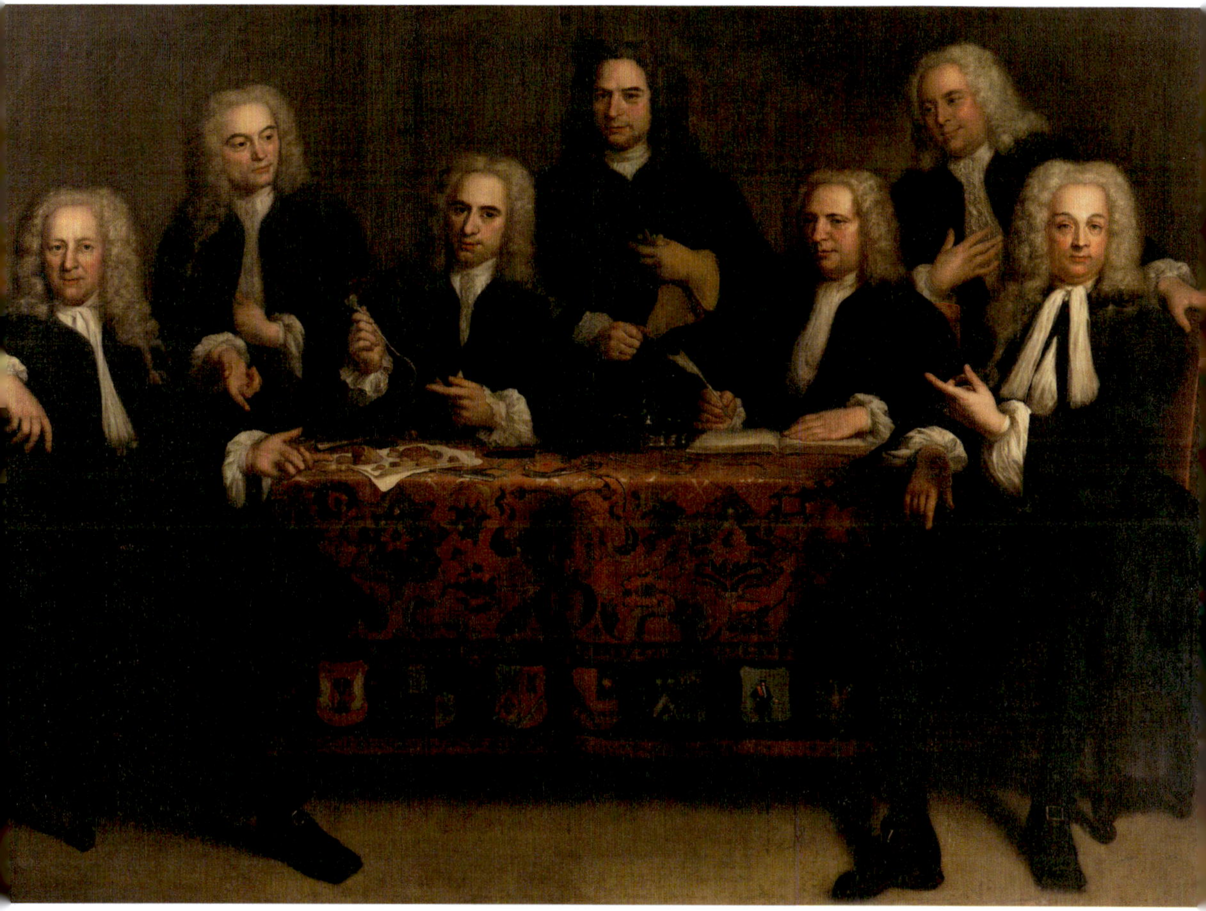

[8]
Jan Maurits Quinkhard, *Seven members of the Surgeons' Guild*, 1737.
From left to right: Pieter Plaatman, Augustinus Graver, Hermannus Meyer, Abraham Titsingh, Jan Bekker, Johannes Lakeman, Leonard Coster.
Collection Amsterdam Museum.

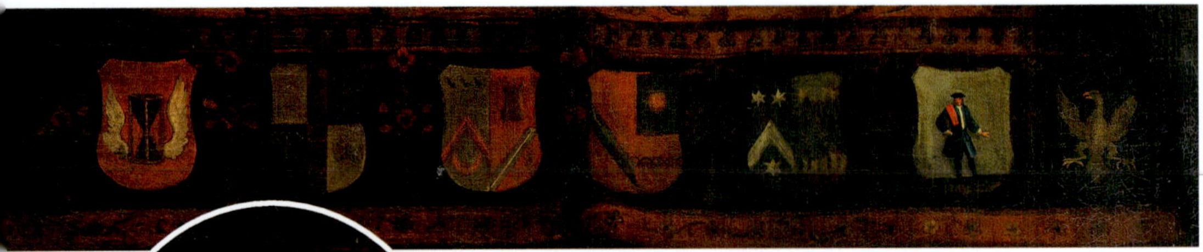

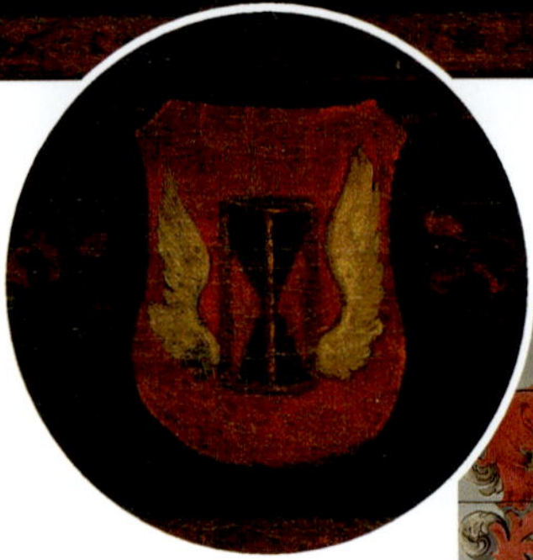

Shown along the border of the table cover are the family crests of the surgeons depicted in the governors' portrait of 1737.

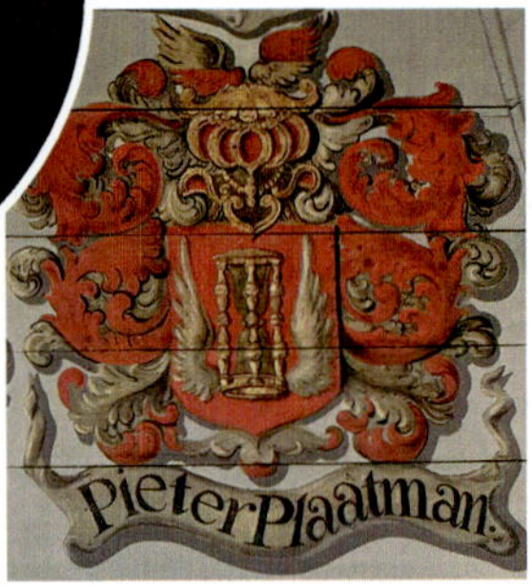

The coat of arms of Pieter Plaatman as painted onto the dome of the *Theatrum Anatomicum* at the Weighing House. It corresponds to the family crest on the far left of the table cover in the governors' portrait from 1737. In the crest's centre, there is an hour-glass flanked by two feathers. The full coat of arms in the vault dome has been adorned, while on the painting, only the family crest is shown.

family crests are shown here, whereas the coats of arms at the *Theatrum Anatomicum* are ornately decorated.

On the table there are a number of bladder stones and the instruments used to extract them. Possible causes of bladder stones are concentrated urine, problems with voiding the bladder and cystitis. The extraction of stones from the bladder was a painful and dangerous operation in those days: it was a surgical procedure not every surgeon could perform. Therefore, Amsterdam had specialist surgeons to extract the stones: these were known as *steensnijders* (stone-cutters or lithotomists). Hermannus Meyer — the third surgeon from the left — was an expert in this field. He is also the one who compiled the *Privilegiën, willekeuren en ordonnantiën, betreffende het Collegium Chirurgicum Amstelaedamense* (Rights, Regulations and Ordinances of the College of Surgeons of Amsterdam), a collection of all the Guild regulations from the period between 1461 and 1736. According to regulations as decreed in 1700, any surgeon about to perform a 'cutting for the stone' had to ask permission from the burgomaster, the Surgeons' Guild's governors and a municipal physician (*doctor*

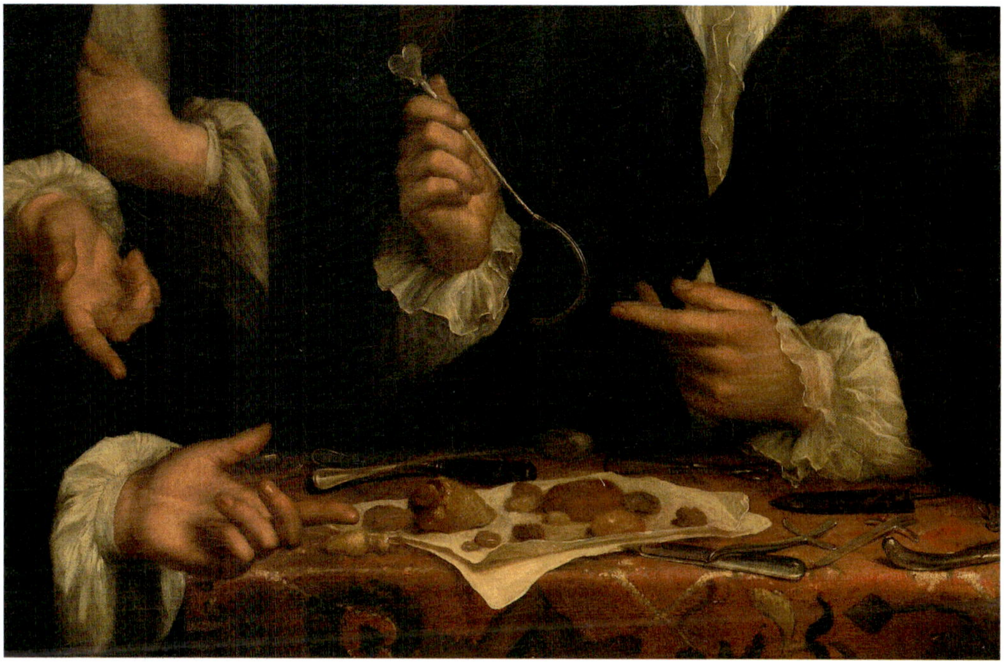

On the table are a number of bladder stones and the instruments used to extract them. In his right hand, Hermannus Meijer (Meyer) is holding a stone extractor.

medicinae) at least twenty-four hours in advance. The procedure had to be done under the supervision of two of the Board's governors and the physician. Furthermore, every 'stone cutting' performed in Amsterdam had to be recorded in what was known as the Guild's *'Steenboek' (Book of Stones)*. According to this book, Hermannus Meyer carried out no fewer than sixty-eight stone-cutting operations in the period between 1732 and 1741. In his right hand he is holding a stone extractor, which was used in such an operation. At the beginning of the procedure, the patient had to draw up both knees. The surgeon then inserted the stone extractor into the bladder via the urethra. Guided by the stone extractor, he would use a scalpel to make an incision across the perineum (in men the area between the scrotum and the anus and in women between the anus and the vagina), until the bladder was reached. Through this open wound, it was then possible for him to remove the bladder stones with 'stone' forceps, also seen on the table. Abraham Titsingh — standing in the middle, behind the table — was also a stone-cutting specialist. In 1731, he published a work entitled *Heelkundige Verhandeling over de Steen*

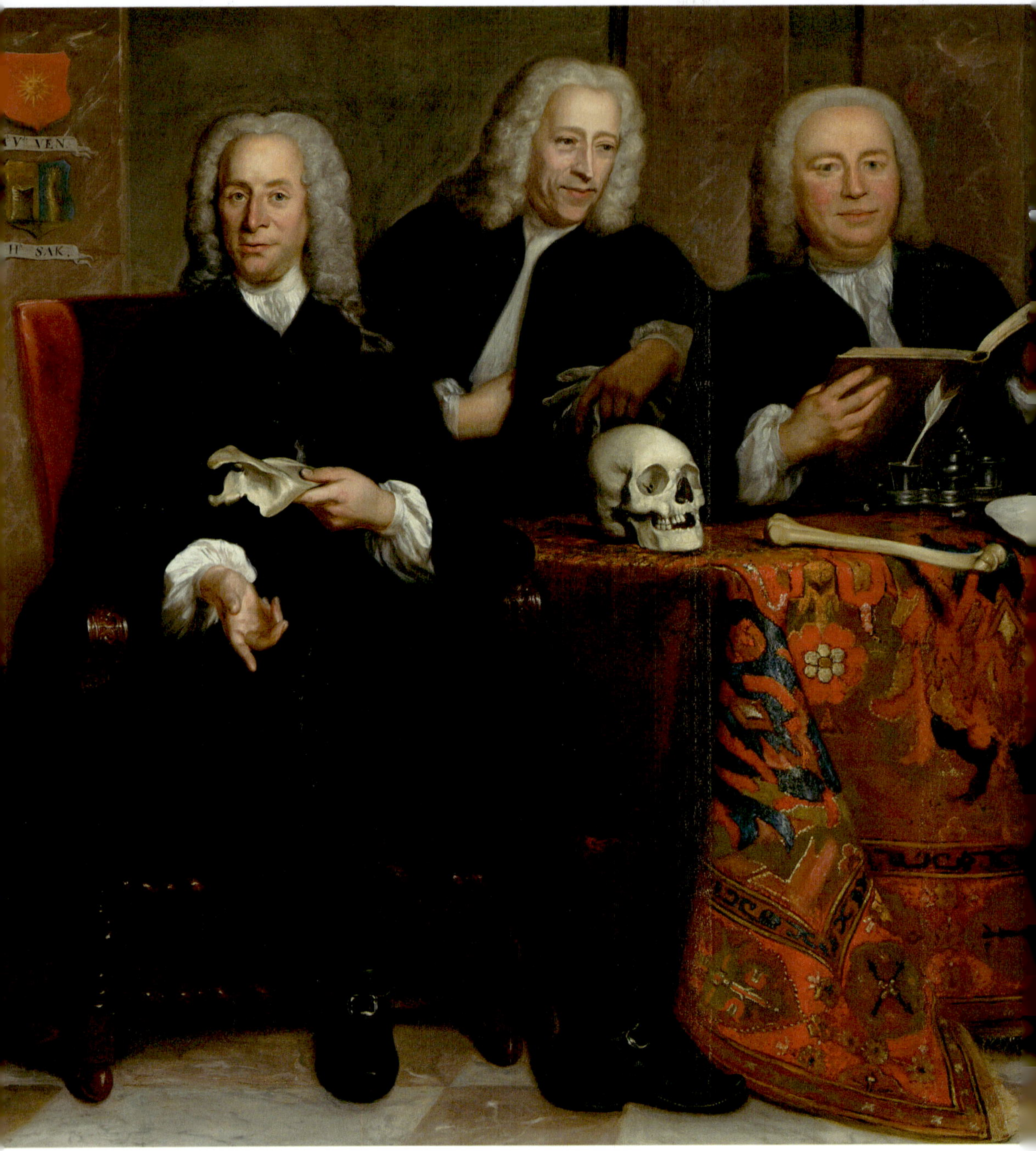

Portraits of the Governors

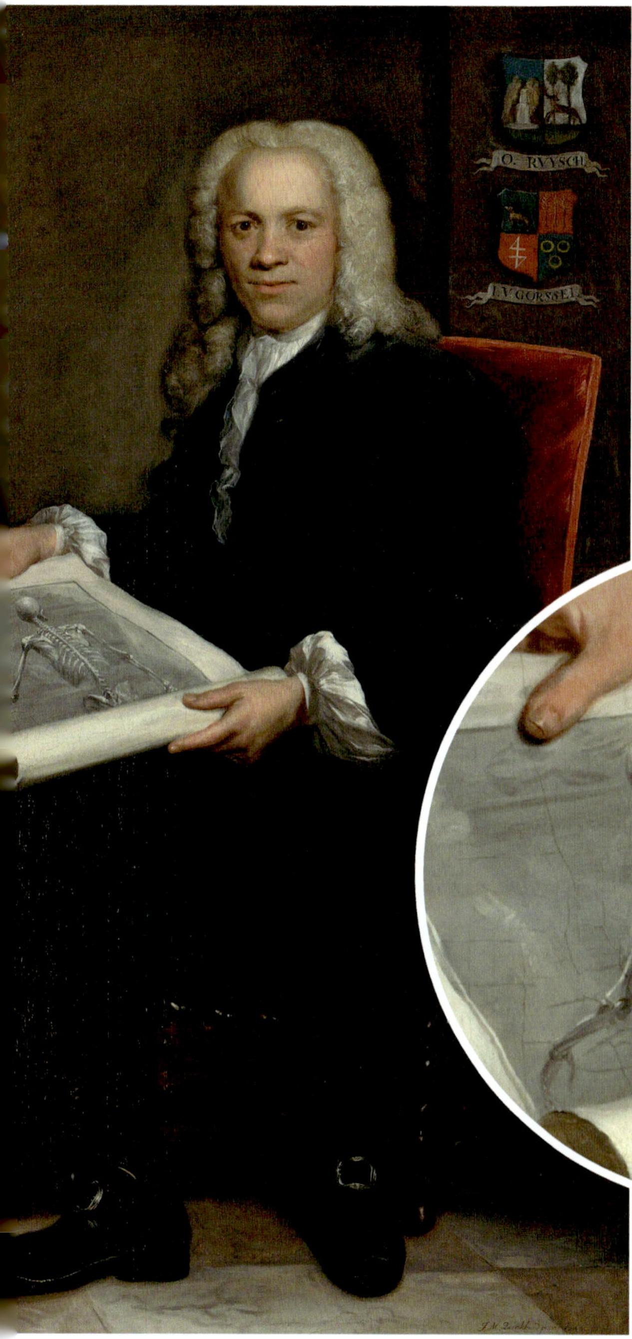

[9]
Jan Maurits Quinkhard, *Four Governors of the Surgeons' Guild*, 1744. From left to right, the governors depicted are: Hendrik van der Ven, Hendrik Sak, Johannes van Gorssel and Otto Ruysch. On the central columns on the rear wall, it is still possible to make out the vague outlines of the coats of arms of Sak and Van Gorssel. Quinkhard had painted over these during the course of his work. Collection Amsterdam Museum.

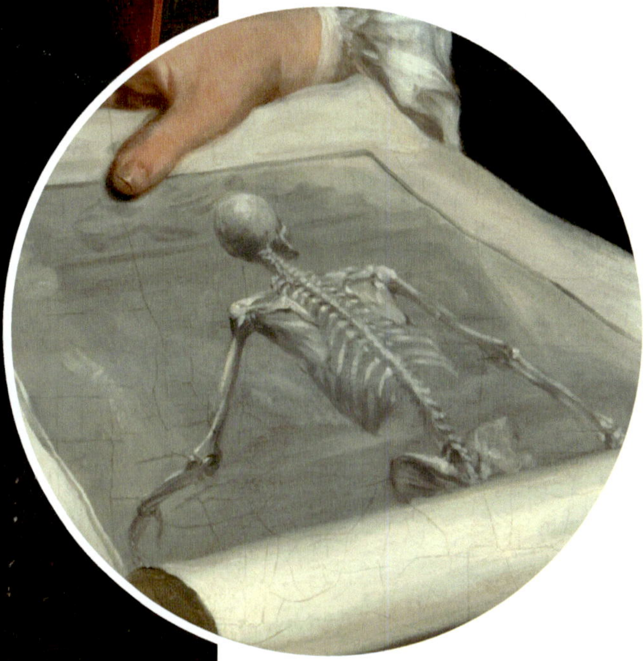

Jan Wandelaar, illustration of a skeleton from the work by Bernard Siegfried Albinus.

en het Steensnyden (Surgical Treatise on the Stone and Stone cutting), a polemic written in response to the recently appeared publication on the subject by his Leiden colleague, Denys.

Of the nine group portraits made for the Amsterdam's Surgeons' Guild, Quinkhard's third group portrait of the Board, painted in 1744, was also the last [9]. The coats of arms of those portrayed, all of whom were Governors of the Guild in the period September 1743 to September 1744, are displayed on the columns on the right and left side of the rear wall. The image of the other two Governors from this period – Abraham Titsingh and Johannes Lakeman – had already been included in the group portrait of the Governors painted in 1737. The coats of arms correspond to those in the vault dome of the *Theatrum Anatomicum* at the Weighing House.

On the table, there is a skull that bears a striking resemblance to the one shown in *The Anatomy Lesson of Johan Fonteijn* (See Chapter 3, p. 77). Next to it, we see an upper arm bone (*humerus*). On the far right sits Otto Ruysch. The illustration he is holding shows a skeleton from the anatomical atlas *De ossibus corporis humani* (On the Bones of the Human Body compiled by Bernard Siegfried Albinus (1697-1770), the incumbent chair of anatomy and surgery in Leiden). This scientific work was published in Leiden in 1726. Johannes Van Gorssel, on Ruysch's left, holds an opened book, with the words 'ALBIN – de Ossibus' on the spine: *De ossibus corporis humani* by Albinus. A skeleton in the same pose as the one on the illustration is also seen in Albinus' famous anatomical atlas *Tabulae sceleti et musculorum corporis humani* (Atlas of the Bones and Muscles of the Human Body) (1747) (see illustration on p. 68).

After the completion of this last portrait of the Board, the Surgeons' Guild was in proud possession of eight 'anatomy lessons' and nine group portraits showing the various Boards of Governors. The one remaining painting that would make the collection complete, was *The Anatomy Lesson of Petrus Camper* (1758), which is discussed further in Chapter 9.

Bibliography

Introduction

Beijer, T., H.A. Bosman-Jelgersma, S.A.C. Dudok van Heel, J.N. Keeman, G. Nolthenius de Man en I.C.E. Wesdorp (1991), *Nicolaes Tulp: Leven en werk van een Amsterdams geneesheer en magistraat.* Amsterdam: Six Art Promotion.

Delprat, C.C. & A. Kummer (1965), *De wording en de geschiedenis van het Genootschap ter Bevordering van Natuur-, Genees- en Heelkunde te Amsterdam 1790–1915. De geschiedenis van het Genootschap ter Bev. van Nat.-, Gen.- en Heelkunde vervolg 1915–1965.* Amsterdam: Genootschap ter Bevordering van Natuur-, Genees- en Heelkunde.

Eeghen, I.H. van (1965), *De gilden: theorie en praktijk.* Bussum: C.A.J. van Dishoeck, 72-100.

Houtzager, H.L. (1997). Een blik in een chirurgijnswinkel. *Geschiedenis der Geneeskunde*, 3(4): 208-214.

Gulik, T.M. van, IJpma, F.F.A., Middelkoop, N.E. (2014), Wapenschilden van het Amsterdamse Chirurgijnsgilde in de koepel van het Theatrum Anatomicum. *Ned Tijdschr Geneeskd*, 158: A6990.

Kooijmans, L. (2004), *De doodskunstenaar: De anatomische lessen van Frederik Ruysch.* Amsterdam: Bert Bakker.

Kurpershoek, E. (1994), *De Waag op de Nieuwmarkt.* Amsterdam: Stadsuitgeverij Amsterdam.

Meyer, H. (1736), *Privilegien, willekeuren en ordonnantiën, betreffende het Collegium Chirurgicum Amstelaedamense.* Amsterdam: Pieter van den Berge.

Middelkoop, N.E., P. Noble, J. Wadum & B. Broos (1998), *Rembrandt onder het mes: De anatomische les van Dr Nicolaes Tulp ontleed.* Amsterdam: Six Art Promotion bv.

Middelkoop, N.E., J. Baptist Bedaux, S.A.C. Dudok van Heel, R. Ekkart & J. van Gent (red.) (2002), *Kopstukken: Amsterdammers geportretteerd 1600/1800.* Bussum: Uitgeverij THOTH / Amsterdams Historisch Museum.

Moulin, D. de (1988), *A history of surgery: with emphasis on the Netherlands.* Dordrecht: Martinus Nijhoff Publishers.

Nuyens, B.W.Th. (1928), Het ontleedkundig onderwijs en de geschilderde Anatomische lessen van het Chirurgijns Gilde te Amsterdam in de jaren 1550 tot 1798. In: Scharp H.J. (red.), *Koninklijk Oudheidkundig Genootschap te Amsterdam: Jaarverslag.* Amsterdam: Koninklijk Oudheidkundig Genootschap, 45-90.

Stadsarchief Amsterdam, Archief van de Gilden en het Brouwerscollege 366/294, *Anatomieboek van het Amsterdamse Chirurgijnsgilde.* Amsterdam: Amsterdamse Chirurgijnsgilde.

IJpma, F.F.A., R.C. van de Graaf, E.G.J.M. Pierik & T.M. van Gulik (2009). De meesterproef in de chirurgijnsopleiding: een historisch concept als voorbeeld voor nu? *Ned Tijdschr Geneeskd*, 153: A795.

IJpma, F.F.A, E.G.J.M Pierik en T.M. van Gulik (2011). De chirurgijnsopleiding van het Amsterdamse Chirurgijnsgilde. *Geschiedenis der Geneeskunde,* 15(6): 380-390.

1

Dodonaeus, R. & S. Egbertszn de Vrij (1616), *Praxis medica Remberti Dodonaei*. Amsterdam: Hendrick Laurensz.

Dodonaeus, R., S. Egbertszn de Vrij & N. van Wassenaar (1624), *Ars Medica, ofte Ghenees-kunst*. Amsterdam: Hans Walschaert.

Dudok van Heel, S.A.C. (1987). Enkele adressen van zestiende eeuwse kunstschilders. *Amstelodamum*, 74: 1-7.

Eeghen, I.H. van (1965), *De gilden: theorie en praktijk*. Bussum: C.A.J. van Dishoeck, 72-100.

Elias, J.E. (1963), *Het vroedschap van Amsterdam 1578–1795*. Amsterdam: N. Israel.

Fernelius, J. & S. Egbertszn de Vrij (1596), *De beschrijvinge der deelen des lichaems van den mensche: In 't Latijnsch door D. Johannem Fernelium ghemaeckt: Ende nu in Neder-duytsche spraecke overghezettet*. Amsterdam: Barendt Adriaenszoon.

Fernelius, J. en S. Egbertszn de Vrij (1649), De beschrijvinge der deelen des menschelijcken lichaems / in 't Latijn beschreven door D. Joh. Fernelium: Ende in 't Nederduyts overgezet door D. Sebastiaen Egbertsz. In: A. Paré en C. Battus, *De chirurgie, ende alle de opera, ofte wercken van Mr. Ambrosius Paré*. Amsterdam: Gerrit Willemsz, 1-43.

Lindeboom, G.A. (1984), *Dutch medical biography: A biographical dictionary of Dutch physicians and surgeons 1475–1975*. Amsterdam: Rodopi.

Meyer, H. (1736), *Privilegien, willekeuren en ordonnantiën, betreffende het Collegium Chirurgicum Amstelaedamense*. Amsterdam: Pieter van den Berge.

Middelkoop, N.E., P. Noble, J. Wadum & B. Broos (1998), *Rembrandt onder het mes: De anatomische les van Dr Nicolaes Tulp ontleed*. Amsterdam: Six Art Promotion bv.

Middelkoop, N.E., J. Baptist Bedaux, S.A.C. Dudok van Heel, R. Ekkart & J. van Gent (red.) (2002), *Kopstukken: Amsterdammers geportretteerd 1600/1800*. Bussum: Uitgeverij THOTH / Amsterdams Historisch Museum.

Moulin, D. de (1988), *A history of surgery: with emphasis on the Netherlands*. Dordrecht: Martinus Nijhoff Publishers.

Nuyens, B.W.Th. (1928), Het ontleedkundig onderwijs en de geschilderde Anatomische lessen van het Chirurgijns Gilde te Amsterdam in de jaren 1550 tot 1798. In: Scharp H.J. (red.), *Koninklijk Oudheidkundig Genootschap te Amsterdam: Jaarverslag*. Amsterdam: Koninklijk Oudheidkundig Genootschap, 45-90.

2

Albinus, B.S. (1747), *Tabulae sceleti et musculorum corporis humani*. Leiden: Lugduni Batavorum, prostant apud Joannem & Hermannum Verbeek.

Albinus, B.S. (1753), *Tabulae ossium humanorum*. Leiden: Joannem & Hermannum Verbeek.

Baruch, J.Z. (1964), *Leven en werk van Andreas Vesalius*. Gravenhage: Kruseman's.

Bidloo, G. (1690), *Ontleding des menschelijken lichaams: Uitgebeeld, naar het leven in honderd en vyf aftekeningen door de Heer Gerard De Lairesse*. Amsterdam: de weduwe van Joannes van Someren, de erfgenamen Joannes van Dijk, Hendrik en de weduwe Dirk Boom.

Bonn, A. (1785), *Tabulae Ossium Morbosorum*. Amsterdam: J.C. Sepp.

Bout, B. de (1693), *'t Nieuwe examen der chirurgie*. Amsterdam: Jan ten Hoorn.

Cheselden, W. (1733), *Osteographia, or the Anatomy of the Bones*. London: William Bowyer.

Herls, C. (1663), *Examen der Chyrurgie*. Middelburg: Françoys Kroock.

Hildebrand, R. (2005). Attic perfection in anatomy: Bernhard Siegfried Albinus (1697–1770) and Samuel Thomas Soemmerring (1755–1830). *Ann Anat*, 187: 555-573.

Lindeboom, G.A. (1982). Cowper's brutale 'plagiaat' van Bidloo's anatomische atlas. *Ned Tijdschr Geneeskd,* 126: 1878-1882.

Loffeld, R.J.L.F. (2002). Het zwevende-ribsyndroom: een veelal niet herkende oorzaak van pijnklachten. *Ned Tijdschr Geneeskd,* 146: 1813–1815.

Meyer, H. (1736), *Privilegien, willekeuren en ordonnantiën, betreffende het Collegium Chirurgicum Amstelaedamense.* Amsterdam: Pieter van den Berge.

Middelkoop, N.E., P. Noble, J. Wadum & B. Broos (1998), *Rembrandt onder het mes: De anatomische les van Dr Nicolaes Tulp ontleed.* Amsterdam: Six Art Promotion bv.

Middelkoop, N.E., J. Baptist Bedaux, S.A.C. Dudok van Heel, R. Ekkart & J. van Gent (red.) (2002), *Kopstukken: Amsterdammers geportretteerd 1600/1800.* Bussum: Uitgeverij THOTH / Amsterdams Historisch Museum.

Molenaar, J.C. (2004). Anatomie als schouwspel. Uit de bibliotheek van de Vereniging Nederlands Tijdschrift voor Geneeskunde. Govard Bidloo: Ontleding des Menschelijken Lichaams; 1689 en William Cowper: The Anatomy of Humane Bodies; 1698. *Ned Tijdschr Geneeskd,* 148: 2594-2602.

Rhijnenburgh, B.I. (1650), *Examen ofte proeve der chirurgijns ende barbieren.* Rotterdam: Pieter van Waesberge, 1650.

Richardson, W.F. & J.B. Carman (1998), *On the Fabric of the Human Body: A Translation of De Humani Corporis Fabrica Libri Septem. Book I: the Bones and Cartilages. Andreas Vesalius.* San Francisco: Norman publishing.

Rifkin, B.A. & M.J. Ackerman (2006), *Menselijke anatomie, van de renaissance tot het digitale tijdperk.* Amsterdam: Mets & Schilt.

Rooy, L. de, H. van den Bogaard, S. Knepper, J. Kortenray & A. Moorman (red.) (2009), *Verzamelaars van vorm.* Amsterdam: Vossiuspers UvA.

Sanders, M.A. (1999). William Cheselden: anatomist, surgeon, and medical illustrator. *Spine,* 24: 2282-2289.

Stadsarchief Amsterdam, Archief van de Gilden en het Brouwerscollege 366/294, *Anatomieboek van het Amsterdamse Chirurgijnsgilde.* Amsterdam: Amsterdamse Chirurgijnsgilde.

Sylvester, D. (ca. 1615), *Ad Clarissimum & Ornatissimum Dominum Doctorem D. Sebastianum Egbertsonum, Consulem & Quaestorem Amstelodamensem, & ibidem in Theatro Anatomico Oratorem publicum.* Amsterdam.

Ulhoorn, H. (1755), *Laurens Heisters heelkundige onderwijzingen.* Amsterdam: Gerrit de Groot en Jan Morterre.

Ulhoorn, H. (ca. 1770), *Ulhoorn's osteologia.* Amsterdam: J. Morterre.

Verbrugge, J. (1677), *Heel-konstige examen ofte instructie der chirurgie begrepen in vier tractaten.* Amsterdam: Jan Claesz Ten Hoorn.

Vesalius, A. (1555), *De humani corporis fabrica libri primus.* Basileae: Ioannem Oporinum.

IJpma, F.F.A., H.J. ten Duis & T.M. van Gulik (2012). Osteology: a cornerstone of orthopaedic education. *Bone & Joint* ^{360}, 1(6): 2-7.

IJpma, F.F.A., T.M. van Gulik (2017), Lessons in osteology using the skeleton of an English pirate. *Br J Surg,* 104(4):316.

3

Beijer, T., H.A. Bosman-Jelgersma, S.A.C. Dudok van Heel, J.N. Keeman, G. Nolthenius de Man & I.C.E. Wesdorp (1991), *Nicolaes Tulp: Leven en werk van een Amsterdams geneesheer en magistraat.* Amsterdam: Six Art Promotion.

Lindeboom, G.A. (1984), *Dutch medical biography: A biographical dictionary of Dutch physicians and surgeons 1475–1975.* Amsterdam: Rodopi.

Middelkoop, N.E., P. Noble, J. Wadum & B. Broos (1998), *Rembrandt onder het mes: De anatomische les van*

Dr Nicolaes Tulp ontleed. Amsterdam: Six Art Promotion bv.

Middelkoop, N.E., J. Baptist Bedaux, S.A.C. Dudok van Heel, R. Ekkart & J. van Gent (red.) (2002), *Kopstukken: Amsterdammers geportretteerd 1600/1800*. Bussum: Uitgeverij THOTH / Amsterdams Historisch Museum.

Nuyens, B.W.Th. (1928), Het ontleedkundig onderwijs en de geschilderde Anatomische lessen van het Chirurgijns Gilde te Amsterdam in de jaren 1550 tot 1798. In: Scharp H.J. (red.), *Koninklijk Oudheidkundig Genootschap te Amsterdam: Jaarverslag*. Amsterdam: Koninklijk Oudheidkundig Genootschap, 45-90.

Tilanus, J.W.R. (1865), *Beschrijving der schilderijen afkomstig van het chirurgijns-gild te Amsterdam: Met enige historische aanteekeningen omtrent het gild, en eene nadere beschouwing der kunstwaarde der verzameling*. Amsterdam: Frederik Muller.

4

Bankl, H.C. & H. Bankl (2000). Dr. Nicolaas Tulp: Rembrandt's Anatomiegemälde kritisch betrachtet. *Wien Klin Wochenschr*, 112: 368-371.

Berichten Binnenland (1986). Nederlandse dokter-dichters in de 15de–19de eeuw. *Ned Tijdschr Geneeskd*, 130: 1774-1776.

Beijer, T., H.A. Bosman-Jelgersma, S.A.C. Dudok van Heel, J.N. Keeman, G. Nolthenius de Man & I.C.E. Wesdorp (1991), *Nicolaes Tulp: Leven en werk van een Amsterdams geneesheer en magistraat*. Amsterdam: Six Art Promotion.

Bezerra, A.J., L.J. DiDio & L. Piva-Junior (1991). Dissection of Rembrandt's 'Anatomy of Dr. Nicolaas Tulp'. *Arch Ital Anat Embriol*, 96: 153-164.

Broos, B. & R. van Leeuwen (1987), *Meesterwerken in het Mauritshuis*. Den Haag: Staatsuitgeverij, 277-288.

Carpentier Alting, M.P. & Tj.W. Waterbok (1976). Nieuw licht op de ontleedkundige fouten in Rembrandt's 'Anatomische les van Dr. Nicolaas Tulp'. *Ned Tijdschr Geneeskd*, 120: 1900-1902.

Carpentier Alting, M.P. & Tj.W. Waterbok (1982). New light on the anatomical errors in Rembrandt's Anatomy lesson of Dr. Nicolaas Tulp. *J Hand Surg [Am]*, 7: 632-634.

Cremone jr, J.C. (1982). The anatomy lesson of Dr. Nicolaas Tulp. *J Hand Surg [Am]*, 7: 530.

Eeghen, I.H. van (1948). De anatomische lessen van Rembrandt. *Amstelodamum*, 35: 34-36.

Eeghen, I.H. van (1969). Rembrandt en de mensenvilders. *Amstelodamum*, 56: 1-11.

Glazenburg, J. (1977). Rembrandt's anatomy of Dr. Nicolaas Tulp. *Arch Chir Neerl*, 29: 83-91.

Glazenburg, J. (1976). Rembrandt's anatomy of Dr. Nicolaas Tulp. *Int Surg*, 61: 586-590.

Goldwyn, R.M. (1961). Nicolaas Tulp (1593–1674). *Med Hist*, 5: 270-276.

Heckscher, W.S. (1958), *Rembrandt's Anatomy of Dr. Nicolaas Tulp: An iconological study*. New York: New York University Press.

Kruger, L. (2005). The scientific impact of Dr. N. Tulp, portrayed in Rembrandt's 'Anatomy lesson'. *J Hist Neurosci*, 14: 85-92.

Light, T.R. (1982). Hands on stamps. *J Hand Surg [Am]*, 7: 20.

Lindeboom, G.A. (1976). Ontleedkundige fouten op Rembrandt's Anatomische Les? *Ned Tijdschr Geneeskd*, 120: 71-73.

Lindeboom, G.A. (1975). Hogarth – Vesalius – Rembrandt. *Ned Tijdschr Geneeskd*, 119: 1869-1870.

Lindeboom, G.A. (1984), *Dutch medical biography: A biographical dictionary of Dutch physicians and surgeons 1475-1975*. Amsterdam: Rodopi.

Lint, J.G. de (1930), *Rembrandt*. Den Haag: J. Philip Kruseman.

Masquelet, A.C. (2005). The anatomy lesson of Dr Tulp. *J Hand Surg [Br]*, 30: 379-381.

Meals, R.A. (1982). The anatomy lesson of Dr. Nicolaas Tulp. *J Hand Surg [Am]*, 7: 530.

Meekeren, J. van (1979), *Heel- en genees-konstige aenmerkingen door Job van Meekeren* (facsimile). Alphen aan den Rijn: Stafleu's wetenschappelijke uitgeversmaatschappij B.V.

Middelkoop, N.E., P. Noble, J. Wadum & B. Broos (1998), *Rembrandt onder het mes: De anatomische les van Dr Nicolaes Tulp ontleed.* Amsterdam: Six Art Promotion bv.

Mills, A.R. (1989). Rembrandt's painting of the Anatomy lesson of Dr Tulp. *Proceedings of the Royal College of Physicians of Edinburgh*, 19: 327-330.

Moulin, D. de, I.H. van Eeghen & R. Meischke (1981), *Vier eeuwen Amsterdams Binnengasthuis.* Wormer: Inmerc B.V., 74-75.

Romanes, G.J. (1989). Rembrandt's painting of the anatomy lesson of dr Tulp. *Proceedings of the Royal College of Physicians of Edinburgh*, 19: 330.

Scherer, H. (1990). Rembrandt's 'Dr. Tulp's anatomy lesson'. *Minn Med*, 73: 24-28.

Schupbach, W. (1982), *The paradox of Rembrandt's 'Anatomy of Dr. Tulp'.* London: Wellcome Institute for the History of Medicine.

Scothorne, R.J. (1989). Rembrandt's painting of the anatomy lesson of dr Tulp. *Proceedings of the Royal College of Physicians of Edinburgh*, 19: 330.

Smeulers, J. (1975). Een samenspraak van clinicus en preclinicus. *Ned Tijdschr Geneeskd*, 119: 1867-1868.

Stadsarchief Amsterdam, Archief van de Gilden en het Brouwerscollege 366/294, *Anatomieboek van het Amsterdamse Chirurgijnsgilde.* Amsterdam: Amsterdamse Chirurgijnsgilde.

Vesalius, A (1555), *De humani corporis fabrica libri septem.* Basileae: Ioannem Oporinum.

Tulp, N. (red.) (1636), *Pharmacopoea Amstelredamensis: Senatus Auctoritata munita.* Amsterdam: apud Guilielmum & Iohannum Blaeu.

Tulp, N. (1641), *Nicolai Tulpii Amstelredamensis Observationes Medicae.* Amsterdam: apud Ludovicum Elzevirium.

Vesalius, A (1555), *De humani corporis fabrica libri septem.* Basileae: Ioannem Oporinum.

Wolf-Heidegger, G. & A.M. Cetto (1967), *Die anatomische Sektion in bildlicher Darstellung.* Bazel: Karger.

Wood Jones, F. (1944), *Principles of anatomy, as seen in the hand.* Londen: Baillière.

IJpma, F.F.A, R.C. van de Graaf, J-P.A. Nicolai & M.F. Meek (2006). The anatomy lesson of Dr. Nicolaes Tulp by Rembrandt (1632): a comparison of the painting with a dissected left forearm of a Dutch male cadaver. *J Hand Surg [Am]*, 31: 882-891.

IJpma, F.F.A., R.C. van de Graaf, J-P.A. Nicolai & M.F. Meek (2006). De anatomische les van dr. Nicolaes Tulp door Rembrandt (1632) en de bevindingen bij de dissectie van de onderarm van een kadaver: anatomische discrepanties. *Ned Tijdschr Geneeskd*, 150: 2756-2765.

IJpma, F.F.A., R.C. van de Graaf, J-P.A. Nicolai & M.F. Meek (2007). De anatomische les van dr. Nicolaes Tulp door Rembrandt (1632) en de bevindingen bij de dissectie van de onderarm van een kadaver: anatomische discrepanties. *Ned Tijdschr Geneeskd*, 151: 562-564.

IJpma, F.F.A., R.C. van de Graaf, M.F. Meek, J-P.A. Nicolai & T.M. van Gulik (2008). The anatomy lesson of Dr. Nicolaes Tulp painted by Rembrandt in 1632. *ANZ J Surg*, 78: 1059-1061.

IJpma, F.F.A., R.C. van de Graaf, M.F. Meek, J-P.A. Nicolai & T.M. van Gulik (2009). 'The Anatomy Lesson of Dr. Nicolaes Tulp': from a group portrait to a true lesson in functional anatomy. *ANZ J Surg*, 79: 496-497.

IJpma, F.F.A. & T.M. van Gulik (2016). The Anatomy Lesson of Nicolaes Tulp, painted by Rembrandt in 1632. *Br J Surg*, 103(11):n/s.

5

Bidloo, G. (1690), *Ontleding des menschelijken lichaams: Uitgebeeld, naar het leven in honderd en vyf aftekeningen door de Heer Gerard De Lairesse.* Amsterdam: de weduwe van Joannes van Someren, de erfgenamen Joannes van Dijk, Hendrik en de weduwe Dirk Boom.

Eeghen, I.H. van (1948). De anatomische lessen van Rembrandt. *Amstelodamum,* 35: 34-36.

Eeghen, I.H. van (1969). Rembrandt en de mensenvilders. *Amstelodamum,* 56: 1-11.

Lakke, J.P. (1998). Autopsy practises for brain dissections and Rembrandt's anatomy lesson of Dr. Deyman. *J Hist Neurosci,* 7: 101-107.

Kooijmans, L. (2004), *De doodskunstenaar: De anatomische lessen van Frederik Ruysch.* Amsterdam: Bert Bakker.

Lindeboom, G.A. (1984), *Dutch medical biography: A biographical dictionary of Dutch physicians and surgeons 1475–1975.* Amsterdam: Rodopi.

Meekeren, J. van (1979), *Heel- en geneeskonstige aenmerkingen door Job van Meekeren* (facsimile). Alphen aan den Rijn: Stafleu's wetenschappelijke uitgeversmaatschappij B.V.

Middelkoop, N.E. (1994), *De anatomische les van Dr. Deijman.* Amsterdam: Amsterdams Historisch Museum.

Middelkoop, N.E. (1994). Rembrandts Anatomische les van Dr. Deijman. *Ned Tijdschr Geneeskd,* 138: 2614-2618.

Middelkoop, N.E., P. Noble, J. Wadum & B. Broos (1998), *Rembrandt onder het mes: De anatomische les van Dr Nicolaes Tulp ontleed.* Amsterdam: Six Art Promotion bv.

Middelkoop, N.E., J. Baptist Bedaux, S.A.C. Dudok van Heel, R. Ekkart & J. van Gent (red.) (2002), *Kopstukken: Amsterdammers geportretteerd 1600/1800.* Bussum: Uitgeverij THOTH / Amsterdams Historisch Museum.

Stadsarchief Amsterdam, Archief van de Gilden en het Brouwerscollege 366/294, *Anatomieboek van het Amsterdamse Chirurgijnsgilde.* Amsterdam: Amsterdamse Chirurgijnsgilde.

Vesalius, A. (1555), *De humani corporis fabrica libri septem.* Basel: Ioannem Oporinum.

IJpma, F.F.A, R.C. van de Graaf, J-P.A. Nicolai & M.F. Meek (2006). The anatomy lesson of Dr. Nicolaes Tulp by Rembrandt (1632): a comparison of the painting with a dissected left forearm of a Dutch male cadaver. *J Hand Surg* [*Am*], 31: 882-891.

IJpma, F.F.A., R.C. van de Graaf, M.F. Meek, J-P.A. Nicolai & T.M. van Gulik (2008). The anatomy lesson of Dr. Nicolaes Tulp painted by Rembrandt in 1632. *ANZ J Surg,* 78: 1059-1061.

IJpma, F.F.A., N.E. Middelkoop & T.M. van Gulik (2013). Rembrandt's anatomy lesson of Dr Deijman of 1656 dissected. *Neurosurgery,* 73(3): 381-385.

IJpma, F.F.A. & T.M. van Gulik (2013). Bidloo's and De Lairesse's early illustrations of the anatomy of the arm (1690): a successful collaboration between a prominent physician and a talented artist. *J Hand Surg Eur Vol,* 38: 94-99.

IJpma F.F.A. & T.M. van Gulik (2018). Anatomy lesson of the brain and cerebral membranes captured on canvas by Rembrandt in 1656. *Br J Surg,* 105: 1–7.

6

Arlebout, Y.G. (red.) (1744), *Alle de ontleed-, genees-, en heelkundige werken van Frederick Ruysch.* Amsterdam: Janssoons van Waesberge.

Asellius, G. (1628), *De lactibus, sive lacteis venis quarto vasorum mesaraicorum genere, novo invento Gasparis Asellii dissertatio: qua sententiae anatomicae multae vel perperam receptae convelluntur, vel parum perceptae illustrantur.* Bazel: Henric-Petrinis.

Berg, N.S. van den, O.R. Brouwer, W.M. Klop, B. Karakullukcu, C.L. Zuur, I.B. Tan, A.J. Balm, M.W. van den Brekel, R.A. Valdés Olmos & F.W. van Leeuwen (2012). Concomitant radio- and fluorescence-guided sentinel lymph node biopsy in squamous cell carcinoma of the oral cavity using ICG-99mTc-nanocolloid. *Eur J Nucl Med Mol Imaging,* 39: 1128-1136.

Bleker, O.P. (2006). Een vroedvrouw gaat 'uyt roeyen': Over Willemtje Cloppenburg en Frederik Ruysch. *Geschiedenis der Geneeskunde,* 11(3): 149-156.

Chikly, B. (1997). Who discovered the lymphatic system. *Lymphology,* 30: 186-193.

Crane, L.M., G. Themelis, K.T. Buddingh, N.J. Harlaar, R.G. Pleijhuis, A. Sarantopoulos, A.G. van der Zee, V. Ntziachristos & G.M van Dam (2010). Multispectral real-time fluorescence imaging for intraoperative detection of the sentinel lymph node in gynecologic oncology. *J Vis Exp,* (44). pii: 2225. doi: 10.3791/2225.

Crane, L.M., G. Themelis, H.J. Arts HJ, K.T. Buddingh, A.H. Brouwers, V. Ntziachristos, G.M. van Dam & A.G. van der Zee (2011). Intraoperative near-infrared fluorescence imaging for sentinel lymph node detection in vulvar cancer: first clinical results. *Gynecol Oncol,* 120: 291-295.

Crane, L.M., G. Themelis, R.G. Pleijhuis, N.J. Harlaar, A. Sarantopoulos, H.J. Arts, A.G. van der Zee, V. Ntziachristos & G.M. van Dam GM (2011). Intraoperative multispectral fluorescence imaging for the detection of the sentinel lymph node in cervical cancer: a novel concept. *Mol Imaging Biol,* 13: 1043-1049.

Dam, G.M. van, G. Themelis, L.M. Crane, N.J. Harlaar, R.G. Pleijhuis, W. Kelder, A. Sarantopoulos, J.S. de Jong, H.J. Arts, A.G. van der Zee, J. Bart, P.S. Low & V. Ntziachristos (2011). Intraoperative tumor-specific fluorescence imaging in ovarian cancer by folate receptor-a targeting: first in-human results. *Nat Med,* 17: 1315-1319.

Driessen-van het Reve, J.J. (2004), *Geloof alleen je eigen ogen: Frederik Ruysch (1638–1731), held van de nieuwe wetenschap.* Amsterdam: Universiteit van Amsterdam.

Driessen-van het Reve, J.J. (2006), *De Kunstkamera van Peter de Grote: De Hollandse inbreng, gereconstrueerd uit brieven van Albert Seba en Johann Daniel Schumacher uit de Jaren 1711–1752.* Hilversum: Verloren.

Dudok van Heel, S.A.C. (1980). Het geboortejaar van de schilder Adriaen Backer (.... — 1684). *Amstelodamum,* 67(6): 138-141.

Hanson, J.V. (1996). Resurrecting death: anatomical art in the cabinet of Dr. Frederik Ruysch. *The Art Bulletin,* 78: 663-679.

Horne, J. van (1652), *Novus ductus chyliferus.* Leiden: Lugduni Batavorum.

Kooijmans, L. (2004), *De doodskunstenaar: De anatomische lessen van Frederik Ruysch.* Amsterdam: Bert Bakker.

Lindeboom, G.A. (1972), *Geschiedenis van de medische wetenschap in Nederland.* Haarlem: Fibula-van Dishoeck.

Loukas, M, S.S. Bellary, M. Kuklinski, J. Ferrauiola, A. Yadav, M.M. Shoja, K. Shaffer & R.S. Tubbs (2011). The lymphatic system: a historical perspective. *Clin Anat,* 24: 807-816.

Middelkoop, N.E., P. Noble, J. Wadum & B. Broos (1998), *Rembrandt onder het mes: De anatomische les van Dr Nicolaes Tulp ontleed.* Amsterdam: Six Art Promotion bv.

Middelkoop, N.E., J. Baptist Bedaux, S.A.C. Dudok van Heel, R. Ekkart & J. van Gent (red.) (2002), *Kopstukken: Amsterdammers geportretteerd 1600/1800.* Bussum: Uitgeverij THOTH / Amsterdams Historisch Museum.

Middelkoop, N.E. (2005). Nieuw leven voor Adriaen Backers Anatomische les van Dr. Frederick Ruysch. *Amstelodamum,* 92-1: 3-16.

Mieog, J.S., S.L. Troyan, M. Hutteman, K.J. Donohoe, J.R. van der Vorst, A. Stockdale, G.J. Liefers, H.S. Choi,

S.L. Gibbs-Strauss, H. Putter, S. Gioux, P.J. Kuppen, Y. Ashitate, C.W. Löwik, V.T. Smit, R. Oketokoun, L.H. Ngo, C.J. van de Velde, J.V. Frangioni & A.L. Vahrmeijer (2011). Toward optimization of imaging system and lymphatic tracer for near-infrared fluorescent sentinel lymph node mapping in breast cancer. *Ann Surg Oncol*, 18: 2483-2491.

Molhuysen, P.C. en P.J. Blok (1911–1937), *Nieuw Nederlandsch Biografisch Woordenboek*. Leiden: A.W. Sijthoff's Uitgevers-maatschappij.

Poel, H.G. van der, T. Buckle, O.R. Brouwer, R.A. Valdés Olmos en F.W. van Leeuwen (2011). Intraoperative laparoscopic fluorescence guidance to the sentinel lymph node in prostate cancer patients: clinical proof of concept of an integrated functional imaging approach using a multimodal tracer. *Eur Urol*, 60: 826-833.

Radziun, A. & Y. Chistov (2012), *The first scientific collections of Kunstkamera*. Sint Petersburg: DITON.

Ruysch, F. (1665), *Dilucidatio valvularum in vasis lymphaticis et lacteis*. Den Haag: Hagæ-com: ex officina Harmani Gael.

Stadsarchief Amsterdam, Archief van de Gilden en het Brouwerscollege 366/294, *Anatomieboek van het Amsterdamse Chirurgijnsgilde*. Amsterdam: Amsterdamse Chirurgijnsgilde.

Vorst, J.R. van der, B.E. Schaafsma, F.P. Verbeek, M. Hutteman, J.S. Mieog, C.W. Lowik, G.J. Liefers, J.V. Frangioni, C.J. van de Velde & A.L. Vahrmeijer (2012). Randomized comparison of near-infrared fluorescence imaging using indocyanine green and 99(m) technetium with or without patent blue for the sentinel lymph node procedure in breast cancer patients. *Ann Surg Oncol*, 19: 4104-4111.

IJpma, F.F.A & H.J. Hoekstra (2012). Van lymfeklierdissectie naar schildwachtklier. In: V.J. de Ru, P.J. van Diest, L.H.J. Looijenga, C.J.H. van de Velde, D.J.Th. Wagener (red.), *Canon van de oncologie*. Haarlem: dchg medische communicatie, 14-15.

IJpma, F.F.A. & T.M. van Gulik (2013). 'Anatomy lesson of Frederik Ruysch' of 1670: A tribute to Ruysch's contributions to lymphatic anatomy. *World J Surg*, 37: 1996-2001.

7

Arlebout, Y.G. (red.) (1744), *Alle de ontleed-, genees-, en heelkundige werken van Frederick Ruysch*. Amsterdam: Janssoons van Waesberge.

Bleker, O.P. (2006). Een vroedvrouw gaat 'uyt roeyen': Over Willemtje Cloppenburg en Frederik Ruysch. *Geschiedenis der Geneeskunde*, 11(3): 149-156.

Driessen-van het Reve, J.J. (2004), *Geloof alleen je eigen ogen: Frederik Ruysch (1638–1731), held van de nieuwe wetenschap*. Amsterdam: Universiteit van Amsterdam.

Hanson, J.V. (1996). Resurrecting death: anatomical art in the cabinet of Dr. Frederik Ruysch. *The Art Bulletin*, 78: 663-679.

Houbraken, A. (1721), *De groote schouburgh der Nederlantsche konstschilders en schilderessen (dl. III)*. Amsterdam: Gedrukt door de Weduwe des autheurs, daar dezelve ook te bekomen zijn, 75.

Kooijmans, L. (2004), *De doodskunstenaar: De anatomische lessen van Frederik Ruysch*. Amsterdam: Bert Bakker.

Luyendijk-Elshout, A.M. (1970). Death enlightened: A study of Frederik Ruysch. *JAMA*, 212: 121-126.

Middelkoop, N.E., P. Noble, J. Wadum & B. Broos (1998), *Rembrandt onder het mes: De anatomische les van Dr Nicolaes Tulp ontleed*. Amsterdam: Six Art Promotion bv.

Radziun, A. & Y. Chistov (2012), *The first scientific collections of Kunstkamera*. Sint Petersburg: DITON.

Stadsarchief Amsterdam, Archief van de Gilden en het Brouwerscollege 366/294, *Anatomieboek van het Amsterdamse Chirurgijnsgilde*. Amsterdam: Amsterdamse Chirurgijnsgilde.

IJpma, F.F.A., A. Radziun & T.M. van Gulik (2013). 'The anatomy lesson of

Frederik Ruysch' of 1683, a milestone in knowledge about obstetrics. *Eur J Obstet Gynecol Reprod Biol*, 170(1): 50-55.

8

Brugmans, H., J.H. Scholte, Ph. Kleintjes & F. Cohen (red.) (1932), *Gedenkboek van het Athenaeum en de universiteit van Amsterdam 1632-1932*. Amsterdam: Stadsdrukkerij.

Dudok van Heel, S.A.C. (1983). Hoe de chirurgijnsweduwe Cleveringh-Schrick in 1710 haar knecht Bernardus van Vijve (1684–1759) tot een huwelijk dwong. *Amstelodamum*, 75: 53-72.

Hulkenberg, A.M. (1975), *Keukenhof.* Dordrecht: Historische Vereniging Holland.

Kooijmans, L. (2004), *De doodskunstenaar: De anatomische lessen van Frederik Ruysch*. Amsterdam: Bert Bakker.

Lindeboom, G.A. (1984), *Dutch medical biography: A biographical dictionary of Dutch physicians and surgeons 1475–1975*. Amsterdam: Rodopi.

Middelkoop, N.E., P. Noble, J. Wadum & B. Broos (1998), *Rembrandt onder het mes: De anatomische les van Dr Nicolaes Tulp ontleed*. Amsterdam: Six Art Promotion bv.

Middelkoop, N.E., J. Baptist Bedaux, S.A.C. Dudok van Heel, R. Ekkart & J. van Gent (red.) (2002), *Kopstukken: Amsterdammers geportretteerd 1600/1800*. Bussum: Uitgeverij THOTH / Amsterdams Historisch Museum.

Niemeijer, J.W. (1973), *Cornelis Troost 1696–1750*. Assen: Van Gorcum & Comp. B.V.

Nierop, L. van (1938). Het dagboek van Jacob Bicker Raye 1732–1772. *Amstelodamum*, 35: 131-178.

Nuyens, B.W.Th. (1928), Het ontleedkundig onderwijs en de geschilderde Anatomische lessen van het Chirurgijns Gilde te Amsterdam in de jaren 1550 tot 1798. In: Scharp H.J. (red.), *Koninklijk Oudheidkundig Genootschap te Amsterdam: Jaarverslag*. Amsterdam: Koninklijk Oudheidkundig Genootschap, 45-90.

Stadsarchief Amsterdam, Archief van de Gilden en het Brouwerscollege 366/294, *Anatomieboek van het Amsterdamse Chirurgijnsgilde*. Amsterdam: Amsterdamse Chirurgijnsgilde.

Teulings, C., F.F.A. IJpma & T.M. van Gulik (2013). Unieke erfstukken van het Amsterdamse chirurgijnsgilde: penningen van de chirurgijns die zijn afgebeeld op de beroemde reeks groepsportretten. *Amstelodamum*, 100-2: 68-86.

Tilanus, J.W.R. (1865), *Beschrijving der schilderijen afkomstig van het chirurgijns-gild te Amsterdam: Met enige historische aanteekeningen omtrent het gild, en eene nadere beschouwing der kunstwaarde der verzameling*. Amsterdam: Frederik Muller.

Titsingh, A. (1731), *De verdonkerde heelkonst der Amsterdammers, uit hunne eigen handvesten, tot nut van de proeve en leerlingen, door redelijke oeffeningen opgehelderd en voor de geleerden, en ervarenen, met aanmerkelyke bevindingen bevestigd door Abraham Titsingh*. Amsterdam: Gysbert Hazemaker.

Wijnands, D.O. , E.J.A. Zevenhuizen & J. Heniger (1994). *Een sieraad voor de stad: De Amsterdamse Hortus Botanicus 1638–1993*. Amsterdam: Amsterdam University Press.

IJpma F.F.A. & T.M. van Gulik (2018). Well-dressed surgeons from Amsterdam portrayed during an anatomy lesson of the knee joint in 1728. *Br J Surg*, 105: 1-6.

9

Bekker, J., J.N. Keeman, M.P. Simons & Th.J. Aufenacker (2007). Een beknopte geschiedenis van de liesbreukoperatie bij volwassenen. *Ned Tijdschr Geneeskd*, 151: 924-931.

Burlet, H.M. de (1939). Petrus Camper als anatoom. *Ned Tijdschr Geneeskd,* 83: 2111-2120.

Camper, P. (1762), *Verhandeling over de oorzaaken der menigvuldige breuken in de eerstgeborene kinderen.* Amsterdam: J.B. Elwe.

Camper, P. (1774), Verhandeling over het toestellen van breukbanden. In: Bataafsch Genootschap der Proefondervindelijke Wijsbegeerte (red.), *Verhandelingen van het Bataafsch Genootschap der Proefondervindelijke Wijsbegeerte te Rotterdam.* Rotterdam: Reinier Arrenberg, 253-276.

Camper, P. (1760), *Demonstrationum anatomico-pathologicarum liber primus continens brachii humani fabricam et morbos.* Amsterdam: Joann Schreuder et Petrum Mortier.

Camper, P. & S.T. von Soemmerring (1801), *Icones herniarum.* Francofurti ad Moenum: Varrentrapp et Wenner.

Engelhard, J.L.B. (1939). Petrus Camper als verloskundige. *Ned Tijdschr Geneeskd,* 83; 2106-2111.

Feyfer, F.M.G. de (1939). Petrus Camper als tekenaar. *Ned Tijdschr Geneeskd,* 83: 2140-2143.

Gool, J. van (1750–1751), *De nieuwe schouburg der Nederlantsche kunstschilders en schilderessen: waer in de levens- en kunstbedryven der tans levende en reets overleedene schilders, die Houbraken, noch eenig ander schryver, zyn aengetekend, verhaelt worden.* Den Haag: gedrukt voor den autheur.

Heuvel, A.J. van den (1883), *Petrus Camper als chirurg beschouwd.* Amsterdam: De Lange.

Korst, J.K. van der (2008), *Het rusteloze bestaan van dokter Petrus Camper.* Houten: Bohn Stafleu van Loghum.

Kuijjer, P.J. (1994), Petrus Camper (1722–1789): chirurg, onderzoeker en hoogleraar te Groningen in de achttiende eeuw. In: Kuijjer, P.J., F.G. Huisman, G.J. Bremer & C.A.E. Volckmann (red.), *Uit de geschiedenis van geneeskunde en verpleging: Petrus Camper Stichting 1984–1994.* Groningen: Universitaire Reproductiedienst, 134-135.

Middelkoop, N.E., P. Noble, J. Wadum & B. Broos (1998), *Rembrandt onder het mes: De anatomische les van Dr Nicolaes Tulp ontleed.* Amsterdam: Six Art Promotion bv.

Molhuysen, P.C. & P.J. Blok (1911–1937), *Nieuw Nederlandsch Biografisch Woordenboek.* Leiden: A.W. Sijthoff's Uitgevers-maatschappij.

Nuyens, B.W.Th. (1928), Het ontleedkundig onderwijs en de geschilderde Anatomische lessen van het Chirurgijns Gilde te Amsterdam in de jaren 1550 tot 1798. In: Scharp H.J. (red.), *Koninklijk Oudheidkundig Genootschap te Amsterdam: Jaarverslag.* Amsterdam: Koninklijk Oudheidkundig Genootschap, 45-90.

Nuyens, B.W.Th (1939). Petrus Camper: Herdenkingsrede gehouden op 29 april 1939 in de aula der Groningsche universiteit. *Ned Tijdschr Geneeskd,* 83: 2073-2084.

Oosterhuis, R.A.B. (1939). De zekerheid der geneeskunde. Inaugureele rede van Petrus Camper, in het openbaar uitgesproken in het Athenaeum Illustre van Amsterdam op 22 juni 1758, bij de plechtige aanvaarding van het gewone professoraat in de geneeskunde I). *Ned Tijdschr Geneeskd,* 83: 2085-2101.

Schuller tot Peursum-Meijer, J. & W.R.H. Koops (red.), *Petrus Camper (1722–1789) onderzoeker van nature.* Groningen: Universiteitsmuseum Groningen.

Schünke, M., E. Schulte & U. Schumacher (red.) (2010), *Anatomische atlas Prometheus, hoofd, hals en neuroanatomie.* Houten: Bohn Stafleu van Loghum.

Teulings, C., F.F.A. IJpma & T.M. van Gulik (2013). Unieke erfstukken van het Amsterdamse chirurgijnsgilde: penningen van de chirurgijns die zijn afgebeeld op de beroemde reeks groepsportretten. *Amstelodamum,* 100-2: 68-86.

Tilanus, J.W.R. (1865), *Beschrijving der schilderijen afkomstig van het chirurgijns-gild te Amsterdam: Met enige historische aanteekeningen omtrent het gild, en eene nadere beschouwing der kunstwaarde der verzameling.* Amsterdam: Frederik Muller.

Vos, J.Th. (1939). Petrus Camper als ziektekundige. *Ned Tijdschr Geneeskd,* 83: 2124-2128.

Wester, J. (1939). Petrus Camper en de geneeskunde der dieren. *Ned Tijdschr Geneeskd,* 83: 2138-2140.

IJpma, F.F.A., R.C. van de Graaf, D. van Geldere & T.M. van Gulik (2009). An early observation on the anatomy of the inguinal canal and the etiology of inguinal hernias by Petrus Camper in the 18th century. *World J Surg,* 33(6): 1318-1324.

IJpma, F.F.A., R.C. van de Graaf & T.M. van Gulik (2010). Petrus Camper's work on the anatomy and pathology of the arm and hand in the 18th century. *J Hand Surg Am,* 35(8): 1382-1387.

Portraits of the Governors

Albinus, B.S. (1726), *De ossibus corporis humani: ad auditors suos.* Leiden: Leidae Batavorum, apud H. Mulhovium.

Albinus, B.S. (1747), *Tabulae sceleti et musculorum corporis humani.* Leiden: Lugduni Batavorum, prostant apud Joannem & Hermannum Verbeek.

Amsterdam Museum, online collectie, zie: http://am.adlibhosting.com.

Arlebout, Y.G. (red.) (1744), *Alle de ontleed-, genees-, en heelkundige werken van Frederick Ruysch.* Amsterdam: Janssoons van Waesberge.

Bidloo, G. (1690), *Ontleding des menschelijken lichaams: Uitgebeeld, naar het leven in honderd en vyf aftekeningen door de Heer Gerard De Lairesse.* Amsterdam: de weduwe van Joannes van Someren, de erfgenamen Joannes van Dijk, Hendrik en de weduwe Dirk Boom.

Kooijmans, L. (2004), *De doodskunstenaar: De anatomische lessen van Frederik Ruysch.* Amsterdam: Bert Bakker.

Meyer, H. (1736), *Privilegien, willekeuren en ordonnantiën, betreffende het Collegium Chirurgicum Amstelaedamense.* Amsterdam: Pieter van den Berge.

Middelkoop, N.E., P. Noble, J. Wadum & B. Broos (1998), *Rembrandt onder het mes: De anatomische les van Dr Nicolaes Tulp ontleed.* Amsterdam: Six Art Promotion bv.

Middelkoop, N.E., J. Baptist Bedaux, S.A.C. Dudok van Heel, R. Ekkart & J. van Gent (red.) (2002), *Kopstukken: Amsterdammers geportretteerd 1600/1800.* Bussum: Uitgeverij THOTH / Amsterdams Historisch Museum.

Teulings, C., F.F.A. IJpma & T.M. van Gulik (2013). Unieke erfstukken van het Amsterdamse chirurgijnsgilde: penningen van de chirurgijns die zijn afgebeeld op de beroemde reeks groepsportretten. *Amstelodamum,* 100-2: 68-86.

Tilanus, J.W.R. (1865), *Beschrijving der schilderijen afkomstig van het chirurgijns-gild te Amsterdam: Met enige historische aanteekeningen omtrent het gild, en eene nadere beschouwing der kunstwaarde der verzameling.* Amsterdam: Frederik Muller.

Titsingh, A. (ca. 1731), *Heelkundige verhandeling over de steen en het steensnyden, van Frere Jacques de Beaulieu uitgevonden, van de Hoogleraar Johan Jacob Rau beschaaft, en door Jacobus Denys verdonkert, nu wederom tot nut voor den weetgierigen opgeheldert door Abraham Titsingh.* Amsterdam: Gerrit Bouman.

Picture acknowledgements

Library of the University of Groningen 55 (LD-25), 61 (uklu KW C 569), 64 (uklu KW C 1150), 65 (uklu KW C 1150), 67 en 68 (uklu KW C 562), 116 (uklu KW C 1150), 118 (uklu KW C 1150), 121 (uklu KW C 569), 140 (LD- 3), 195, 215 (left and right, uklu KW C 1150). [Photography by Dirk Fennema, Haren.]

Special Collections, University of Amsterdam 37 (OTM: O 62-7274), 38 (left, OTM: O 73-16), 39 (OTM: O 73-16), 58 (UBM: Br. M.G. 4to 58: 17), 85, 198 (OTM O 62-2672), 199 (OTM OL 63-946), 200 (left and right, OTM OL 63-946), 201 (UBM DT 839: 1 (5)), 202-203 (OTM: OL 63-1402), 205 (OTM: OL 63-1402)

Collection Amsterdam Museum 9 (SA 2121), 17 (SB 5749), 30-31 (SA 7387), 33 (SA 7387), 34 (above, SA 7386), 46-47 (SA 7352), 70-72 (SA 2048), 77 (above, SA 7390), 106-107 (SA 7394), 109 (above, TA 7395), 109 (under, A 41060), 122-123 (SA 2000), 125 left (SA 2000), 148-149 en 151 (SA 2644, J & M Zweerts Photography), 172-173 (SA 7412), 190-192 (SA 7391), 206 (KA 22098), 209 (PA 18), 216-217 (SA 7541), 218 (above, SA 3035), 218 (under, SA 3031), 221 (above, SA 3012), 222 (SA 2067), 224 (SA 7415), 226-227 (SA 454), 229 (SA 453), 232-233 (SA 7390)

Collection Dick van Geldere 87 (left and right), 88 (left and right), 89

Collection Hans van den Boogaard 51, 52-53

Collection Frank IJpma 16, 62, 63, 66, 100, 105, 119 (above and under), 135, 204

Collection Laurens de Rooy 54

Collection Matthanja Bieze 18, 19 (above and under), 127 (right), 182, 187 (mid), 225 (under right), 230 (under)

Collectie Rijksmuseum, Amsterdam 23 (RP-P-OB-22.436), 26 (RP-P-1887-A-12041), 34 (under, SK-C-455), 49 (SK-C-381-00), 176 (SK-A-1635), 177 (above, SK-A-4225), 177 (under, SK-C-87), 186 (RP-P-OB-83.678), 221 (under, NG-VG-7-47)

Collection Six, Amsterdam 83 (above and under), 86 (left and right), 92 (left and right)

Collection Thomas van Gulik 127 (left), 131, 132, 145-147, 154-157, 159 (above and under), 167, 219 (right)

Koninklijk Kabinet van Schilderijen Mauritshuis (Royal Cabinet of Paintings Mauritshuis) 78-79 (149), 103

Koninklijk Oudheidkundig Genootschap (Royal Antiquarian Society) 175 (KOG-0000288)

Museum Boerhaave, Leiden 36 (under, P03239)

Index

Bold page numbers refer to an image.

Acknowledgements

We thank Norbert **Middelkoop** of the **Amsterdam Museum** for his valuable advice and his contribution to the research into Jan Deijman's anatomy lesson; Jhr Jan **Six van Hillegom** for making photo material available of the **Collection Six**; Doede **Hardeman** and his colleagues from the **Gemeentemuseum** (now **Kunstmuseum**) in The Hague for the collaboration on the occasion of the exhibition 'From Rembrandt to Damien Hirst'; Anna **Radziun** and Yuri **Chistov** of the **Peter the Great Museum of Anthropology and Ethnography (Kunstkamera)** in St Petersburg for their help in researching the anatomical collection of Frederik Ruysch.

We are grateful to the **Amsterdam Museum, Library of the University of Groningen**, the **Special Collections Department of the University of Amsterdam**, the **Royal Cabinet of Paintings Mauritshuis** in The Hague, the **Royal Antiquarian Society (Koninklijk Oudheidkundig Genootschap)**, **Museum Boerhaave** in Leiden, **Museum Vrolik** (Academic Medical Center, Amsterdam), the **National Bureau for Art Historical Documentation**, the **Rijksmuseum** in Amsterdam and the **Amsterdam City Archives**, for the use of archive documents, anatomical atlases, medical manuals and images for this book.

We thank Robert **Pierik** for his valuable advice and contribution to research into surgical training; Dick van **Geldere** for his contribution to the research into 'Camper and inguinal hernias'; Robert **van de Graaf**, Marcel **Meek**, Jean-Philippe **Nicolai** and Aris **Sterodimas** for their efforts in researching the dissected arm in Nicolaes Tulp's anatomy lesson. Robert **van de Graaf** also for his contributions to the studies of surgical training, 'Camper and inguinal hernias' and the 'chiasma tendinum' of Camper; Henk Jan **ten Duis** for his contribution to the chapter on the Osteology lesson of Sebastiaen Egbertszn; Chris **Teulings** for the input of his expertise in the research into surgeons' tokens; Otto **Bleker**, Jozien **Driessen-van het Reve**, Cisca **Griffioen**, Wim **Mulder**, Roelof-Jan **Oostra**, Laurens **de Rooy** of the 'Ruysch research group' for their input in the chapters on Ruysch; and Kees **ter Horst** for his enthusiasm to support our projects.

We are very grateful to the photographers for making their photo material available: Matthanja **Bieze** took the photos of the coats-of-arms in the vault of the dome in the Weighing House (Waag). We would like to thank Hans **van den Bogaard** and Laurens **de Rooy** for unique images of the Hovius' Cabinet at the Vrolik museum. Dirk **Fennema** made the reproductions of the anatomical atlases and textbooks from the Library of the University of Groningen. Phil **Nijhuis** made a portrait photo of the authors at Nicolaes Tulp's Anatomy Lesson (1632).

Many have helped with the creation of this book: Vera **Bertheux**, Marlies **Enklaar**, Gerda **Huisman**, Jacqueline **IJpma**, Yep **IJpma**, Maarten **Jansen**, Marcel **Levi**, Simon **Knepper**, Johan **Kortenray**, Andrea **de Leeuw**, Klaas van Linschoten, May **Meurs**, Ron **van der Lugt**, Mireille **van der Meij**, Emma **van Proosdij**, Rutger **Schimmelpenninck**, Benno **Tempel** and Ludwich **Verberne**.

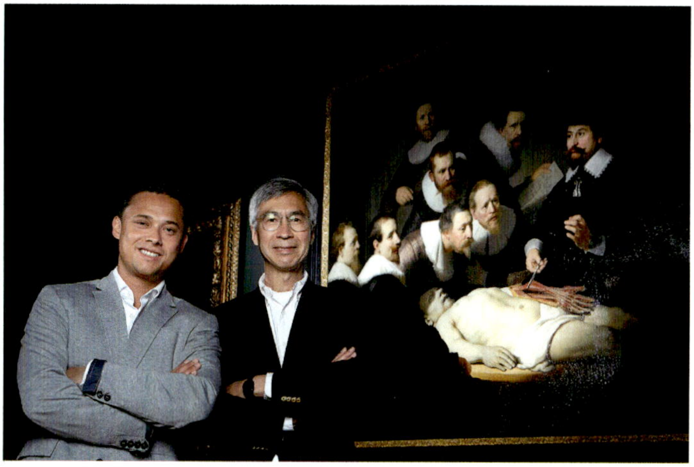

About the authors **Frank IJpma** is surgeon at the University Medical Center Groningen, The Netherlands. **Thomas van Gulik** is em. professor of surgery at the Amsterdam University Medical Center (location AMC), The Netherlands. This edition is the result of the PhD research of Frank IJpma concerning the 'Anatomy lessons' painted for the Amsterdam Surgeons' Guild in the seventeenth and eighteenth century. The PhD thesis of Frank IJpma came out in June 2014 at the University of Amsterdam.

End note This book initially appeared on November 14, 2013, on the occasion of the twentieth edition of the 'Anatomy Lesson' in Amsterdam, a medical public lecture on the intersection of medicine and society, annually organized by the Amsterdam University Medical Center.

For Product Safety Concerns and Information please contact our EU representative GPSR@taylorandfrancis.com Taylor & Francis Verlag GmbH, Kaufingerstraße 24, 80331 München, Germany

Batch number: 10722658

Printed by Printforce, the Netherlands